Erectile Dysfunction in Hypertension and Cardiovascular Disease

Margus Viigimaa
Charalambos Vlachopoulos
Michael Doumas
Editors

Erectile Dysfunction in Hypertension and Cardiovascular Disease

A Guide for Clinicians

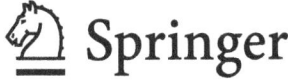

Editors
Margus Viigimaa
North Estonia Medical Centre
Tallinn University of Technology
Tallinn
Estonia

Michael Doumas
Internal Medicine
Aristotle University
Thessaloniki
Greece

Charalambos Vlachopoulos
Athens Medical School
Athens
Greece

ISBN 978-3-319-08271-4   ISBN 978-3-319-08272-1   (eBook)
DOI 10.1007/978-3-319-08272-1
Springer Cham Heidelberg New York Dordrecht London

Library of Congress Control Number: 2014956269

© Springer International Publishing Switzerland 2015
This work is subject to copyright. All rights are reserved by the Publisher, whether the whole or part of the material is concerned, specifically the rights of translation, reprinting, reuse of illustrations, recitation, broadcasting, reproduction on microfilms or in any other physical way, and transmission or information storage and retrieval, electronic adaptation, computer software, or by similar or dissimilar methodology now known or hereafter developed. Exempted from this legal reservation are brief excerpts in connection with reviews or scholarly analysis or material supplied specifically for the purpose of being entered and executed on a computer system, for exclusive use by the purchaser of the work. Duplication of this publication or parts thereof is permitted only under the provisions of the Copyright Law of the Publisher's location, in its current version, and permission for use must always be obtained from Springer. Permissions for use may be obtained through RightsLink at the Copyright Clearance Center. Violations are liable to prosecution under the respective Copyright Law.
The use of general descriptive names, registered names, trademarks, service marks, etc. in this publication does not imply, even in the absence of a specific statement, that such names are exempt from the relevant protective laws and regulations and therefore free for general use.
While the advice and information in this book are believed to be true and accurate at the date of publication, neither the authors nor the editors nor the publisher can accept any legal responsibility for any errors or omissions that may be made. The publisher makes no warranty, express or implied, with respect to the material contained herein.

Printed on acid-free paper

Springer is part of Springer Science+Business Media (www.springer.com)

Preface

Erectile dysfunction is defined as the persistent inability to attain and/or maintain erection sufficient for a satisfactory sexual intercourse. Erectile dysfunction is frequently encountered in the general population, and its frequency increases with age. Erectile dysfunction exerts a major impact on patients' and their sexual partners' quality of life and significantly affects self-confidence and self-esteem with substantial psychological consequences. Erectile dysfunction has been considered for very long the territory of psychiatrists and urologists. However, advances in the pathophysiology and treatment of erectile dysfunction during the last two decades uncovered a strong vascular component, rendering erectile dysfunction a primarily vascular disease in most cases.

Erectile dysfunction is more prevalent in patients with cardiovascular disease than in the general healthy population. The vascular origin of erectile dysfunction and its frequent coexistence with cardiovascular disease and/or cardiovascular risk factors and shared pathophysiological process set the basis for the in-depth examination of the association between erectile dysfunction and cardiovascular disease.

Assessing the association between erectile dysfunction and cardiovascular disease is a reciprocal, bidirectional task. Cardiovascular disease has to be proactively and thoroughly searched in patients with erectile dysfunction, since erectile dysfunction may precede coronary artery disease by 3–5 years. Erectile dysfunction can thus be considered as an "early diagnostic window" for the detection of asymptomatic coronary artery disease. On the other hand, patients with overt cardiovascular disease or cardiovascular risk factors (hypertension, diabetes mellitus, dyslipidemia, obesity, metabolic syndrome) need to be assessed for erectile dysfunction, since erectile dysfunction is highly prevalent in these disease conditions and affects significantly patients' quality of life, and the therapeutic management of these patients needs caution in some cases.

The European Society of Hypertension has acknowledged the significance of erectile dysfunction in the management of patients with arterial hypertension during the last decade, and relevant newsletters were published. A working group on sexual dysfunction and arterial hypertension was formed on 2009, and its inaugural session took place in Oslo during the 2010 annual meeting of the society. Since then, this group published a position paper regarding the association between erectile dysfunction and arterial hypertension, continued the intense efforts in clinical research, and tried to spread current knowledge in this field not only to the European hypertension community but to other international societies as well.

This book aims to provide a comprehensive and up-to-date presentation of the strong and clinically meaningful association between erectile dysfunction and cardiovascular disease. It gives us a great pleasure and honor that some of the most eminent, widely recognized, and highly respected experts in the field of erectile dysfunction and cardiovascular disease from both sides of the Atlantic joined this project and provided valuable contributions. Moreover, we would like to emphasize the multidisciplinary nature of this book, since contributing authors come from a wide variety of medical specialties (cardiology, internal medicine, nephrology, endocrinology, urology, family medicine). In addition, health-care professionals who are strongly involved in the management of patients with erectile dysfunction such as psychologists have been also involved in the authorship. It is with great honor that a distinguished team of basic research from the École Polytechnique Fédérale de Lausanne (EPFL) has also joined this effort and provided a different view on current research and future directions.

This book is actually divided into three parts. The first part covers the epidemiology and the pathophysiology of erectile dysfunction, highlighting the connection between erectile dysfunction and cardiovascular disease and unveiling the role of erectile dysfunction as a marker of silent coronary artery disease and as a predictor of future cardiovascular events. The second part discusses the presence of erectile dysfunction in the various diseases of the cardiovascular continuum and associated conditions. The last part deals with the broad spectrum of erectile dysfunction therapy, while the assessment and management of patients with erectile dysfunction represent the "grand finale" of this book.

We would like to express our sincere gratitude to all contributing authors for embracing this effort and providing well-written chapters of the highest scientific quality. We would also like to cordially thank the contributing authors for complying with our wish of presenting a book which will be easy to read and appropriate for a wide variety of practicing physicians, such as general practitioners and primary health physicians, cardiologists, internists, nephrologists, endocrinologists, pneumonologists, urologists, and psychiatrists. Finally, we cannot forget Roberto Garbero for his continuous efforts and the valuable help during all stages of book production, and Springer for providing the chance to present this book.

Tallinn, Estonia	Margus Viigimaa
Athens, Greece	Charalambos Vlachopoulos
Thessaloniki, Greece	Michael Doumas

Contents

1 **Definition and Assessment of Erectile Dysfunction** 1
  Charalambos Vlachopoulos

2 **Epidemiology of Erectile Dysfunction in Hypertension** 9
  Charalampos A. Grassos, Charalampos I. Liakos,
  Eirini Papadopoulou, Theodosia Papadopoulou, and Michael Doumas

3 **Pathophysiology of Erectile Dysfunction** 19
  Dragan Lovic

4 **Erectile Dysfunction and Testosterone** 29
  Charalambos Vlachopoulos

5 **The Role of the Renin-Angiotensin System in Erectile Dysfunction: Present and Future** 39
  Rodrigo Araujo Fraga-Silva and Nikolaos Stergiopulos

6 **Erectile Dysfunction and Target Organ Damage** 51
  Nikolaos Ioakeimidis

7 **Erectile Dysfunction in Coronary Artery Disease and Heart Failure** 59
  Giorgio Gandaglia, Alberto Briganti, Piero Montorsi,
  Francesco Montorsi, and Charalambos Vlachopoulos

8 **Erectile Dysfunction as an 'Early Diagnostic Window' for Asymptomatic Coronary Artery Disease** 73
  Graham Jackson

9 **The Prognostic Role of Erectile Dysfunction for Cardiovascular Events** 83
  Dimitrios Terentes-Printzios, and Charalambos Vlachopoulos

10 **Erectile Dysfunction in Chronic Kidney Disease** 97
  Bojan Jelaković, Margareta Fištrek Prlić, and Mario Laganović

11 **Erectile Dysfunction and Sleep Apnea** 109
  Jacek Wolf and Krzysztof Narkiewicz

12 Diabetes Mellitus and Erectile Dysfunction.   119
    Barbara Nikolaidou, Christos Nouris, Antonios Lazaridis,
    Christos Sampanis, and Michael Doumas

13 The Association Between Dyslipidemia and Its Treatment
    with Erectile Dysfunction   129
    Andreas Pittaras, Konstantinos Avranas, Konstantinos Imprialos,
    Charles Faselis, and Peter Kokkinos

14 Endocrine Disorders and Erectile Dysfunction.   139
    Konstantinos Tziomalos and Vasilios G. Athyros

15 The Metabolic Investigation of Erectile Dysfunction:
    Cardiometabolic Risk Stratification.   145
    Martin Miner

16 Erectile Dysfunction in the Elderly   159
    Siegfried Meryn

17 Lifestyle Modification in Erectile Dysfunction
    and Hypertension.   167
    Margus Viigimaa

18 Antihypertensive Drug Therapy and Erectile Dysfunction   175
    Vasilios Papademetriou, Antonios Lazaridis, Eirini Papadopoulou,
    Theodosia Papadopoulou, and Michael Doumas

19 PDE5 Inhibitors for the Treatment of Erectile Dysfunction
    in Patients with Hypertension.   185
    Peter Kokkinos, Apostolos Tsimploulis, and Charles Faselis

20 Management of Erectile Dysfunction Beyond PDE-5 Inhibitors. . . .   195
    Konstantinos Rokkas

21 Cognitive Behavioral Therapy in Sexual Dysfunction   205
    Penelope-Alexia Avagianou

22 Basic Principles of the Princeton Recommendations   213
    Patrick S. Whelan and Ajay Nehra

23 Sexual Counseling for Patients with Cardiovascular Disease   231
    Athanasios Manolis, Andreas Pittaras, Antonios Lazaridis,
    and Michael Doumas

24 Management of Erectile Dysfunction: Therapeutic Algorithm.   241
    Charalambos Vlachopoulos and Nikolaos Ioakeimidis

Definition and Assessment of Erectile Dysfunction

Charalambos Vlachopoulos

1.1 Definition of Erectile Dysfunction

Erectile dysfunction (ED) is the most common sexual problem in men. Inadequate penile erection, otherwise known as ED, is defined as the inability to attain or maintain a penile erection sufficient for successful vaginal intercourse [1]. This symptom must be present for at least 3 months before a diagnosis can be made. In some instances of surgically induced ED (e.g., following radical prostatectomy) or trauma, the diagnosis may be made prior to 3 months [2]. Objective testing (or partner reports) may be used to support the diagnosis of ED, but these measures cannot substitute for the patient's self report in classifying the dysfunction or establishing the diagnosis [2]. ED often causes serious distress, prompting men to seek medical attention they may not otherwise seek. It affects intimate relationship, self-esteem, and quality of life and has significant unfavorable consequences.

1.2 Distinction Between Organic and Psychogenic ED

Normal erectile function has been described as a process that involves the coordination of psychological, vascular, endocrine, and neurological systems. For clinical purposes, ED is categorized into three types according to their etiology: type I, psychogenic; type II, organic; and type III, mixed [3]. Types II and III differ according to the absence or presence of significant mental (cognitive) or emotional (affect) distress. In type II ED, resolution of the main symptom adequately

---

C. Vlachopoulos
1st Cardiology Department, Athens Medical School,
Hippokration Hospital, Profiti Elia 24, Athens 14575, Greece
e-mail: cvlachop@otenet.gr

Table 1.1 Differential characteristics of psychogenic versus organic ED

Characteristic	Predominantly psychogenic ED	Predominantly organic ED
Onset	Acute	Gradual
Circumstances	Situational	Global
Course	Intermittent	Constant
Noncoital erection	Rigid	Poor
Nocturnal/early AM erections	Normal	Inconsistent
Psychosexual problems	Long history	Secondary to ED
Partner problems	At onset	Secondary to ED
Anxiety/fear	Primary	Secondary to ED

From Persu et al. [4]

diminishes mental and/or emotional distress, whereas in type III ED complementary psychotherapy is indicated. Usual type II (organic) etiologies are vasculogenic, hormonal, and neurogenic. Due to the relationship of vasculogenic ED with cardiovascular disease, it is important to distinguish men with predominantly vasculogenic ED from those with predominantly psychogenic ED (type I) or non-vasculogenic organic ED.

Table 1.1 offers elements for distinction between type I (psychogenic) and type II (organic) ED [4]. The most common organic etiology of ED is vasculogenic. Coexistense of vascular disease, advancing age, and the presence of cardiovascular risk factors and metabolic disorders increase the likelihood that ED is of vasculogenic etiology. The etiology of predominantly psychogenic ED is multifactorial, and components may include psychiatric disorders (especially depression), interpersonal problems with the sexual partner, or misconceptions about normal sexual activity. Identifying and getting treatment for those patients with psychogenic causes of ED such as depression that may also increase cardiovascular risk is also important [4].

1.3 The Importance of the Medical History

While additional workup is usually necessary, the medical and sexual history is essential and frequently the most revealing aspect of the ED assessment process [5]. Although not always definitive, a detailed history may provide suggestive evidence for or against the role of specific organic or psychogenic factors and should be obtained in all cases of ED. A detailed description should be made of the rigidity and duration of both erotic and morning erections and of problems with arousal, ejaculation, and orgasm [6]. Documenting a medical history has several goals [6–8]. First, it is important to evaluate the potential role of underlying comorbidities. ED may be symptomatic of an underlying comorbidity, such as atherosclerosis or diabetes. Second, a possible association with cardiovascular conditions to differentiate among potential organic and psychogenic causes in the etiology of a patient's sexual problem must be investigated. Third, the history helps to assess the use of concomitant medications. Some of these medications can either cause or contribute to ED, and a change in medication may result in an improvement in sexual function.

Additionally, the use of certain medications (e.g. nitrates) may be important contraindications for specific treatments. Interviewing the patient's partner during the ED assessment is also usually advisable.

Standardized questionnaires are frequently used to confirm that the disorder is truly ED and to measure its severity. They are also valuable research aids that help assess the response to different treatments of ED. Several questionnaires are available. Two of the most practical and easily administered are the International Index of Erectile Function (IIEF) and the Sexual Health Inventory for Men (SHIM) [9, 10]. The IIEF, a 15-item, self-evaluation questionnaire is a validated instrument for assessing erectile function, orgasmic function, desire, and satisfaction after sexual relations [9]. An abridged version of the IIEF is a five-item questionnaire the SHIM or IIEF-5 (Table 1.2). Responses to the five questions range from 1 (worst) to 5 (best). Questions 2–4 may be graded 0 if there is no sexual activity, or no sexual intercourse attempt) and the final score ranges from 1 to 25 points; a descending score indicates worsening of erectile function, with values ≤21 being diagnostic of ED [10]. Importantly, validated questionnaires correlate with the extend of coronary artery disease and improve the predictive value of ED for total cardiovascular events compared to a single-question ED diagnosis [11]. It cannot be overemphasized that the SHIM can be effectively used not only by andrologists and urologists but by a wide array of medical specialists, such as cardiologists, diabetologists, primary care physicians, etc.

1.4 Physical Examination

The physical examination may corroborate aspects of the medical history and can sometimes reveal unsuspected physical findings (e.g., decreased peripheral pulses, atrophic testes, penile plaque). In addition to identifying specific etiologies or comorbidities, the physical examination may provide an opportunity to inform the patient about aspects of his sexual anatomy or physiology as well as to provide reassurance about body appearance and function [5, 6]. It should be recognized that the physical examination can also be a source of shame, embarrassment, or discomfort for many patients. Every effort should be made to ensure the patient's privacy, confidentiality, and personal comfort during the examination. It is important to review the major findings of the examination and address any questions or concerns of the patient regarding his physical appearance or normality.

1.5 Biochemical and Hormonal Testing

The laboratory investigation for ED depends on information gathered during the medical history. Laboratory testing is necessary for most patients, though not for all. On the basis of laboratory tests, it is crucial to determine the medical status of the patient, to identify and characterize the type of dysfunction, and to determine the need for additional specialized testing (e.g., penile or pelvic blood flow studies, nocturnal penile tumescence testing, or other blood tests).

Table 1.2 The Sexual Health Inventory for Men (SHIM) or IIEF-5 over the past 6 months

		Very low	Low	Moderate	High	Very high
1. How did you rate your confidence that you could get and keep an erection?		1	2	3	4	5
		Almost never or never	A few times	Sometimes	Most times	Almost always or always
2. When you had erections with sexual stimulation, how often were your erections hard enough for penetration?	No sexual activity 0	1	2	3	4	5
3. During sexual intercourse, how often were you able to maintain your erection after you had penetrated your partner?	Did not attempt intercourse 0	Almost never or never 1	A few times 2	Sometimes 3	Most times 4	Almost always or always 5
4. During sexual intercourse, how difficult was it to maintain your erection to completion of intercourse?	Did not attempt intercourse 0	Extremely difficult 1	Very difficult 2	Difficult 3	Slightly difficult 4	Not difficult 5
5. When you attempted sexual intercourse, how often was it satisfactory to you?	Did not attempt intercourse 0	Almost never or never 1	A few times 2	Sometimes 3	Most times 4	Almost always or always 5

The IIEF-5 is administered as a screening instrument for the presence and severity of ED in conjunction with the clinical assessment. The score is the sum of the responses to the five items, so that overall score may range from 1 to 25
No ED (total score, 22–25), mild (17–21), mild to moderate (12–16), moderate (8–11), and severe ED (1–7)

All patients must undergo a fasting glucose and lipid profile if not assessed in the previous 12 months. Total (and free) testosterone should be measured in all ED patients because there is documented evidence of a high incidence of impairment in pathways of cavernosal homeostasis and penile vascular remodeling related to low androgen level [12]. Tests that measure bioavailable or calculated-free testosterone are preferred to total testosterone tests because they are better at establishing testosterone deficiency [13]. There are many studies showing a significant association of low testosterone levels with the presence and extent of vasculogenic ED; however, age-adjusted cutoff testosterone values for exclusion of vasculogenic ED presence or severity have not been identified yet [12–14]. Additional hormonal tests, e.g., prolactin, follicle-stimulating hormone (FSH), and luteinizing hormone (LH), must be carried out when low testosterone levels are detected [13]. If any abnormality is observed, referral to an endocrinologist may be necessary.

The rationale for assaying proinflammatory markers is the potential bidirectional association between endothelial dysfunction and inflammation [15]. The majority of these markers are upregulated in men with ED, irrespective of the etiology resulting in ED [16, 17], but most importantly, combining proinflammatory markers such as fibrinogen or interleukin-6 has been shown to have a satisfactory negative-predictive value for ED (few false-negative results), and perhaps they may comprise a useful tool to rule out ED in high-risk profile patients. Among a wide range of proinflammatory and endothelial-prothrombotic markers, the negative-predictive value of the combination of fibrinogen <225 mg/dL with interleukin-6 <1.24 pg/mL for excluding ED was 91.7 % [16].

1.6 Specialized Testing

Table 1.3 lists the most common specific diagnostic tests for ED and their benefits and limitations. The classical specialized tests such as penile color Doppler ultrasound accurately assess cavernous artery inflow and venous leakage [18]. Neurological testing (penile biothesiometry, dorsal nerve conduction velocity) is useful to assess somatic pathways [8]. However, these tests frequently do not add to data already available from the medical history and assessments based on patient self-report, physical examination, and laboratory testing [3]. Furthermore, it should be born in mind that these tests are expensive, time consuming, invasive, prone to complications (prolonged erections), and prone to error except in experienced hands.

Nevertheless, evaluation by color Doppler ultrasound still remains the cornerstone of the diagnostic workup of the patients with vasculogenic ED. The measurement of peak systolic velocity by using a dynamic penile Doppler ultrasound (with intracavernous injection of alprostadil and audiovisual stimulation) alone represents a reliable marker for detecting penile vascular damage and diagnosis of vasculogenic ED in patients with CV risk factors because this is a parameter that strongly correlates with functional erection [18]. Criteria for evaluating the study results vary to some degree. A peak systolic velocity lower than 25 cm/s is generally agreed to

Table 1.3 Advantages and disadvantages of commonly used specific ED tests

	Advantages	Disadvantages
Color Doppler ultrasound	A definitive and accurate diagnosis for arteriogenic ED	Incomplete smooth muscle relaxation due to anxiety or sympathetic overtone might lead to false-positive results
	Peak systolic velocity is related to incident major cardiovascular events. Association with the degree and distribution of atherosclerotic lesions in other vascular beds	
Pharmaco-arteriography	Mandatory prior to revascularization procedures. Outlines anatomy of pudendal and penile arteries before arterial surgery in post-traumatic and congenital cases	Invasive. Affected by methodology and timing
Pharmaco-cavernosometry or cavernosography	Suggests veno-occlusive dysfunction. It is recommended before venous surgery to confirm the diagnosis and to locate the site of venous leakage	Moderately invasive. Incomplete smooth muscle relaxation due to anxiety or sympathetic overtone might lead to false-positive results
Neurological testing	Detect somatic motor pathways, sensory pathways, reflexes	Does not directly assess autonomic nerve function. Complex and time consuming
Nocturnal penile tumescence monitoring	One of the most commonly used tests to distinguish psychogenic from organic ED	Age dependent, it does not detect sensory deficit impotence. False-positive results can occur if patients do not sleep well. Assesses only radial, not axial rigidity. Does not correlate well with IIEF domain scores

indicate arterial insufficiency. The proposed value for the lower limit of normal ranges from 25 to 35 cm/s, but a peak systolic velocity of 35 cm/s or higher clearly rules out arterial insufficiency. End-diastolic velocity serves as a proxy for venous outflow; a velocity of 5 cm/s or lower when the penis is at full rigidity indicates the absence of abnormal venous leakage.

Nocturnal penile tumescence and rigidity testing using Rigiscan should take place for at least two nights. A functional erectile mechanism is indicated by an erectile event of at least 60 % rigidity recorded on the tip of the penis lasting for ≥10 min.

Recent research-based techniques that attempt to assess penile endothelial dysfunction [19] and to differentiate men with vasculogenic ED from those without include the penile nitric oxide release test and Endo-PAT2000 [20].

> **Conclusions** (Fig. 1.1)
> A comprehensive evaluation of ED is the foundation of the management plan. The initial assessment should focus on identification of the actual presence of the consensus definition of ED. Administration of various questionnaires focused on ED could be a part of the initial assessment. A further step includes a detailed

1 Definition and Assessment of Erectile Dysfunction

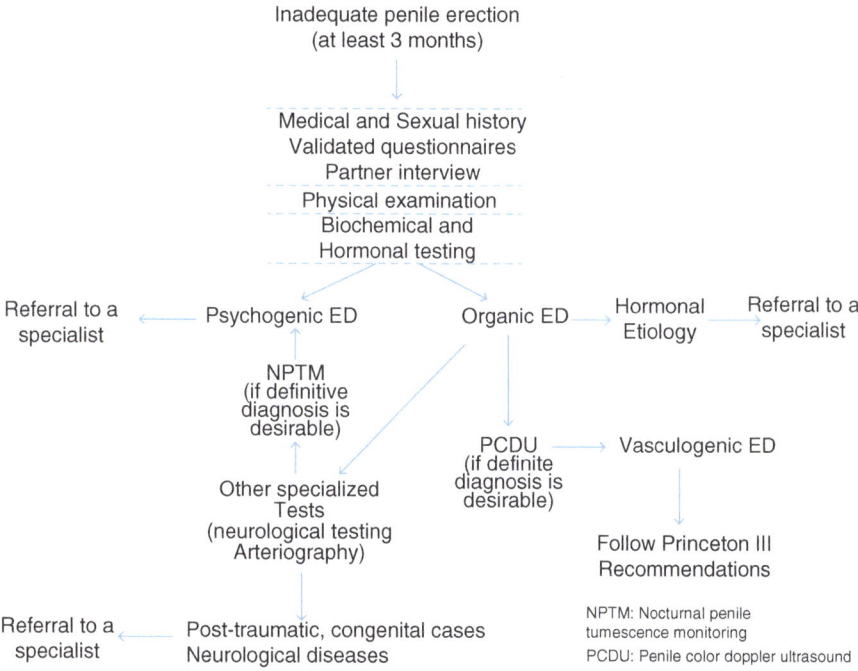

Fig. 1.1 Proposed stepwise algorithm for the initial assessment of men with erectile dysfunction

medical history, psychiatric history, psychosocial assessment, assessment of lifestyle factors, and medication review. Physical examination should be comprehensive, with a focus on genitourinary, vascular, and neurological systems and inspection of secondary sexual characteristics. Biochemical and hormonal testing should be tailored to the individual patient and should focus on the possible etiological factors of ED. Additionally, proinflammatory biomarkers with good performance characteristics (i.e., sensitivity, specificity, positive- and negative-predictive values) can assist in the diagnosis of ED, discriminate the cause of ED, and estimate the severity of ED. Further focused, specialized testing could include penile vascular assessment and neurological testing.

References

1. NIH Consensus Conference. Impotence (1993) NIH consensus development panel on impotence. JAMA 270:83–90
2. Lewis R, Fugl-Meyer K, Corona G et al (2010) Definitions epidemiology/risk factors for sexual dysfunction. J Sex Med 7:1598–1607
3. Montorsi F, Adaikan G, Becher E et al (2010) Summary of the recommendations on sexual dysfunctions in men. J Sex Med 7:3572–3588
4. Persu C, Cauni V, Gutue S et al (2009) Diagnosis and treatment of erectile dysfunction–a practical update. J Med Life 2:394–400

5. The Process of Care Consensus Panel (1999) The process of care model for evaluation and treatment of erectile dysfunction. Int J Impot Res 11:59–70
6. Hatzichristou D, Rosen RC, Derogatis LR et al (2010) Recommendations for the clinical evaluation of men and women with sexual dysfunction. J Sex Med 7:337–348
7. Hatzimouratidis K, Amar E, Eardley I et al; for the European Association of Urology (2010) Guidelines on male sexual dysfunction: erectile dysfunction and premature ejaculation. Eur Urol 57:804–814
8. Shamloul R, Ghanem H (2013) Erectile dysfunction. Lancet 381(9861):153–165
9. Rosen RC, Riley A, Wagner G et al (1997) The international index of erectile function (IIEF): a multidimensional scale for assessment of erectile dysfunction. Urology 49:822–830
10. Cappelleri JC, Rosen RC (2005) The Sexual Health Inventory for Men (SHIM): a 5-year review of research and clinical experience. Int J Impot Res 17:307–319
11. Vlachopoulos C, Jackson G, Stefanadis C et al (2013) Erectile dysfunction in the cardiovascular patient. Eur Heart J 34:2034–2046
12. Corona G, Maggi M (2010) The role of testosterone in erectile dysfunction. Nat Rev Urol 7:46–56
13. Sansone A, Romanelli F, Gianfrilli D et al (2014) Endocrine evaluation of erectile dysfunction. Endocrine 46:423–430
14. Corona G, Mannucci E, Fisher AD et al (2008) Low levels of androgens in men with erectile dysfunction and obesity. J Sex Med 5:2454–2463
15. Vlachopoulos C, Ioakeimidis N, Terentes-Printzios D et al (2008) The triad: erectile dysfunction–endothelial dysfunction-cardiovascular disease. Curr Pharm Des 14:3700–3714
16. Vlachopoulos C, Aznaouridis K, Ioakeimidis N et al (2006) Unfavourable endothelial and inflammatory state in erectile dysfunction patients with or without coronary artery disease. Eur Heart J 27:2640–2648
17. Billups KL, Kaiser DR, Kelly AS et al (2006) Relation of C-reactive protein and other cardiovascular risk factors to penile vascular disease in men with erectile dysfunction. Int J Impot Res 15:231–236
18. Aversa A, Sarteschi LM (2007) The role of penile color-duplex ultrasound for the evaluation of erectile dysfunction. J Sex Med 4:1437–1447
19. Vardi Y, Dayan L, Apple B et al (2009) Penile and systemic endothelial function in men with and without erectile dysfunction. Eur Urol 55:969–976
20. Kovac JR, Gomez L, Smith RP et al (2014) Measurement of endothelial dysfunction via peripheral arterial tonometry predicts vasculogenic erectile dysfunction. Int J Impot Res. Epub ahead print

Epidemiology of Erectile Dysfunction in Hypertension

Charalampos A. Grassos, Charalampos I. Liakos,
Eirini Papadopoulou, Theodosia Papadopoulou,
and Michael Doumas

2.1 Introduction

Erectile dysfunction has been called the "prima ballerina" of hypertension-related, quality-of-life complications. This is because erectile dysfunction is frequently encountered in hypertensive patients and exerts a major impact on the quality of life of patients and their sexual partners [1, 2]. Several mechanisms have been implicated in the pathogenesis of erectile dysfunction in hypertensive patients. Studies of Doppler ultrasonography of the penile arteries, with or without papaverine injections, suggested that in 89 % of these hypertensive patients, the cause of erectile dysfunction was penile circulation disability, probably due to atherosclerosis [3].

Erectile dysfunction may actually be a risk marker of cardiovascular complications in hypertensive patients [4] as well as an early diagnostic indicator for asymptomatic organ damages (higher common carotid intima-media thickness, higher carotid-femoral pulse-wave velocity, and lower flow-mediated dilation of

---

C.A. Grassos • C.I. Liakos
Cardiology Department, KAT General Hospital,
2, Nikis Street, Kifissia, Athens 14561, Greece
e-mail: harigrass@yahoo.gr; bliakos@med.uoa.gr

E. Papadopoulou • T. Papadopoulou
2nd Propedeutic Department of Internal Medicine, Aristotle University,
49, Konstantinoupoleos Street, Thessaloniki 54643, Greece
e-mail: eirini.papadopoulou@yahoo.it; sissipapth@yahoo.gr

M. Doumas (✉)
Hippokration Hospital, 49, Konstantinoupoleos Street,
Thessaloniki 54643, Greece

2nd Propedeutic Department of Internal Medicine, Aristotle University, Thessaloniki, Greece

George Washington University, Washington, DC, USA
e-mail: michalisdoumas@yahoo.co.uk

the brachial artery) [5]. Treatment of erectile dysfunction with phosphodiesterase-5 inhibitors may also improve adherence to antihypertensive therapy [6].

This review aims to present epidemiological data regarding the impact of hypertension on erectile function, the prevalence of erectile dysfunction in hypertensive patients compared to normotensive individuals; critically evaluate available data; and summarize the determinants of erectile dysfunction in hypertensive patients.

2.2 The Impact of Hypertension on Erectile Dysfunction

Available data on the risk for erectile dysfunction in the presence of hypertension come mainly from large studies in community-based populations that include subgroups of hypertensive men [7–16]. In these studies, the odds ratio for erectile dysfunction in hypertensive individuals ranges from 1.30 to 2.79 (Table 2.1).

Specifically, Derby et al. [7] reevaluating the results of the Massachusetts Male Aging Study (MMAS) found an 80 % greater risk for erectile dysfunction in hypertensive individuals aged 40–70 years (age-adjusted odds ratio 1.80). In the Cologne Male Survey which was performed by Braun et al. [8] in 4,489 men, 30–80 years of age in the Cologne urban district, an age-adjusted odds ratio 1.58 (95 % confidence intervals 1.29–1.93) was found for erectile dysfunction in the subgroup of hypertensives. Martin-Morales et al. [9] conducted a large cross-sectional study in 2,476 individuals in Spain including 850 hypertensives. The International Index of Erectile Function (IIEF) questionnaire was used for the assessment of erectile dysfunction. The study included both younger and older patients (age range 25–70 years) with a mean ± SD age of 48 ± 12 years. It has to be noted, however, that the majority of study participants was of older age (50–70 years: 68 %). Hypertension was associated with a 58 % increased risk for erectile dysfunction (odds ratio 1.58). Marumo et al. [10] evaluated the significance of

Table 2.1 Odds ratio for erectile dysfunction in hypertensive subgroups from larger cohorts studied [7–16]

Study (authors – year)	Age of participants (years)	Odds ratio for erectile dysfunction in hypertensives
Derby et al. 2000 [7]	40–70	1.80[a]
Braun et al. 2000 [8]	30–80	1.58[a]
Martin-Morales et al. 2001 [9]	25–70	1.58
Marumo et al. 2001 [10]	40–79	2.79
Nicolosi et al. 2003 [11]	40–70	1.45[a]
Mirone et al. 2004 [12]	17–98	1.30
Ponholzer et al. 2005 [13]	20–80	2.05
Saigal et al. 2006 [14]	≥20	1.56
Laumann et al. 2007 [15]	≥40	1.60
Selvin et al. 2007 [16]	≥20	2.22[a]

[a]Adjusted for age

several risk factors for erectile dysfunction in 1,014 men aged 40–79 years, according to a univariate logistic regression analysis and found a 48 % prevalence of erectile dysfunction and a 2.79 odds ratio (95 % confidence intervals 2.05–3.80) for erectile dysfunction in the 223 hypertensives included in the study.

Nicolosi et al. [11] assessed the epidemiology of erectile dysfunction in community-based populations in four countries (Brazil, Italy, Japan, and Malaysia). It was a cross-national study performed in a random sample of approximately 600 men in each country aged 40–70 years. An age- and country-adjusted odds ratio for erectile dysfunction 1.45 (95 % confidence intervals 1.15–1.84) was found in the group of 540 hypertensives included in the study. Mirone et al. [12] sought to assess determinants of erectile dysfunction in men aged 17–98 years who asked for a free of charge andrologic consultation during a week focused on andrologic prevention in Italy. They found an increased risk of ED (odds ratio 1.30, 95 % confidence intervals 1.10–1.40) in men with hypertension. Ponholzer et al. [13] assessed the prevalence and risk factors for erectile dysfunction in 2,869 men aged 20–80 years participating in a health-screening project in the area of Vienna. Participants completed the IIEF questionnaire for the evaluation of erectile dysfunction. Risk factors for erectile dysfunction included hypertension with an odds ratio 2.05 (95 % confidence intervals 1.61–2.60). Saigal et al. [14] analyzed data from the 2001–2002 National Health and Nutrition Examination Survey (NHANES) to evaluate predictors and prevalence of erectile dysfunction in a racially diverse population (3,566 men, 20 years and older). They found several modifiable risk factors that were independently associated with erectile dysfunction, including hypertension (odds ratio 1.56). Laumann et al. [15] conducted in the United States the Male Attitudes Regarding Sexual Health (MARSH) study, a cross-sectional, nationally representative probability survey of 1,955 men aged 40 years or older that oversampled blacks and Hispanics. They aimed to estimate, by race/ethnicity, the prevalence of erectile dysfunction and the impact of sociodemographic, health, relationship, psychological, and lifestyle variables. An odds ratio for erectile dysfunction 1.60 (95 % confidence intervals 1.00–2.40) was found in the subgroup of patients with hypertension. Selvin et al. [16] also performed a cross-sectional analysis of data from 2,126 adult male participants in the 2001–2002 National Health and Nutrition Examination Survey (NHANES) to assess the prevalence of erectile dysfunction and to quantify associations between putative risk factors and erectile dysfunction in the US adult male population (20 years and older). Slightly less than half of individuals with treated hypertension (44.1 %) were affected by erectile dysfunction (age-adjusted odds ratio 2.22, 95 % confidence intervals 1.30–3.80).

2.3 Prevalence of Erectile Dysfunction in Hypertensive Patients

The prevalence of erectile dysfunction in patients with essential hypertension, either treated or untreated, has been evaluated in studies dedicated to that purpose and was compared to the prevalence of erectile dysfunction in normotensive individuals in

Table 2.2 Prevalence of erectile dysfunction in hypertensive and normotensive individuals from respective studies [17–23]

Study (authors – year)	Prevalence of erectile dysfunction (%)		
	Treated hypertensives	Untreated hypertensives	Normotensives
Bulpitt et al. 1976 [17]	25	17	7
Croog et al. 1988 [18]	58	44	–
Düsing 2003 [19]	45	65	–
Doumas et al. 2006 [20]	40	20	14
Bener et al. 2007 [21]	72	65	24
Baumhäkel et al. 2008 [22]	64	79	–
Cordero et al. 2010 [23]	71	–	–

some of these studies [17–23]. According to these studies, some degree of erectile dysfunction is present with a prevalence that ranges from 17 to 79 % in untreated hypertensives, from 25 to 72 % in patients under blood pressure-lowering treatment while from 7 to 24 % in normotensive subjects (Table 2.2).

Specifically, Bulpitt et al. [17] described a study of 302 patients in which erectile dysfunction was observed in 7 % of normotensive men, 17 % of men with untreated hypertension, and 25 % of men with treated hypertension. The effects of antihypertensive medications on reported distress over sexual symptoms over a 24-week treatment period were examined by Croog et al. [18] as part of a multicenter, randomized, double-blind clinical trial in which 626 men with mild to moderate hypertension participated. On entry into the clinical trial, 58 % of patients taking antihypertensive medications and 44 % of men not receiving antihypertensive drugs reported some degree of erectile dysfunction. Düsing [19] designed an open, prospective study to investigate the effect of the angiotensin II receptor blocker valsartan on sexual function in hypertensive males. The patients' sexual function was assessed before valsartan and after 6 months of treatment using the IIEF questionnaire. At baseline, 65.0 % of the 952 patients without previous antihypertensive treatment could be diagnosed as having erectile dysfunction, according to the IIEF. Valsartan therapy markedly reduced the prevalence of erectile dysfunction to 45 %. In a sample of 634 Greek young and middle-aged men (31–65 years), erectile dysfunction was at least twice as common in treated hypertensives compared to untreated hypertensives and normotensives (40 % versus 20 % and 14 %, respectively), as reported by Doumas et al. [20].

A matched case-control study was conducted by Bener et al. [21] at primary health-care clinics with 296 Qatari hypertensive participants and 298 normotensive men aged 30–75 years. The mean ± SD age was 54.8 ± 11.5 years for hypertensives as compared to 54.5 ± 12.1 years for non-hypertensives. Sexual function was evaluated with the IIEF questionnaire. Among the 298 non-hypertensive participants, only 71 had erectile dysfunction (24 %), while of the 296 hypertensive patients, 196 participants reported erectile dysfunction (66 %). Moreover, among the 53 treated hypertensives, 38 were found with erectile dysfunction (72 %), while of the remaining 243 untreated hypertensives, 158 reported an erectile dysfunction (65 %). Of the 296 hypertensive participants studied, 25 % had severe, 29 % had moderate, and 12 % had mild erectile dysfunction. Frequency and severity of erectile dysfunction increased with advancing age. Baumhäkel et al. [22] aimed to determine the influence of irbesartan on erectile dysfunction in a total of 1,069 consecutive hypertensive patients with a metabolic syndrome recruited from the documentation of hypertension and metabolic syndrome in patients with irbesartan treatment (DO-IT) survey. Erectile dysfunction was assessed using the IIEF questionnaire. Erectile function increased significantly after 6 months of treatment with irbesartan, irrespective of dosage and independent of additional treatment with hydrochlorothiazide. Prevalence of erectile dysfunction declined to 64 % from 79 % at baseline. Cordero et al. [23] designed a cross-sectional and observational study in 1,007 high-risk hypertensive male subjects treated with any beta-blockade agent for at least 6 months (mean ± SD age of participants 57.9 ± 10.6 years). Erectile dysfunction was assessed by the IIEF questionnaire. The prevalence of any category of erectile dysfunction was 71 % (38.1 % mild, 16.8 % moderate, and 16.1 % severe erectile dysfunction, respectively). Patients with erectile dysfunction had longer time since the diagnosis of hypertension and higher prevalence of risk factors and comorbidities. The prevalence of ED increased linearly with age. ED patients received more medications and were more frequently treated with carvedilol and less frequently with nebivolol.

The prevalence of erectile dysfunction in hypertensive men is even higher when diabetes mellitus coexists (77 % versus 67 %), as reported by Giuliano et al. [24]. Moreover, the previous studies clearly demonstrate that the severity of erectile dysfunction is worse in patients with hypertension than in the general population.

2.4 Comments on Variation in Odds Ratio and Prevalence of Erectile Dysfunction in Hypertensive Patients

The large variation in the reported odds ratio and prevalence may reflect different sample populations, different assessment methods (e.g., telephone interviews, face-to-face interviews, mailed questionnaires, in-office questionnaires), different severity of erectile dysfunction, different medications, cultural differences in the willingness of individuals to discuss such issues and accept the social stigma of erectile dysfunction, as well as ethnic differences (genetic and environmental factors affecting erectile function) [2]. Considering the various methods for the assessment of erectile dysfunction, some trials have used a single question about sexual satisfaction while others have adopted multiple-scale validated questionnaires like the IIEF that checks all five major domains of sexuality: sexual desire, erectile function, orgasmic function, intercourse satisfaction, and overall satisfaction with sexual life.

The aforementioned factors may explain the lower prevalence of erectile dysfunction in hypertensive patients (12.2 %) reported in the Treatment of Mild Hypertension Study (TOMHS) [25], one of the first large-scale studies in the field: (i) the study included only mildly hypertensive patients since diabetic and severely hypertensive individuals were excluded; (ii) patients' age ranged from 45 to 69 years, excluding older patients; and (iii) there was only one question assessing sexual dysfunction.

2.5 The Role of Antihypertensive Drugs

An interesting and perhaps paradoxical observation among the previous studies is that treated hypertensive patients often were no better or perhaps even demonstrated higher prevalence of erectile dysfunction. This paradox is explained, in part, by the concept that some of the antihypertensive medicines that are used may actually worsen erectile dysfunction. Specifically, older antihypertensive drugs (diuretics, traditional beta-blockers, centrally acting) exert negative results [1, 17, 18, 20, 26], whereas newer agents have either neutral (calcium antagonists, angiotensin-converting enzyme inhibitors) [1, 18, 20] or even beneficial effects (angiotensin receptor blockers) [1, 19, 20, 22, 26]. In regard with the vasodilating beta-blockers, it seems that they do not share the unfavorable effects of traditional beta-blockers though precise data on this issue are lacking [1, 27]. Development of erectile dysfunction in connection with beta-blockers might be biased by psychological effects derived from the awareness of being treated with a certain substance [28]. This is an important point since patient's concerns about the adverse effects of drugs on erectile function might limit the use of essential medications in high-risk patients [28]. Available data point towards significant benefits in sexual function when prior antihypertensive therapy is switched to either nebivolol or angiotensin receptor blockers [19, 22, 29].

2.6 Determinants of Erectile Dysfunction in Hypertensive Patients

Major determinants of the frequency and severity of erectile dysfunction in hypertensive men include the duration and severity of hypertension, the age, and the type of antihypertensive therapy [1, 20, 21, 23]. No difference in the prevalence of erectile dysfunction was found among hypertensive and pre-hypertensive men aged 25–40 years compared with normotensive controls, pointing that the damage caused by hypertension may take years to become evident [30]. Long-standing hypertension (>5–6 years) has been associated with more frequent and more severe erectile dysfunction compared to hypertension of recent onset [20]. The results of a recent study further suggest that non-dipping status is a risk indicator for early deterioration of erectile function in hypertensive patients [31]. No definite data exist regarding the role of smoking, alcohol intake, and the level of physical activity on erectile function in patients with essential hypertension [20, 27]. The effect of lifestyle modification on erectile function has not been adequately addressed but there are reports for beneficial results: an interval exercise program implemented for 8 weeks in hypertensive patients with severe erectile dysfunction had positive effects on sexual functioning [32]. A recent meta-analysis suggests a beneficial effect of lifestyle modification on erectile function [33]; however, available data in patients with hypertension is not of adequate power and quality to permit for definite conclusions [34].

Conclusions

Patients with essential hypertension present with erectile dysfunction more frequently than matched normotensive individuals, a condition with a major effect on their quality of life. Because erectile dysfunction is a topic of potential embarrassment, doctors must be motivated to discuss such issues. Main determinants of the prevalence and severity of erectile dysfunction in hypertensive individuals are the age, the severity and duration of hypertension, and the type of antihypertensive therapy. Blood pressure-lowering treatment may even increase the prevalence of erectile dysfunction, with older drugs (diuretics, traditional beta-blockers, centrally acting) showing a worse profile than newer drugs (vasodilating beta-blockers, calcium antagonists, angiotensin-converting enzyme inhibitors, angiotensin receptor blockers). By identifying hypertensive individuals with erectile dysfunction, a cautious antihypertensive drug selection is mandatory. Changing the antihypertensive drug class in a treated patient with erectile dysfunction may also improve his sexual function.

References

1. Manolis A, Doumas M (2008) Sexual dysfunction: the "prima ballerina" of hypertension-related quality-of-life complications. J Hypertens 26:2074–2084
2. Doumas M, Douma S (2006) Sexual dysfunction in essential hypertension: myth or reality? J Clin Hypertens 8:269–274
3. Jensen J, Lendorf A, Stimpel H, Frost J, Ibsen H, Rosenkilde P (1999) The prevalence and etiology of impotence in 101 male hypertensive outpatients. Am J Hypertens 12:271–275
4. Burchardt M, Burchardt T, Anastasiadis AG, Kiss AJ, Shabsigh A, de La Taille A, Pawar RV, Baer L, Shabsigh R (2001) Erectile dysfunction is a marker for cardiovascular complications and psychological functioning in men with hypertension. Int J Impot Res 13:276–281
5. Vlachopoulos C, Aznaouridis K, Ioakeimidis N, Rokkas K, Tsekoura D, Vasiliadou C, Stefanadi E, Askitis A, Stefanadis C (2008) Arterial function and intima-media thickness in hypertensive patients with erectile dysfunction. J Hypertens 26:1829–1836
6. Scranton RE, Lawler E, Botteman M, Chittamooru S, Gagnon D, Lew R, Harnett J, Gaziano JM (2007) Effect of treating erectile dysfunction on management of systolic hypertension. Am J Cardiol 100:459–463
7. Derby CA, Araujo AB, Johannes CB, Feldman HA, McKinlay JB (2000) Measurement of erectile dysfunction in population-based studies: the use of a single question self-assessment in the Massachusetts Male Aging Study. Int J Impot Res 12:197–204
8. Braun M, Wassmer G, Klotz T, Reifenrath B, Mathers M, Engelmann U (2000) Epidemiology of erectile dysfunction: results of the "Cologne Male Survey.". Int J Impot Res 12:305–311
9. Martin-Morales A, Sanchez-Cruz JJ, de Saenz Tejada I, Rodriguez-Vela L, Jimenez-Cruz JF, Burgos-Rodriguez R (2001) Prevalence and independent risk factors for erectile dysfunction in Spain: results of the Epidemiologia de la Disfuncion Erectil Masculina Study. J Urol 166:569–575

10. Marumo K, Nakashima J, Murai M (2001) Age-related prevalence of erectile dysfunction in Japan: assessment by the International Index of Erectile Function. Int J Urol 8:53–59
11. Nicolosi A, Moreira ED Jr, Shirai M, Bin Mohd Tambi MI, Glasser DB (2003) Epidemiology of erectile dysfunction in four countries: cross-national study of the prevalence and correlates of erectile dysfunction. Urology 61:201–206
12. Mirone V, Ricci E, Gentile V, Basile Fasolo C, Parazzini F (2004) Determinants of erectile dysfunction risk in a large series of Italian men attending andrology clinics. Eur Urol 45:87–91
13. Ponholzer A, Temml C, Mock K, Marszalek M, Obermayr R, Madersbacher S (2005) Prevalence and risk factors for erectile dysfunction in 2869 men using a validated questionnaire. Eur Urol 47:80–86
14. Saigal CS, Wessells H, Pace J, Schonlau M, Wilt TJ, Urologic Diseases in America Project (2006) Predictors and prevalence of erectile dysfunction in a racially diverse population. Arch Intern Med 166:207–212
15. Laumann EO, West S, Glasser D, Carson C, Rosen R, Kang JH (2007) Prevalence and correlates of erectile dysfunction by race and ethnicity among men aged 40 or older in the United States: from the male attitudes regarding sexual health survey. J Sex Med 4:57–65
16. Selvin E, Burnett AL, Platz EA (2007) Prevalence and risk factors for erectile dysfunction in the US. Am J Med 120:151–157
17. Bulpitt CJ, Dollery CT, Carne S (1976) Changes in symptoms in hypertensive patients after referral to hospital clinic. Br Heart J 38:121–128
18. Croog SH, Levine S, Sudilovsky A, Baume RM, Clive J (1988) Sexual symptoms in hypertensive patients. A clinical trial of antihypertensive medications. Arch Intern Med 148:788–794
19. Düsing R (2003) Effect of the angiotensin II antagonist valsartan on sexual function in hypertensive men. Blood Press Suppl 12:29–34
20. Doumas M, Tsakiris A, Douma S, Grigorakis A, Papadopoulos A, Hounta A, Tsiodras S, Dimitriou D, Giamarellou H (2006) Factors affecting the increased prevalence of erectile dysfunction in Greek hypertensive compared to normotensive individuals. J Androl 27:469–477
21. Bener A, Al-Ansari A, Al-Hamaq AO, Elbagi IE, Afifi M (2007) Prevalence of erectile dysfunction among hypertensive and nonhypertensive Qatari men. Medicina 43:870–878
22. Baumhäkel M, Schlimmer N, Böhm M, DO-IT Investigators (2008) Effect of irbesartan on erectile function in patients with hypertension and metabolic syndrome. Int J Impot Res 20:493–500
23. Cordero A, Bertomeu-Martínez V, Mazón P, Fácila L, Bertomeu-González V, Conthe P, González-Juanatey JR (2010) Erectile dysfunction in high-risk hypertensive patients treated with beta-blockade agents. Cardiovasc Ther 28:15–22
24. Giuliano FA, Leriche A, Jaudinot EO, de Gendre AS (2004) Prevalence of erectile dysfunction among 7689 patients with diabetes or hypertension, or both. Urology 64:1196–1201
25. Grimm RH, Grandits GA, Priueas RJ et al (1997) Long-term effects on sexual function of five antihypertensive drugs and nutritional hygienic treatment in hypertensive men and women in the Treatment of Mild Hypertension Study. (THOMS). Hypertension 29:8–14
26. Fogari R, Zoppi A, Poletti L, Marasi G, Mugellini A, Corradi L (2001) Sexual activity in hypertensive men treated with valsartan or carvedilol: a crossover study. Am J Hypertens 14:27–31
27. Ker JA (2012) Hypertension and sexual dysfunction. S Afr Fam Pract 54:117–118
28. Silvestri A, Galetta P, Cerquetani E, Marazzi G, Patrizi R, Fini M, Rosano GM (2003) Report of erectile dysfunction after therapy with beta-blockers is related to patient knowledge of side effects and is reversed by placebo. Eur Heart J 24:1928–1932
29. Manolis A, Doumas M (2012) Antihypertensive treatment and sexual dysfunction. Curr Hypertens Rep 14:285–292
30. Heruti RJ, Sharabi Y, Arbel Y, Shochat T, Swartzon M, Brenner G, Justo D (2007) The prevalence of erectile dysfunction among hypertensive and prehypertensive men aged 25–40 years. J Sex Med 4:596–601
31. Erden I, Ozhan H, Ordu S, Yalcin S, Caglar O, Kayikci A (2010) The effect of non-dipper pattern of hypertension on erectile dysfunction. Blood Press 19:249–253

32. Lamina S, Okoye CG, Dagogo TT (2009) Therapeutic effect of an interval exercise training program in the management of erectile dysfunction in hypertensive patients. J Clin Hypertens 11:125–129
33. Gupta BP, Murad MH, Clifton MM, Prokop L, Nehra A, Kopesky SL (2011) The effect of lifestyle modification and cardiovascular risk factor reduction on erectile dysfunction: a systematic review and meta-analysis. Arch Intern Med 171:1797–1803
34. Doumas M, Anyfanti P, Triantafyllou A (2012) Management of erectile dysfunction: do not forget hypertension. Arch Intern Med 172:597–598

Pathophysiology of Erectile Dysfunction

Dragan Lovic

Erectile dysfunction (ED) is a major problem in a life of the modern men. It affects 10–25 % of middle-aged and elderly men. ED is the failure to achieve erection, ejaculation, or both. Normal erectile function requires the involvement and coordination of multiple regulatory systems and is thus subject to the influence of psychological, hormonal, neurological, vascular, and cavernosal factors. An alteration in any of these factors may be sufficient to cause erectile dysfunction (ED), but in many cases a combination of several factors is involved [1]. Some conditions such as diabetes, atherosclerotic, and drug-related causes account for 80 % of causes of ED in elderly.

Evidence suggests that ED may result from three basic mechanisms:

1. Failure to initiate (psychogenic, endocrinologic, or neurogenic)
2. Failure to fill arteriogenic (atherogenic)
3. Failure to store adequate blood volume within the lacunars network (veno-occlusive dysfunction)

Psychological factors are involved in a significant number of cases of erectile dysfunction alone or in combination with organic causes. An important psychogenic factor related to erectile dysfunction is performance anxiety (fear of failure during intercourse).

There is a lot theory explaining psychological factors in erectile dysfunction have described multiple developmental, cognitive, affective, and interpersonal factors that predispose men to sexual dysfunction [2]. At present, psychogenic erectile dysfunction is thought to be primarily related to a group of predisposing, precipitating, and maintaining factors.

D. Lovic
Cardiology Department, Hypertension Centre, Clinic for Internal
Medicine Intermedica, Jovana Ristica 20/2, Nis 18000, Serbia
e-mail: draganl1@sbb.rs

3.1 Neurogenic Erectile Dysfunction

Certain neurological disorders are frequently associated with erectile dysfunction, including multiple sclerosis, temporal lobe epilepsy, Parkinson's disease, stroke, Alzheimer's disease, and spinal cord injury [3].

Events that disrupt central neural networks or the peripheral nerves involved in sexual function can cause ED. Evidence suggest that this form of ED has been termed "neurogenic impotence" [4].

The etiologies of neurogenic ED can be classified as:

- Peripheral (peripheral ED)
- Spinal (sacral-peripheral ED, suprasacral-central ED)
- Supraspinal (suprasacral ED)

3.1.1 Peripheral ED

Peripheral ED can be secondary to the disruption of sensory nerves that bring local information to the brain and contribute the afferent arm of reflex erection or to the disruption of autonomic nerves which mediate arterial dilation and trabecular smooth muscle relaxation.

3.1.2 Erectile Dysfunction in Spinal Cord Injury

Patients with lesions above the sacral parasympathetic center maintain reflexogenic erection. In these patients, minimal tactile stimulation can trigger erection, although of short duration requiring continuous stimulation to maintain erection. If the lesion is incomplete patients can receive input from psychogenic erection and maintain erectile function. Patients with significant lesions affecting the sacral parasympathetic center do not have reflex erections and have severe ED [5].

3.1.3 Erectile Dysfunction After Radical Pelvic Surgery (Supraspinal)

The neurologic lesion occurs in the pelvic plexus or in the cavernosal nerves located in the posterolateral aspect of the prostate. Maintenance of erectile capacity with nerve-sparing procedures varies between 35 and 68 % depending on the surgical technique, the clinical and pathological staging of the tumor, and the age of the patient [5]. Recovery of erectile function after radical pelvic surgery can be slow over the course of 12–18 months. Intracavernosal administration of vasoactive agents improves the probability of recovering erectile function, probably by preventing prolonged ischemia.

However, recent advances in surgical techniques have significantly lowered the incidence of post-pelvic-surgery erectile dysfunction [6].

3.2 Atherosclerosis and Erectile Dysfunction

Most important risk factors are connected with penile arterial insufficiency, including atherosclerosis, hyperlipidaemia, hypertension, diabetes mellitus, cigarette smoking, and pelvic irradiation.

Consistency of evidence association of ED to systemic vascular diseases is clear. There is notice a high prevalence of ED in patients having cardiovascular disease (CAD), peripheral arterial disease, and cerebrovascular disease [7]. The prevalence of ED looks to be increased with severity of vascular disease. Patients with lesions in two or more coronary arteries had worse erectile function than patients with normal coronary arteries or single vessel CAD. However, cardiovascular diseases are also prevalent among patients with ED. Furthermore, CAD has been revealed in patients reporting ED without any other symptomatology of vascular disease [8]. ED has also been associated to the presence of peripheral atherosclerotic lesions. Among patients with ED, 66.4 % presented atherosclerotic lesions, while lesions were only present in 36.5 % of patients without ED. In rabbit's chronic ischemia provoked by atherosclerotic stenosis of the proximal iliac artery is also associated with functional changes in the distal part of the penile vasculature such as nitric oxide synthase (NOS) activity. Neurogenic contractions were potentiated, while endothelium-dependent and neurogenic NO-mediated relaxations were reduced in cavernosal tissue. Reduced NOS activity and impaired endothelium-dependent and neurogenic NO-mediated relaxation of cavernosal tissue have been confirmed in a rabbit model of cavernosal ischemia without hyperlipidemia. An elevation of the cavernosal content of endogenous inhibitors of NOS was proposed to be responsible for these effects.

Inman and colleagues in their studies suggested that erectile dysfunction shares the same risk factors as CAD, with endothelial dysfunction being an important underlying pathological change in both diseases. Other potential mechanisms involved in the development of endothelial dysfunction that can lead to erectile dysfunction and CAD include a dysfunctional L-arginine NO pathway, increased peripheral sympathetic activity, vascular structural alterations leading to decreased vascular dilatation capacity, and increased specific [9].

Evidence from studies of Montorsi suggested that inflammatory phenomenon might be related to the caliber of the blood vessels. Whereas the penile artery has a diameter of 1–2 mm, the proximal left anterior descending coronary artery is 3–4 mm in diameter. Thus, an equally sized atherosclerotic plaque developing in the smaller penile arteries would more likely compromise flow, presenting itself as an erectile dysfunction complaint much earlier than if the same amount of plaque developed in the larger coronary artery, causing angina. Inadequate venous occlusion is another important cause of vasculogenic erectile dysfunction [9]. Inadequate venous occlusion can occur as a result of the development of large venous channels draining the cavernous tissue. It might also be caused by severe degenerative, functional, or anatomical changes in the tunica albuginea, such as those that occur in Peyronie's disease [10].

The present Princeton III Consensus guidelines recognize erectile dysfunction as a strong predictor of CVD. This association between CVD and erectile dysfunction was confirmed in a study that reported that erectile dysfunction is a potent predictor of adverse cardiovascular events in high-risk cardiovascular patients [11].

Recent findings that erectile dysfunction is a strong predictor of CAD and that the development of symptomatic erectile dysfunction might precede the occurrence of a cardiovascular event by 2–3 years have led to stricter measures during the assessment of patients who present with poor erections [12, 13]. A strong recommendation is that all men with erectile dysfunction who are free from any cardiac symptoms should be considered to be cardiac (or vascular) patients until proven otherwise (Fig. 3.1).

3.3 Hyperlipidemia and ED

It is an important association of ED and hyperlipidemia which has been found in several clinical studies. Most of them suggest that hypercholesterolemia at baseline was also shown as a predictor of ED. High concentrations of low-density lipoprotein seem to be related to ED, although low levels of high-density lipoproteins have been shown to be predictive of ED [15].

The selective action of the endothelial NO/cGMP pathway in hypercholesterolemia could be due to increased superoxide production by nicotinamide adenine dinucleotide phosphate (NADPH) oxidase or to increased plasma levels of asymmetric dimethylarginine, an endogenous inhibitor of NOS [16].

3.4 Hypertension and ED

High blood pressure is an independent risk factor for development of ED [17, 18]. Cardiovascular complications following hypertension such as ischemic heart disease and renal failure are associated with an even higher prevalence of ED.

Hypertension affects blood vessels by shear stress, which can lead to endothelial abnormalities such as an altered production and activity of vasoactive substances. It has been proposed that in hypertension, the increased blood pressure per se does not induce an impairment of erectile function; therefore, it is thought that the resultant dysfunction could be caused by the associated arterial stenotic lesions [19].

In hypertensive population, ED was associated to older age, longer duration of hypertension, and a more severe hypertension. ED was also related to the antihypertensive therapy [20].

Together with high blood pressure, it should be emphasize that some endocrinological disorders and hormone irregularity can lead to ED.

Endocrinological erectile dysfunction thru androgens plays important parts in enhancing sexual desire and maintaining adequate sleep-related erections but have a limited effect on visually induced erections. It is spot that testosterone is important in the regulation of the expression of NO synthase (NOS) and PDE5 inside the penis [21]. Testosterone deficiency or hypogonadism has been recently associated with cardiovascular morbidity and mortality. Hyperprolactinemia leads to sexual dysfunction, due to low testosterone concentrations. Increased prolactin concentration leads to the inhibition of gonadotropin-releasing hormones, which, in turn, decreases the secretion of luteinizing hormone, which is responsible for testosterone secretion [22].

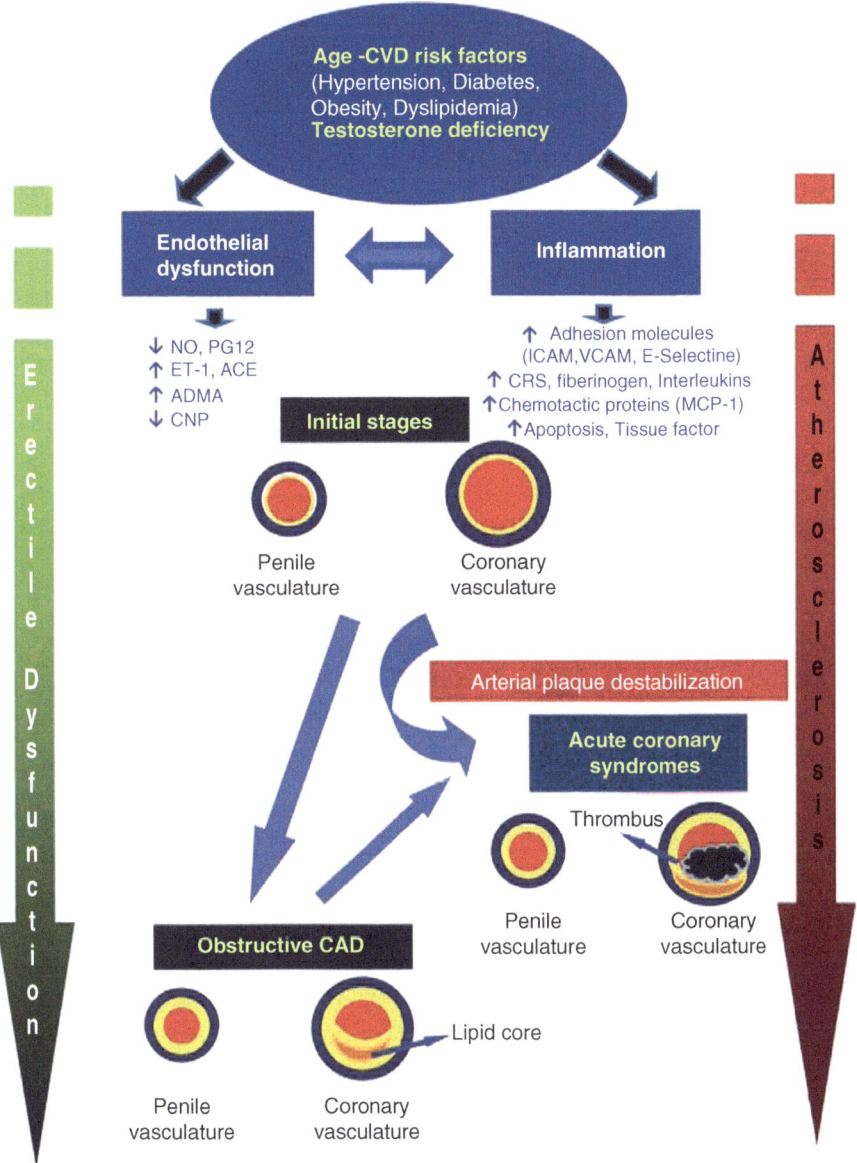

Fig. 3.1 Pathophysiological links between endothelial dysfunction, inflammation, testosterone deficiency, and acute or chronic coronary artery disease (Modified with permission by Vlachopoulos et al. [14]). *ACE* angiotensin-converting enzyme, *ADMA* asymmetric dimethylarginine, *CAD* coronary artery disease, *CNP* C-type natriuretic peptide, *CRP* C-reactive protein, *ET-1* endothelin-1, *ICAM-1* intercellular adhesion molecule, *MCP-1* monocyte chemotactic protein-1, *NO* nitric oxide, *PGI2* prostaglandin, *VCAM* vascular cell adhesion molecule

3.5 Cigarette Smoking and ED

Cigarette smoking is an important independent modifiable risk factor and it appears to have a deleterious effect on penile hemodynamic integrity. Mannino showed an odds ratio (OR) of 1.4 for smokers vs. nonsmokers. Some researchers furthermore demonstrated an OR of 1.7 and also that the risk of ED increases with duration of this habit [23]. Cigarette smoking showed also to increase the age-adjusted risk of ED in addition to increasing the relative risk for antihypertensive medications, cardiac drugs, and systemic illness as diabetes mellitus (50 vs. 45.4 % of complete ED, smokers vs. nonsmokers, respectively). The authors reported that there are strong parallelisms and shared risks among smoking, CAD, atherosclerosis, and ED [7]. Clinical and basic science studies provide strong indirect evidence that smoking may affect penile erection by the impairment of endothelium-dependent smooth muscle relaxation. They also confirmed that the association of ED with risk factors such as CAD and hypertension appears to be amplified by cigarette smoking [24].

From a pathophysiological point of view, nicotine may inhibit smooth muscle function or the neurovascular mediators, such as prostacyclin, causing many types of hemodynamic alterations. Hypercoagulability and increased platelet aggregation, the release of fatty acids and catecholamines, or direct toxic effects on the vascular endothelium have also been considered as possible mechanisms. Recently, literature data showed that smoking may act as a risk factor for ED by reducing high-density lipoprotein (HDL) and increasing fibrinogen concentrations [25].

3.6 Increased Vasoconstriction and ED

Enhanced basal and myogenic tone has been observed in arteries from hypertensive rats [26]. It is unclear whether enhanced myogenic constriction reflects a primary pathological defect contributing to the hypertensive state or a secondary adaptive process protecting the exchange vessels from elevated pressures [27]. Although the role of myogenic tone in the penile vasculature for erection remains to be clarified, the increased vasoconstriction could contribute to decreased arterial inflow and erectile response [28].

Enhanced adrenergic activity keeping the penile smooth muscle contracted is expected to result in ED. Sympathetic nerve activity accompanies hypertension in man and hypertensive animals [29]. However, in corpus cavernosum from spontaneously hypertensive rats, the content of sympathetic neurotransmitters was found to be unchanged [30]. Neither the contractions evoked by the α1-adrenoceptor agonist, phenylephrine, nor the contractions induced by electrical field stimulation were enhanced in arteries or erectile tissue from renal hypertensive compared to normotensive rats.

In view of these findings, it is unlikely that changes in the peripheral sympathetic neuro-effectors junction or responsiveness to α-adrenoceptor agonists play a role for the decreased erectile function observed in hypertensive rats [31].

3.7 Impaired Neurogenic Vasodilatation and ED

Immunohistochemical and functional studies of isolated penile small arteries indicate that NO is the main neurotransmitter mediating nonadrenergic noncholinergic relaxations to electrical field stimulation [32].

In patients with essential hypertension, endothelium-dependent vasodilatation elicited by infusion of agonists such as acetylcholine, bradykinin, or flow is diminished [33, 34].

There is a lack for studies addressing whether endothelium-dependent vasodilatation in the penile circulation is altered in hypertensive men.

3.8 Diabetes and ED

Diabetes mellitus type 2 is the second most common risk factor for erectile dysfunction, which in turn develops in 50–75 % of diabetics. The prevalence of ED is three times higher in diabetic men (28 % vs. 9.6 %), occurs at an earlier age, and increases with disease duration, being approximately 15 % at age 30 rising to 55 % at 60 years [35]. Diabetes mellitus may cause ED through a number of pathophysiological changes affecting psychological function, central nervous system (CNS) function, androgen secretion, peripheral nerve activity, endothelial cell function, and smooth muscle contractility [36].

In diabetic patients, insulin is thought to enhance nitric oxide synthase (NOS) activity by increasing transport of L-arginine into the cell and furnishing greater quantities of the essential cofactor NADPH. These effects are reversed in the insulin lack or insulin resistance of diabetes. Plasmatic concentration and vascular content of L-arginine are reduced in diabetic rats [37]. Arginase is an enzyme that competes with NOS for the 30 substrate, L-arginine. The inducible form of the enzyme, arginase II, is overexpressed in corpus cavernosum from diabetic patients, where inhibition of arginase restores NOS activity. Intracellular availability of L-arginine in diabetic cavernosal tissue could be reduced not only by transport impairment but also by excessive metabolization through arginase pathway.

The ratio of reductase cofactors NADH/NAD + is increased in diabetes. This reduces the levels of NADPH, an essential cofactor for NOS, and increases the levels of calcium-elevating second messengers such as diacylglycerol and protein kinase C (PKC) thus increasing smooth muscle contractility [38].

3.9 Chronic Renal Failure and ED

Men suffering chronic renal failure (CRF) requiring renal replacement therapy have a high prevalence of sexual dysfunction (20–50 %) [39]. Many of the pathophysiological effects of persistent uremia can potentially contribute to the development of ED including disturbance of the hypothalamic-pituitary-testis sex hormonal axis, hyperprolactinemia, accelerated atheromatous disease, and psychological factors [40].

Uremia results in a decrease in bioavailable NO in erythrocytes. Sarioglu and coworkers demonstrated that a chronic uremic state resulted in impaired nerve and endothelial-mediated relaxation of rabbit cavernosal smooth muscle while relaxation induced by NO donors or purinergic activation was preserved [41].

Cavernosal vascular function in men undergoing renal replacement therapy showed that 80 % had both arterial insufficiency and veno-occlusive dysfunction. A link with possible impairment of the NO/cGMP pathway relating to failure of cavernosal relaxation is provided by the finding of increased serum levels of endogenous inhibitors of NO synthesis in uremic patients [42].

3.10 Drug-Induced Erectile Dysfunction

Treatment using higher doses of a thiazide showed a significant increase in ED compared to placebo [43]. Addition of a thiazide to existing treatment with propanolol or methyldopa also increased the prevalence of ED, while this effect did not occur when the thiazide was combined with an ACE inhibitor [44]. Data from a large UK trial showed that twice as many men taking thiazides for treatment of mild hypertension reported ED compared to those treated with propanolol or placebo, this being the commonest reason for withdrawal from the bendrofluazide arm of the study [45]. In the Treatment of Mild Hypertension Study (TOMHS), the prevalence of ED at 2 years in men taking low-dose thiazide was twice that of both the placebo group and those on alternative agents [46].

Psychotropic drugs are among the most common drug classes involved in the development of erectile dysfunction. In a first place, antidepressants are the most common psychotropic drugs associated with significant rates of erectile dysfunction, including the selective serotonin reuptake inhibitors and venlafaxine. Antipsychotics such as risperidone and olanzapine have the highest likelihood of all psychotropic drugs of causing erectile dysfunction [47].

In conclusion, several mechanisms related with ED are well done, described, and known. Despite the fact that some conditions joined with ED increase risk for cardiovascular disease, we need some more evidence to have clear picture on how to bring a gap between potential in distinctions in pathophysiology of ED.

References

1. Braumvald F, Hauser K, Loskalso J et al (2008) Erectile dysfunction in Harrison's manual of medicine. 17:950–952
2. Carson C, Dean J, Wylie M (2006) Management of erectile dysfunction in clinical practice. Springer Medical Publishing, New York
3. Siddiqui MA, Peng B, Shanmugam N et al (2012) Erectile dysfunction in young surgically treated patients with lumbar spine disease: a prospective follow-up study. Spine (Phila Pa 1976) 37:797–801
4. Chuang AT, Steers WD (1999) Neurophysiology of penile erection. In: Carson CC, Kirby R, Goldstein I (eds) Textbook of erectile dysfunction. ISIS Medical Media, Oxford, pp 59–72

5. Quinlan DM, Epstein JI, Carter BS (1991) Sexual function following radical prostatectomy: influence of preservation of neurovascular bundles. J Urol 145:998
6. Mulhall JP (2008) Penile rehabilitation following radical prostatectomy. Curr Opin Urol 18:613–620
7. Virag R, Bouilly P, Frydman D (1985) Is impotence an arterial disorder? A study of arterial risk factors in 440 impotent men. Lancet 1:181–184
8. Mittawae B, El-Nashaar AR, Fouda A et al (2006) Incidence of erectile dysfunction in 800 hypertensive patients: a multicenter Egyptian national study. Urology 67:575–578
9. Burchardt M, Burchardt T, Baer L et al (2000) Hypertension is associated with severe erectile dysfunction. J Urol 164:1188–1191
10. Corona G, Rastrelli G, Monami M et al (2011) Hypogonadism as a risk factor for cardiovascular mortality in men: a meta-analytic study. Eur J Endocrinol 165:687–701
11. Nehra A, Jackson G, Miner M et al (2012) The Princeton III consensus recommendations for the management of erectile dysfunction and cardiovascular disease. Mayo Clin Proc 87:766–778
12. Böhm M, Baumhäkel M, Teo K, ONTARGET/TRANSCEND Erectile Dysfunction Substudy Investigators et al (2010) Erectile dysfunction predicts cardiovascular events in high-risk patients receiving telmisartan, ramipril or both: the ONgoing Telmisartan Alone and in combination with Ramipril Global Endpoint Trial/Telmisartan Randomized AssessmeNt Study in ACE iNtolerant subjects with cardiovascular Disease (ONTARGET/TRANSCEND) Trials. Circulation 121:1439–1446
13. Montorsi P, Montorsi F, Schulman CC (2003) Is erectile dysfunction the "tip of the iceberg" of a systemic vascular disorder? Eur Urol 44:352–354
14. Vlachopoulos C, Jackson G, Stefanadis C et al (2013) Erectile dysfunction in the cardiovascular patient. Eur Heart J 34:2034–2046
15. Kim JH, Klyachkin ML, Svendsen E et al (1994) Experimental hypercholesterolemia in rabbits induces cavernosal atherosclerosis with endothelial and smooth-muscle cell dysfunction. J Urol 151:198–205
16. Kim SC, Kim IK, Seo KK et al (1997) Involvement of superoxide radical in the impaired endothelium-dependent relaxation of cavernous smooth muscle in hypercholesterolemic rabbits. Urol Res 25:341–346
17. Effects on sexual function of five antihypertensive drugs and nutritional hygienic treatment in hypertensive men and women: Treatment of Mild Hypertension Study (TOMHS) (1997) Hypertension 29:8–14
18. Aranda P, Ruilope LM, Calvo C et al (2004) Erectile dysfunction in essential arterial hypertension and effects of sildenafil: results of a Spanish national study. Am J Hypertens 17:139–145
19. Jensen J, Lendorf A, Stimpel H et al (1999) The prevalence and etiology of impotence in 101 male hypertensive outpatients. Am J Hypertens 12:271–275
20. Toblli JE, Stella I, Mazza ON et al (2004) Protection of cavernous tissue in male spontaneously hypertensive rats: beyond blood pressure control. Am J Hypertens 17:516–522
21. Hale TM, Okabe H, Bushfield TL et al (2002) Recovery of erectile function after brief aggressive antihypertensive therapy. J Urol 168:348–354
22. Ushiyama M, Morita T, Kuramochi T et al (2004) Erectile dysfunction in hypertensive rats results from impairment of the relaxation evoked by neurogenic carbon monoxide and nitric oxide. Hypertens Res 27:253–261
23. Salonia A (2003) Blackwell Publishing Ltd. Int J Androl 26:129–136
24. Shabsigh R, Fishman IJ, Schum C et al (1991) Cigarette smoking and other vascular risk factors in vasculogenic impotence. Urology 38:227–231
25. Jaffe A, Chen Y, Kisch ES et al (1996) Erectile dysfunction in hypertensive subjects: assessment of potential determinants. Hypertension 28:859–862
26. Schubert R, Mulvany MJ (1999) The myogenic response: established facts and attractive hypotheses. Clin Sci (Colch) 96:313–326
27. Davis MJ, Hill MA (1999) Signaling mechanisms underlying the vascular myogenic response. Physiol Rev 79:387–423

28. Simonsen U, Garcia-Sacristan A, Prieto D (2002) Penile arteries and erection. J Vasc Res 39:283–303
29. Norman RA Jr, Dzielak DJ (1986) Immunological dysfunction and enhanced sympathetic activity contribute to the pathogenesis of spontaneous hypertension. J Hypertens Suppl 4:S437–S439
30. Mancia G, Grassi G, Giannattasio C et al (1999) Sympathetic activation in the pathogenesis of hypertension and progression of organ damage. Hypertension 34:724–728
31. Tong YC, Hung YC, Lin SN et al (1996) The norepinephrine tissue concentration and neuropeptide Y immunoreactivity in genitourinary organs of the spontaneously hypertensive rat. J Auton Nerv Syst 56:215–218
32. Simonsen U, Contreras J, Garcia-Sacristan A (2001) Effect of sildenafil on non adrenergic non-cholinergic neurotransmission in bovine penile small arteries. Eur J Pharmacol 412:155–169
33. Panza JA, Quyyumi AA, Brush JE Jr, Epstein SE (1990) Abnormal endothelium-dependent vascular relaxation in patients with essential hypertension. N Engl J Med 323:22–27
34. Taddei S, Virdis A, Ghiadoni L et al (1998) Vitamin C improves endothelium dependent vasodilation by restoring nitric oxide activity in essential hypertension. Circulation 97:2222–2229
35. Koldny RC, Kahn CB, Goldstein HH (1973) Sexual function in diabetic men. Diabetes 23:306–309
36. McCulloch DK, Young RJ, Prescott RJ et al (1984) The natural history of impotence in diabetic men. Diabetologia 26:437–440
37. Pieper GM, Dondlinger LA (1997) Plasma and vascular tissue arginine are decreased in diabetes: acute arginine supplementation restores endothelium-dependent relaxation by augmenting cGMP production. J Pharmacol Exp Ther 283:684–691
38. Bivalacqua TJ, Hellstrom WJG, Kadowitz PJ (2001) Increased expression of arginase II in human diabetic corpus cavernosum: in diabetic associated erectile dysfunction. Biochem Biophys Res Commun 283:923–927
39. Carson CC, Patel MP (1999) The epidemiology, anatomy, physiology, and treatment of erectile dysfunction in chronic renal failure patients. Adv Ren Replace Ther 6:296–309
40. Rosas SE, Joffe M, Franklin E et al (2001) Prevalence and determinants of erectile dysfunction in haemodialysis patients. Kidney Int 59:2259–2266
41. Ayub W, Fletcher S (2000) End-stage renal disease and erectile dysfunction. Is there any hope? Nephrol Dial Transplant 15:1525–1528
42. Mendes Ribeiro AC, Brunini TM, Ellory JC (2001) Abnormalities in L arginine transport and nitric oxide biosynthesis in chronic renal and heart failure. Cardiovasc Res 49:697–712
43. Chang SW, Fine R, Siegel D et al (1991) The impact of diuretic therapy on reported sexual function. Arch Intern Med 151:2402–2408
44. Croog SH, Levine S, Sudilovsky A et al (1988) Sexual symptoms in hypertensive patients. A clinical trial of antihypertensive medications. Arch Intern Med 148:788–794
45. Medical Research Council Working Party on Mild to Moderate Hypertension. Adverse reactions to bendrofluazide and propanolol for the treatment of mild hypertension (1981) Lancet 2:539–543
46. Grimm RH Jr, Grandits GA, Prineas RJ et al (1997) Long term effects on sexual function of five antihypertensive drugs and nutritional hygienic treatment in hypertensive men and women: Treatment of mild hypertension study (TOMHS). Hypertension 29:8–14
47. Serretti A, Chiesa A (2011) A meta-analysis of sexual dysfunction in psychiatric patients taking antipsychotics. Int Clin Psychopharmacol 26:130–140

Erectile Dysfunction and Testosterone

Charalambos Vlachopoulos

4.1 Testosterone and Hypertension

There has been some debate about testosterone levels and high blood pressure (BP). Studies in experimental animals and in men with withdrawal of sex hormones indicate that androgens may be important determinants of the sex-specific differences in arterial BP (higher BP in men compared to women till menopause) [1–3]. On the other hand, in most of the observational studies in humans, levels of testosterone (when below normal limits) relate inversely to systolic blood BP [4–7]. Men with low levels of testosterone have a greater risk (up to 20 %) of developing high blood pressure over the next 5 years when compared to men with the higher testosterone levels [7]. Testosterone deficiency defined as total testosterone (TT) below 300 ng/mL is highly prevalent among hypertensive men (42.3 %), and the relative risk for having testosterone deficiency is significantly higher in men with hypertension (relative risk = 1.84) than in normotensive individuals [8]. Notably, testosterone levels undergo age-related decline; risk factors, such as high BP or insulin resistance, may hasten this age-related fall [4, 9]. A number of hypotheses have been proposed to explain the finding that hypertension is associated with lower levels of plasma testosterone as compared to normotensive controls: (1) serum testosterone influences BP regulation; (2) elevated BP can negatively affect steroidogenesis or clearance, and (3) there are genes involved in the regulation of BP that also affect steroidogenesis [4, 10]. Finally, this inverse relationship of testosterone and BP may be partly due to reduction in the testosterone levels because of antihypertensive medications that are known to affect the sexual function in hypertensive men on therapy. Indeed, decreased testosterone levels have been reported in hypertensive patients under treatment with β-blockers or spironolactone [11, 12] (see below).

C. Vlachopoulos
1st Cardiology Department, Athens Medical School, Hippokration Hospital, Athens, Greece
e-mail: cvlachop@otenet.gr

4.2 Testosterone and Erectile Dysfunction in Hypertension

Although the mechanisms are to a certain extent unclear, hypertension itself is associated with sexual dysfunction and the incidence of sexual problems is considerably higher among untreated hypertensive men than among normotensive ones [13, 14]. The relationship between hypertension and decreased testosterone levels may be partly responsible for the impaired sexual function observed in hypertensive men [4]. Indeed, increasing attention is focused on the effect of testosterone on penile arterial function. On one hand, testosterone deficiency leads to erectile dysfunction (ED). Testosterone is required for maintenance of penile structure and functional integrity [15]. Doppler studies show that penile arterial insufficiency is frequent, and of higher severity, in men with testosterone deficiency [16]. Appropriate testosterone levels are necessary for maintenance of intrapenile nitric oxide (NO) synthase levels [17]. On the other hand, testosterone deficiency and penile arterial dysfunction appear to be pathophysiologically interrelated through endothelial dysfunction and activation of inflammatory state [18]. These associations have led to the hypothesis that testosterone deficiency contributes to the onset and progression of penile vascular disease, a hypothesis that is continuously gaining grounds in terms of evidence. Thus, testosterone deficiency which is frequent in aged males with hypertension [8] may be also implicated in the common pathogenetic pathways of hypertension and vasculogenic ED.

While hypertension per se seems to be related to ED, in many patients the onset of erectile dysfunction is related to the initiation of antihypertensive therapy [11, 13, 19]. Decreased levels of testosterone and, in part, of the follicle-stimulating hormone by metoprolol, pindolol, atenolol, and propranolol have been suggested to be involved in reduction of sexual function and desire [11, 12]. Thiazide diuretics are reported to have unfavorable effect on erectile function; however, their influence on sex-related hormones is not likely, because there was no effect on testosterone in humans [11, 13]. Spironolactone decreases erectile function and sexual desire supposedly due to androgen suppression by competing with testosterone and dihydrotestosterone for peripheral androgen-binding sites [20]. Additionally, spironolactone seems to be a weak inhibitor of testosterone synthesis [11]. Regarding statins, the largest body of evidence point towards a beneficial effect on erectile function [21]. A negative effect has been reported in high statin doses, possibly related to a potential reduction in serum testosterone levels, which directly needs cholesterol as its main substrate, but this dose dependency warrants further investigation [22].

4.3 Testosterone and CVD Risk

4.3.1 Testosterone and CV Events

There is a significant inverse association between low testosterone levels and CV events [23–34] (Table 4.1), although not all studies confirm this [35, 36]. Seen from a different angle, there is a protective link between higher endogenous

Table 4.1 Low testosterone levels and increased all-cause mortality/CVD events in recent publications [23–32]

Reference	HR	Men (n)	CVD (%)	Hypertension (%)	Mean follow-up (years)	All-cause mortality/CVD
Shores et al. [23]	1.88	858	20.7	NA	8.0	All cause
Khaw et al. [24]	2.29	2,314	0	20	10	All cause and CVD
Laughlin et al. [25]	1.40 1.38	794	35	75	20	All cause CVD
Tivesten et al. [26]	1.65	3,014	26.5	NA	4.5	All cause
Vikan et al. [27]	1.24	1,568	17	NA	11.2	All cause
Haring et al. [28]	2.32 2.56	1,954	9	29	7.2	All cause CVD
Malkin et al. [29]	2.27	930	100	42.6	6.9	All cause
Menke et al. [30]	1.43	1,114	0	NA	9.0	All cause
Corona et al. [31]	7.10	1,687	11.6	27.4	4.3	CVD
Vlachopoulos et al. [32]	3.83	228	0	100	3.8	CVD

CAD coronary artery disease, *CVD* cardiovascular disease, *HR* hazard ratio, *NA* no data available

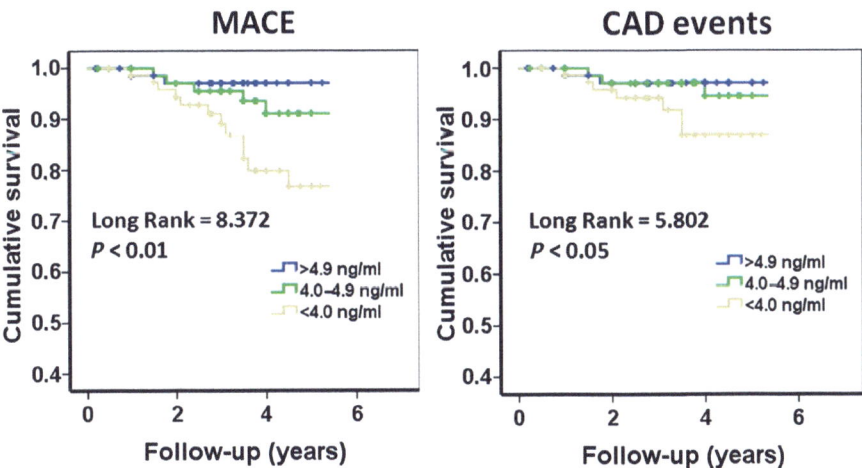

Fig. 4.1 Kaplan-Meier curves for major adverse cardiovascular events (*MACE*) and coronary artery disease (*CAD*) events by tertile group of total testosterone (TT). Cut-offs of the TT tertiles were 4.0 and 4.9 ng/mL (With permission from Vlachopoulos et al. [32])

testosterone levels and CV events as it was reported in a prospective study in males aged 61–80 years [37]. Interestingly, androgen-deprivation therapy in prostate cancer patients increases CV risk [38]. In a recent study we demonstrated a significant association of low testosterone with increased risk for major adverse cardiovascular events in hypertensive males without clinical atherosclerosis (Fig. 4.1) [32].

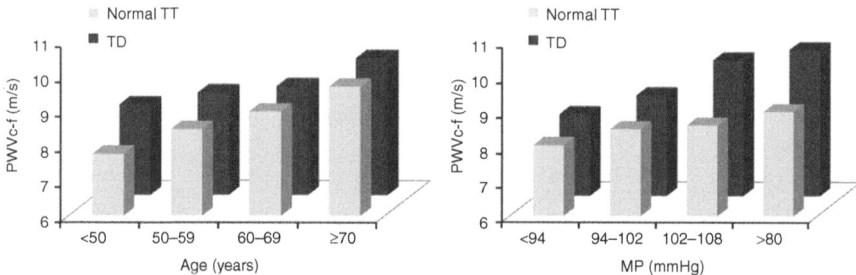

Fig. 4.2 Impact of the relation between (**a**) age groups, (**b**) BP (mean pressure) groups, and testosterone deficiency (*TD*) on carotid-femoral pulse wave velocity (*PWVc–f*). In younger categories (<50 year and 50–59 years), patients with TD had higher blood pressure-adjusted PWVc–f compared to subjects with normal TT, indicating an "aging effect" of 10 years, whereas in older age categories such a difference was not observed. In men with a higher mean pressure (102–108 mmHg and >108 mmHg), patients with TD had higher age-adjusted PWVc–f compared to subjects with normal TT, indicating a synergistic unfavorable effect of TD and blood pressure on aortic stiffness (With permission from Vlachopoulos et al. [41])

This predictive ability of low testosterone was independent of hypertension severity and related metabolic components. Importantly, when added to standard risk models such as the Framingham Risk Score, total testosterone reclassifies correctly a considerable percentage (38.8 %) of patients to a higher or lower-risk category in the whole population. A particular strength of this study is that it excluded patients with a history of cardiovascular disease and diabetes; this allowed assessing the level and predictive role of testosterone more likely related to hypertension itself and not to other conditions or risk factors. Also, the mean age of patients in this study (56 years) underscores the clinical importance of measuring plasma testosterone in middle-aged patients, an age group that is in need of a potent biomarker.

4.3.2 Testosterone and Target Organ Damage

Screening for subclinical organ damage is of paramount importance, because asymptomatic alterations of the cardiovascular system and the kidney are crucial intermediate stages in the disease continuum that links hypertension to cardiovascular events and death [39]. Low testosterone may be implicated in the common pathogenetic pathways of ED and CVD through changes in vascular function and structure. Testosterone has been reported to inhibit vascular smooth muscle cell proliferation and neointima formation, suggesting a direct action of testosterone on the vasculature [40]. Indeed, testosterone has been associated with increased *arterial stiffness* [41], *carotid intima-media thickness* (*IMT*) [42], and *ankle-brachial index* [43]. Interestingly, in a recent study we reported a more prominent effect of testosterone deficiency on aortic stiffness in young men and in subjects with higher blood pressure levels (Fig. 4.2) [41]. This finding identifies testosterone as a marker of arterial damage with special emphasis on young and hypertensive individuals and supports its role as predictor of events. Of particular importance is the finding that aortic stiffness is a potent biomarker within the context of ED that identifies patients who are at higher risk [44]. Finally, changes in cardiac function may also be involved: low testosterone has been associated with *left ventricular hypertrophy* [6].

4.4 Measurement of Testosterone in the Evaluation of ED Hypertensive Men

In the ED patient, measurement of testosterone levels is justified to be included in the clinical evaluation of the patient because it serves the following purposes: (1) to assist in the diagnosis of ED, discriminate the cause of ED, and estimate the severity of ED; (2) to identify patients at higher cardiovascular risk and predict CV events in ED patients (i.e., to predict CVD incidence); (3) to identify hypertensive males with subclinical organ damage; and (4) to enhance the ability of the clinician to optimally choose the correct treatment for patients in whom phosphodiesterase-5 (PDE5) inhibitors have failed [45–47]. Importantly, it has been integrated as first tool in the most recent, third (2012) Princeton Consensus for the assessment and management of patients with hypertension of organ ED [48].

4.5 Testosterone Therapy

To whom: Testosterone therapy (TTh) should be reserved for patients who (i) are symptomatic (ED or reduced libido) of testosterone deficiency and (ii) they have biochemical evidence of low testosterone (TT <8 nmol/L or 2.3 ng/mL) [49]. In men with borderline TT levels (8–12 nmol/L or 2.3–3.5 ng/mL), a TTh trial (for 3–6 months and continuation if effective) may be envisaged. Improvement is dependent on the testosterone levels with best results being obtained when TT is below 10.4 nmol/L (3 ng/mL). Men treated with testosterone require long-term, careful follow-up. There should be careful follow-up of men with severe obstructive sleep apnea and men with severe hypertension, due to the risk of fluid retention in case of overdosing [49].

Effect on BP: Currently, available evidence derived from a meta-analysis of 30 trials supported a neutral effect of testosterone supplementation on systolic (0.8 mmHg; 95 % CI, −4 to 5 mmHg, $P=NS$) and diastolic (2 mmHg; 95 % CI, −2 to 6 mmHg, $P=NS$) BP that was consistent across trials [50]. However, in a recent prospective, observational study of the use of injectable long-acting testosterone undecanoate in men during routine clinical care (of them, 26 % were hypertensives), blood pressure changed in a significant and favorable manner [51]. Data on the impact of TTh on BP levels in treated and untreated hypogonadic essential hypertensive patients with no other conditions or risk factors are not yet available.

Effect on lipids: The majority of prospective clinical studies indicate that TTh within physiologic limits has beneficial or neutral effects on lipid profile other than HDL-C, beneficial or neutral effects on inflammatory mediators, and generally beneficial effects on glycemic state [52, 53]. Lean body mass is typically increased in hypogonadal subjects, and visceral adiposity is decreased in several studies and unchanged in the remainder [54]. Such metabolic effects have raised interest on the potential impact on cardiovascular health.

Effect on TOD: Regarding the effect of TTh on markers of organ damage, a decrease in aortic stiffness measured as pulse wave velocity was evident after 48 weeks; likewise, a decrease in large artery compliance was found after 3 months [55]. A reduction on carotid artery intimal thickness was observed at 12 months in one study, but this did not reach significance because of the small cohort size [56]. The effect of TTh in men with left ventricular hypertrophy or microalbuminuria has not been examined yet.

Effect on CV risk: Most studies have shown neutral [57] or even beneficial [58] effect of TTh on cardiovascular risk. However, in two recent studies there was an increase in cardiovascular events with TTh [59, 60]. In both of these studies, hypertension was highly prevalent (~90 %). The increase in adverse events with TTh reported in the Testosterone in Older Men with Mobility Limitations (TOM) trial may have been related to a high rate of comorbidities and the use of high and rapid escalation dosing regimens [59]. The study by Vigen et al. retrospectively compared rates of death, myocardial infarction, and stroke from a dataset of 8,709 men who had undergone coronary angiography with prior documentation of serum T concentration <300 ng/dL; however, credibility of this article is deeply compromised by major errors, and subsequent attempts to correct, in values presented [60]. It cannot be overemphasized, therefore, that prospective data from large, well-designed, long-term trials of TTh in hypertensive males without clinical atherosclerosis are warranted.

Conclusions

Human studies indicate that men with lower testosterone levels tend to have higher blood pressure levels and incidence of hypertension. Testosterone deficiency is a common pathogenetic mechanism linking hypertension and vasculogenic ED. The relationship between hypertension and ED may also be due to reductions in testosterone levels due to antihypertensive drugs such as β-blockers and spironolactone that are known to affect the sexual function in hypertensive men on therapy. Emerging evidence supports that lower androgen levels are associated with indices of organ damage and predict poor cardiovascular risk profile. Measurement of testosterone also allows better prediction of CV risk compared with conventional risk assessment and identifies high-risk individuals in whom a more intense treatment is needed. Increased recognition of the potential of looking for testosterone deficiency in hypertensive men with ED, followed by appropriate replacement therapy, can improve sexual function and may decrease blood pressure levels and affect incidence of adverse CV events. We recommend that measurement of testosterone is part of cardiovascular risk assessment in all hypertensive males.

References

1. Reckelhoff J (2001) Gender differences in the regulation of blood pressure. Hypertension 37:1199–1208
2. Kaushik M, Sontineni SP, Hunter C (2010) Cardiovascular disease and androgens: a review. Int J Cardiol 142:8–14
3. Kelly DM, Jones TH (2013) Testosterone: a vascular hormone in health and disease. J Endocrinol 217:R47–R71
4. Fogari R, Zoppi A, Preti P et al (2002) Sexual activity and plasma testosterone levels in hypertensive males. Am J Hypertens 15:217–221
5. Fogari R, Preti P, Zoppi A et al (2005) Serum testosterone levels and arterial blood pressure in the elderly. Hypertens Res 28:625–633
6. Svartberg J, von Mühlen D, Schirmer H et al (2004) Association of endogenous testosterone with blood pressure and left ventricular mass in men. The tromsø study. Eur J Endocrinol 150:65–71
7. Torkler S, Wallaschofski H, Baumeister SE et al (2011) Inverse association between total testosterone concentrations, incident hypertension and blood pressure. Aging Male 14:176–182
8. Mulligan T, Frick MF, Zuraw QC et al (2006) Prevalence of hypogonadism in males aged at least 45 years: the HIM study. Int J Clin Pract 60:762–769
9. Gray A, Feldman HA, McKinlay JB et al (1991) Age, disease, and changing sex hormone levels in middle-aged men: results of the Massachusetts male aging study. J Clin Endocrinol Metab 73:1016–1025
10. Endre T, Mattiason I, Berglund G et al (1996) Low testosterone and insulin resistance in hypertension prone men. J Hum Hypertens 10:755–761
11. Baumhäkel M, Schlimmer N, Kratz M et al (2011) Cardiovascular risk, drugs and erectile function–a systematic analysis. Int J Clin Pract 65:289–298
12. Fogari R, Preti P, Derosa G et al (2002) Effect of antihypertensive treatment with valsartan or atenolol on sexual activity and plasma testosterone in hypertensive men. Eur J Clin Pharmacol 58:177–180
13. Manolis A, Doumas M (2012) Antihypertensive treatment and sexual dysfunction. Curr Hypertens Rep 14:285–292
14. Manolis A, Doumas M (2008) Sexual dysfunction: the 'prima ballerina' of hypertension-related quality-of-life complications. J Hypertens 26:2074–2084
15. Mirone V, Imbimbo C, Fusco F et al (2009) Androgens and morphologic remodeling at penile and cardiovascular levels: a common piece in complicated puzzles? Eur Urol 56:309–316
16. Corona G, Maggi M (2010) The role of testosterone in erectile dysfunction. Nat Rev Urol 7:46–56
17. Khalil RA (2005) Sex hormones as potential modulators of vascular function in hypertension. Hypertension 46:249–254
18. Kupelian V, Chiu GR, Araujo AB et al (2010) Association of sex hormones and C-reactive protein levels in men. Clin Endocrinol (Oxford) 72:527–533
19. Doumas M, Viigimaa M, Papademetriou V (2013) Combined antihypertensive therapy and sexual dysfunction: terra incognita. Cardiology 125:232–234
20. Rastogi S, Rodriguez JJ, Kapur V et al (2005) Why do patients with heart failure suffer from erectile dysfunction? A critical review and suggestions on how to approach this problem. Int J Impot Res 17:S25–S36
21. Cui Y, Zong H, Yan H et al (2014) The effect of statins on erectile dysfunction: a systematic review and meta-analysis. J Sex Med 11(6):1367–1375
22. La Vignera S, Condorelli RA, Vicari E et al (2012) Statins and erectile dysfunction: a critical summary of current evidence. J Androl 33:552–558
23. Shores MM, Matsumoto AM, Sloan KL et al (2006) Low serum testosterone and mortality in male veterans. Arch Intern Med 166:1660–1665

24. Khaw KT, Dowsett M, Folkerd E et al (2007) Endogenous testosterone and mortality due to all causes, cardiovascular disease, and cancer in men: European prospective investigation into cancer in Norfolk (EPIC-Norfolk) prospective population study. Circulation 116:2694–2701
25. Laughlin GA, Barrett-Connor E, Bergstrom J (2008) Low serum testosterone and mortality in older men. J Clin Endocrinol Metab 93:68–75
26. TivestenA VL, Labrie F et al (2009) Low serum testosterone and estradiol predict mortality in elderly men. J Clin Endocrinol Metab 94:2482–2488
27. Vikan T, Schirmer H, Njolstad I et al (2009) Endogenous sex hormones and the prospective association with cardiovascular disease and mortality in men: the tromso study. Eur J Endocrinol 161:435–442
28. Haring R, Volzke H, Steveling A et al (2010) Low serum testosterone levels are associated with increased risk of mortality in a population-based cohort of men aged 20–79. Eur Heart J 31:1494–1501
29. Malkin CJ, Pugh PJ, Morris PD (2010) Low serum testosterone and increased mortality in men with coronary heart disease. Heart 96:1821–1825
30. Menke A, Guallar E, Rohrmann S et al (2010) Sex steroid hormone concentrations and risk of death in US men. Am J Epidemiol 171:583–592
31. Corona G, Monami M, Boddi V et al (2010) Low testosterone is associated with an increased risk of MACE lethality in subjects with erectile dysfunction. J Sex Med 7:1557–1564
32. Vlachopoulos C, Ioakeimidis N, Terentes-Printzios D et al (2013) Plasma total testosterone and incident cardiovascular events in hypertensive patients. Am J Hypertens 26:373–381
33. Ruige JB, Mahmoud AM, De Bacquer D et al (2011) Endogenous testosterone and cardiovascular disease in healthy men: a meta-analysis. Heart 97:870–875
34. Corona G, Rastrelli G, Monami M et al (2011) Hypogonadism as a risk factor for cardiovascular mortality in men: a meta-analytic study. Eur J Endocrinol 165:687–701
35. Araujo AB, Kupelian V, Page ST et al (2007) Sex steroids and all-cause and cause specific mortality in men. Arch Intern Med 167:1252–1260
36. Smith GD, Ben-Shlomo Y, Beswick A et al (2005) Cortisol, testosterone, and coronary heart disease: prospective evidence from the Caerphilly study. Circulation 112:332–340
37. Ohlsson C, Barrett-Connor E, Bhasin S et al (2011) High serum testosterone is associated with reduced risk of cardiovascular events in elderly men. The MrOS (Osteoporotic Fractures in Men) study in Sweden. J Am Coll Cardiol 58:1674–1681
38. Nguyen PL, Je Y, Schutz FA, Hoffman KE et al (2011) Association of androgen deprivation therapy with cardiovascular death in patients with prostate cancer: a meta-analysis of randomized trials. JAMA 306:2359–2366
39. Mancia G, Laurent S, Agabiti-Rosei E et al (2009) Reappraisal of European guidelines on hypertension management: a European society of hypertension task force document. J Hypertens 27:2121–2158
40. Hanke H, Lenz C, Hess B et al (2001) Effect of testosterone on plaque development and androgen receptor expression in the arterial vessel wall. Circulation 103:1382–1385
41. Vlachopoulos C, Ioakeimidis N, Miner M et al (2014) Testosterone deficiency: a determinant of aortic stiffness in men. Atherosclerosis 233:278–283
42. Muller M, van den Beld AW, Bots ML et al (2004) Endogenous sex hormones and progression of carotid atherosclerosis in elderly men. Circulation 109:2074–2079
43. Tivesten A, Mellström D, Jutberger H et al (2007) Low serum testosterone and high serum estradiol associate with lower extremity peripheral arterial disease in elderly men. The MrOS Study in Sweden. J Am Coll Cardiol 50:1070–1076
44. Vlachopoulos C, Ioakeimidis N, Aznaouridis K et al (2014) Prediction of cardiovascular events with aortic stiffness in patients with erectile dysfunction. Hypertension 64:672–678
45. Vlachopoulos C, Jackson G, Stefanadis C et al (2012) Erectile dysfunction in the cardiovascular patient. Eur Heart J 34:2034–2046
46. Gandaglia G, Briganti A, Jackson G et al (2014) A systematic review of the association between erectile dysfunction and cardiovascular disease. Eur Urol 65:968–978

47. Viigimaa M, Doumas M, Vlachopoulos C et al (2011) European society of hypertension working group on sexual dysfunction. Hypertension and sexual dysfunction: time to act. J Hypertens 29:403–407
48. Nehra A, Jackson G, Miner M et al (2012) The princeton III consensus recommendations for the management of erectile dysfunction and cardiovascular disease. Mayo Clin Proc 87:766–778
49. Buvat J, Maggi M, Guay A et al (2013) Testosterone deficiency in men: systematic review and standard operating procedures for diagnosis and treatment. J Sex Med 10:245–284
50. Haddad RM, Kennedy CC, Caples SM et al (2007) Testosterone and cardiovascular risk in men: a systematic review and meta-analysis of randomized placebo-controlled trials. Mayo Clin Proc 82:29–39
51. Zitzmann M, Mattern A, Hanisch J et al (2013) IPASS: a study on the tolerability and effectiveness of injectable testosterone undecanoate for the treatment of male hypogonadism in a worldwide sample of 1,438 men. J Sex Med 10:579–588
52. Corona G, Monami M, Rastrelli G et al (2011) Testosterone and metabolic syndrome: a meta-analysis study. J Sex Med 8(1):272–283
53. Miner MM (2012) Men's health in primary care: an emerging paradigm of sexual function and cardiometabolic risk. Urol Clin N Am 39:1–23
54. Saad F, Haider A, Doros G et al (2013) Long-term treatment of hypogonadal men with testosterone produces substantial and sustained weight loss. Obesity (Silver Spring) 21:1975–1981
55. Yaron M, Greenman Y, Rosenfeld JB et al (2009) Effect of testosterone replacement therapy on arterial stiffness in older hypogonadal men. Eur J Endocrinol 160:839–846
56. Mathur A, Malkin C, Saeed B et al (2009) Long-term benefits of testosterone replacement therapy on angina threshold and atheroma in men. Eur J Endocrinol 161:443–449
57. Carson CC 3rd, Rosano G (2012) Exogenous testosterone, cardiovascular events, and cardiovascular risk factors in elderly men: a review of trial data. J Sex Med 9:54–67
58. Shores M, Smith N, Forsberg C, Anawalt B et al (2012) Testosterone replacement therapy and mortality in men with low testosterone levels. J Clin Endocrinol Metab 97:2050–2058
59. Basaria S, Coviello AD, Travison TG et al (2010) Adverse events associated with testosterone administration. N Engl J Med 363:109–122
60. Vigen R, O'Donnell CI, Barón AE et al (2013) Association of testosterone therapy with mortality, myocardial infarction, and stroke in men with low testosterone levels. JAMA 310:1829–1836

The Role of the Renin-Angiotensin System in Erectile Dysfunction: Present and Future

5

Rodrigo Araujo Fraga-Silva and Nikolaos Stergiopulos

5.1 Introduction

The renin-angiotensin system (RAS) is a peptidergic hormone system that plays a central role in cardiovascular hemostasis [1, 2]. In fact, the relevance of this system became evident in the last decades due to the therapeutic success achieved by the angiotensin-converting enzyme inhibitors (ACEi) and AT1 receptor blockers (ARBs) [1, 2].

In a classical view, the RAS is an endocrine system orchestrated by a sequential enzymatic reactions culminating in a linear generation and actions of angiotensin II (Ang II), the primary system effector [3]. However, this classical concept, taken purely as an endocrinal system, has greatly expanded over the years. Several organs express all the major RAS components, suggesting paracrine actions [3–5]. Therefore, the RAS may be locally autonomous, capable of significant regulatory functions and potential pathophysiological impact [3, 6]. For instance, the existence of a local RAS in the heart, kidney, blood vessels, and brain has been shown by numerous studies [3, 5–7]. Likewise, evidence has indicated the existence of relevant RAS directly within erectile tissue [8], where most RAS components have been identified, specifically in cavernosal tissue [8, 9]. Interestingly, the physiological quantity of Ang II produced in the corpus cavernosum is significantly higher than those found in the systemic circulation [10], suggesting an augmented role and intense activity of RAS-based erectile tissue. Under pathological conditions, exacerbated stimulation of Ang II produced contraction of corpus cavernosum smooth muscle, cellular proliferation, oxidative stress, inflammation, and fibrosis [8], which collectively mediates a direct influence on erectile dysfunction (ED) initiation and progression [8].

R.A. Fraga-Silva, PhD (✉) • N. Stergiopulos, PhD
Institute of Bioengineering, Ecole Polytechnique Fédérale de Lausanne,
Station 17, BM 5115, Lausanne CH-1007, Switzerland
e-mail: fragasilvar@gmail.com; nikolaos.stergiopulos@epfl.ch

© Springer International Publishing Switzerland 2015
M. Viigimaa et al. (eds.), *Erectile Dysfunction in Hypertension and Cardiovascular Disease: A Guide for Clinicians*,
DOI 10.1007/978-3-319-08272-1_5

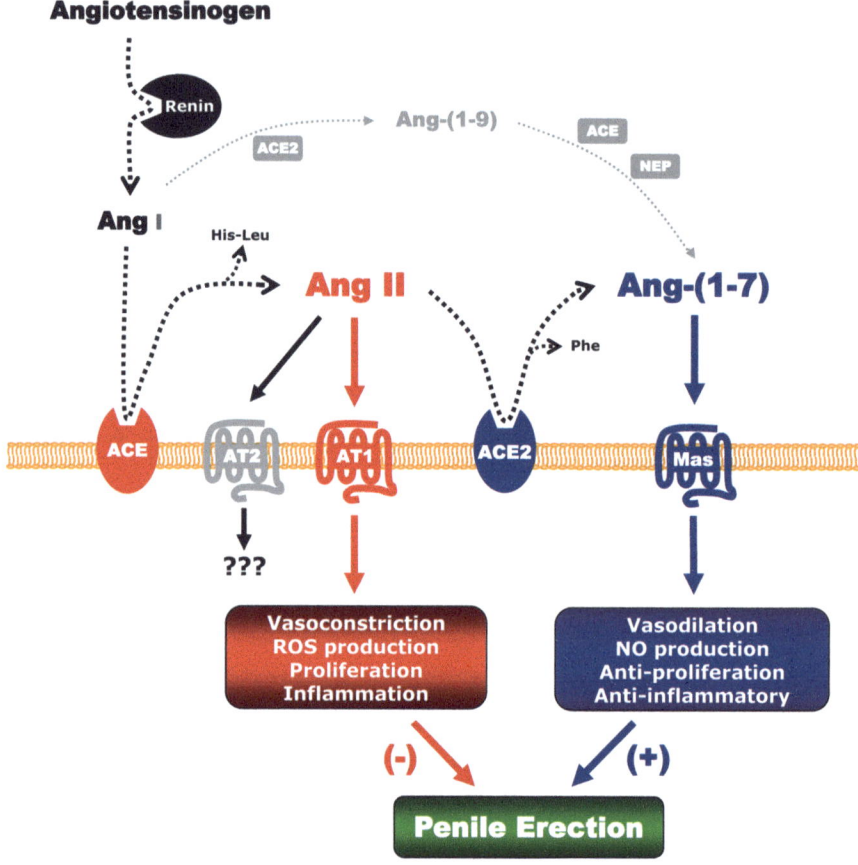

Fig. 5.1 Schematic representation of the current RAS cascade: focusing on the two major axes and its main effects on erectile tissues. *Ang I*, angiotensin I, *Ang II*, angiotensin II, *Ang-(1–7)* angiotensin-(1–7), *Ang-(1–9)* angiotensin-(1–9), *ACE* angiotensin-converting enzyme, *AT2* angiotensin II type 2 receptor, *AT1* angiotensin II type 1 receptor, *ACE2* angiotensin-converting enzyme 2, *Mas* Mas receptor, *His-Leu* amino acid residues histidine and leucine, *Phe* phenylalanine, *NEP* neutral endopeptidase

Another transformation of the classical RAS view has been observed in peptide cascade, effectors, and functions. The simplistic paradigm of the RAS as a linear cascade leading to a unique main effector has expanded into a complex and multi-regulated system. In the last decade, findings have demonstrated the existence of previously unknown signal transduction pathways, alternative metabolic cascades, and the discovery of additional components [3, 11, 12]. For instance, in addition to the Ang II/AT1 receptor axis actions, the RAS has a counter-regulatory axis composed of angiotensin-(1–7) [Ang–(1–7)] and the Mas receptor. Within the corpus cavernosum, the Ang-(1–7)/Mas axis increases nitric oxide (NO) production and facilitates penile erection [13]. Overall, it is well accepted that the RAS is modulated by two major axes, one deleterious triggered by Ang II and another protective triggered by Ang-(1–7) [11, 12]. Furthermore, it is known that disturbances between these two major axes are associated with several cardiovascular diseases [3, 11], as well as ED [8] (Fig. 5.1).

This chapter will summarize the most current literature, addressing the pathophysiological role of RAS on erectile function. Moreover, it highlights the recent suggesting that the protective axis of RAS may represent a therapeutic target for ED treatment.

5.2 Renin-Angiotensin System: Current Paradigm

Traditionally, RAS biosynthesis is comprised of a sequential linear enzymatic cascade initiated by renin, an enzyme released from the juxtaglomerular cells in response to a reduction in blood pressure [3]. When found in the circulation, renin cleaves the zymogen angiotensinogen, which is synthesized and secreted mainly by the liver, forming the inactive decapeptide angiotensin I (Ang I). Ang I is sequentially cleaved by ACE, an enzyme mainly expressed on the surface of vascular endothelial cells, forming the octapeptide Ang II [3, 14]. Ang II demonstrates a high affinity with two distinct G protein-coupled receptors, AT1 and AT2 receptors. Under both physiological and pathological condition, AT1 receptor activation leads to blood pressure increase by stimulating vasoconstriction and sodium retention. Moreover, chronic AT1 receptor activation induces cellular proliferation, fibrosis, and inflammation [3, 15]. The relevance of Ang II/AT1 receptor actions on the cardiovascular system is underscored by the remarkable achievement of ACEi and ARBs, which inhibit Ang II formation and AT1 receptor stimulation, respectively. Nowadays, these drugs are considered the main class of pharmacotherapy in the treatment of hypertension and cardiovascular diseases [2, 15].

Ang II also binds to the AT2 receptor, producing effects that often opposite those produced by AT1, such as vasodilation and antiproliferative and anti-inflammatory actions [16, 17]. During Ang II stimulation, AT1 receptor actions mask that of the AT2 receptor, principally due to increased expression and high distribution of AT1. Although a comprehensive understanding of the role of the AT2 receptor has yet to be fully elucidated, evidence indicates that AT2 receptors may participate in mechanisms where ARBs induce cardiovascular protection [17]. This suggests that AT2 receptor agonists are a potential therapeutic tool for the treatment of cardiovascular diseases [18, 19].

The recent discovery of novel RAS components has illuminated alternative metabolic cascades and actions, thus expanding the traditional RAS paradigm [11, 12]. ACE2, an ACE homologous enzyme, acts as key enzyme by cleaving the C-terminal phenylalanine of Ang II, leading to Ang-(1–7) formation [20, 21]. Ang-(1–7) is a heptapeptide with biological actions that frequently oppose those attributed to Ang II [12, 22]. Acting via the G protein-coupled Mas receptor [23], Ang-(1–7) mediates vasodilation [11, 12], NO release [24], and antiproliferative [25], antifibrotic [26], and anti-inflammatory [27] effects. Therefore, Ang-(1–7) is well accepted in the scientific community as the primary endogenous counter-regulator of Ang II [3, 11, 12, 22]. ACE2 appears to be the major Ang-(1–7)-forming enzyme; however, additional pathways, such as neutral endopeptidase (prolylcarboxypeptidase [PCP] and prolylendopeptidase [PEP]), are also involved in the generation of Ang-(1–7) [21, 28, 29] (Fig. 5.1).

In the current scenario, RAS is regulated by two opposing axes, one deleterious branch composed of ACE/Ang II/AT1 receptor, and the other, a protective branch formed by ACE2/Ang-(1–7)/Mas receptor [11, 12]. Recent studies suggest that these two axes modulate cardiovascular homeostasis, while a chronic and sustained imbalance may contribute pathological etiologies [11]. For instance, in erectile tissues, elevated Ang II production has been observed in humans with ED [10]. Additionally, deletion of the Mas receptor gene significantly impaired erectile function and augmented collagen deposition within the corpus cavernosum in mice [13].

5.3 ACE/Ang II/AT1 Receptor on Erection Function

The RAS is highly involved in disturbances of the cardiovascular system, as well; it is considerably involved in ED pathophysiology [8, 9, 13, 30, 31]. The existence of a local RAS within the penis has been confirmed by several studies [9, 10, 13], suggesting a paracrinal modulation independent of systemic circulation. In fact, ACE, AT1 receptor, Ang I, and Ang II were detected in human corpus cavernosum [32]. In 1997, Kifor et al. found that human corpus cavernosum produces and secretes physiologically relevant amounts of Ang II [32]. Moreover, in the same study, intracavernosal injection of Ang II resulted in cavernosal smooth muscle contraction and eliminated spontaneous erection in anesthetized dog. On the other hand, when administered the Ang II receptor antagonist, losartan, a consistent and prolonged increase in cavernosal pressure was observed [32]. Interestingly, other studies have observed that human corpus cavernosum produces and secretes physiological amounts of Ang II in greater quantities than those found in the systemic plasma [8, 10], indicating an intense local modulation of erectile function by RAS. Supporting these reports, Iwamoto and coworkers demonstrated that ACE activity in canine corpus cavernosum was 30-fold higher than in canine common carotid artery [33].

Physiologically, Ang II mediates tonus contraction of the smooth muscle in the corpus cavernosum [8, 9, 30]. In fact, the local blockage of AT1 receptor by intracavernosal losartan administration increased the cavernosal pressure, suggesting the fundamental role of Ang II in the maintenance of the penile flaccid state [32]. Furthermore, Becker et al. compared the level of Ang II in blood samples acquired from the corpus cavernosum during various stages: penile flaccidity, tumescence, rigidity, and detumescence [9]. They found that Ang II cavernosal level was significantly higher in the detumescence stage, suggesting an essential role of this peptide on the detumescence process [9].

The main actions of Ang II are mediated by AT1 receptor. This receptor is expressed on the cavernosal smooth muscle and endothelial cells [3]. The activation of AT1 receptor initiates multiple intracellular signal transduction pathways that are complex and specific but converge, yielding multiple short- or long-term responses [34, 35]. One of the major pathways trigger by AT1 stimulation involves the classical phospholipase C (PLC) activation, resulting in the generation of inositol trisphosphate IP3 and diacylglycerol (DAG). IP3 and DAG regulate two distinct pathways that lead to an increase in intracellular Ca^{2+}, culminating in the activation of myosin light chain kinase and smooth muscle contraction [35]. Additionally, AT1 activation may also stimulate the RhoA/Rho-kinase pathway prompting inhibition of myosin light chain phosphatase (MLCP), thereby regulating smooth muscle contraction [36]. These independent pathways make Ang II one of the most powerful endogenous vasoconstrictors. Therefore, its action on the tonus and contraction of the corpus cavernosum might be critical to erectile pathophysiology [8].

The activation of AT1 receptor also produces additional actions with critical repercussion for erectile function. Stimulation of this receptor can activate nicotinamide adenine dinucleotide phosphate (NADPH) oxidase, the main enzyme responsible for reactive oxygen species (ROS) production [34]. ROS is involved in the physiologic redox of cellular function; however its overproduction is closely associated with the development of vasculogenic ED [37]. In fact, Jin et al. reported that the development of hypertension-associated ED caused by Ang II infusion was associated with an increased NADPH oxidase expression and ROS production into the corpus cavernosum [38]. In addition, during long-term stimulation, AT1 activation may also induce a proinflammatory response, cell proliferation, hypertrophy, increased collagen deposition in the extracellular matrix by regulating mitogen-activated protein (MAP) kinases, and transcription factors [39, 40].

Ang II also can activate the AT2 receptor, resulting in cardiovascular consequences often opposite to that of the AT1 receptor. The AT2 receptor is highly expressed in fetal tissues, then production quickly declines following birth [16]. In light of this, the receptor still remains present and can be detected in various adult tissues. Nevertheless, its role in cardiovascular hemostasis is not completely established. To date, the role of AT2 in erectile tissues remains unknown. Previous reports have demonstrated that the specific binding of Ang II in the corpus cavernosum of rabbit was displaced by a selective AT1 antagonist, but not by an AT2 antagonist, suggesting a marginal role of AT2 in erectile tissues [30]. However, to the best of our knowledge, this is the only study addressing AT2 in the corpus cavernosum, and therefore future studies are needed to further explore the role of this receptor erection pathophysiology. Evidences point out that following injury, the AT2 receptor can be upregulated and its actions become more relevant during the pathological condition [16, 41]. Therefore, an in depth investigation of AT2 during ED would be relevant to compliment the overall understanding of RAS in this pathology.

Several reports indicate a positive correlation between increased Ang II activity and ED [8]. Indeed, Ang II plasma levels were elevated in the cavernous blood of patients with an organogenic etiology of ED [10]. This was complimented by the observation that ACE mRNA expression was upregulated in the penis of rats with arteriogenic ED [42], while Ang II-induced contraction was significantly increased in the cavernosum strips from older and diabetic rabbits [43]. Additionally, diabetic ED rats demonstrated a significant increase in Ang II intrapenile levels [44]. Reinforcing these reports, continuous subcutaneous infusion of Ang II has become a common method to produce an ED animal model, underscoring the central role of Ang II/AT1 receptor in the pathophysiology of ED [8].

The link between the ACE/Ang II/AT1 receptor axis hyperactivity and ED suggests that the application of ACEi and ARBs would be an interesting strategy to treat vasculogenic ED. In fact, several preclinical and clinical studies report beneficial outcomes on the sexual function by ACEi and ARB treatment [45–53]. In a hypertension-induced ED rat model, captopril treatment normalized both the blood pressure and erectile response, completely restoring the impaired erectile function [46]. Accordingly, in a rat model of diabetes-induced ED, losartan treatment markedly improved the erectile response [47]. Additionally, in a mouse model of hypercholesterolemia-induced ED, both telmisartan and ramipril (ARBs and ACEi respectively) restored the impaired cavernosal endothelial function by reducing the oxidative stress and normalizing the endothelial nitric oxide synthase expression [48].

Importantly, the beneficial effects produced by ACEi and ARBs on erectile function have also been documented in humans. Several antihypertensive drugs possess the undesirable adverse effect of causing or worsening ED [49], while ACEi and ARBs may have less of an effect to merely improve erectile function [50–53]. In a comparative study between different antihypertensive agents, trichlormethiazide, atenolol, and nifedipine all negatively influenced the sexual activity, with the exception of captopril [54]. Supporting that finding, a study of hypertensive men without a history of sexual dysfunction found that atenolol treatment significantly worsened erectile function, as assessed by the number of sexual intercourse episodes per month, while lisinopril showed minimal influence during the first month which was later fully recovered [55]. In a cohort of 124 diabetic patients with ED, it was observed that losartan has significantly improved sexual activity, assessed by International Index of Erectile Function-5 [45]. Interestingly, the combination of losartan and tadalafil was more effective in improving sexual satisfaction than the single use of one of these drugs [45]. In another study, 12 weeks of losartan treatment significantly improved satisfaction and frequency of sexual activity in hypertensive patients with ED [51]. Interestingly, the positive effect of ABR has also been documented in patients with ED caused by nerve-sparing radical prostatectomy. In a retrospective cohort, it was found that irbesartan treatment significantly increased sexual activity and avoided early loss of stretched penile length, an important common adverse issue in post-prostatectomy patients [56]. Contrary to these reports, a retrospective cohort study from 1990 to 2006 that was based on spontaneous reports in the Swedish adverse drug reaction database indicated a relatively high prevalence of ED in patients treated with ARBs, suggesting these drugs may have a negative effect on ED [57]. Several limitations of a retrospective exist and therefore should be taken into account, especially when interpreting data from spontaneous reports; however this contradictory finding demonstrates that large and well-controlled clinical trials are indeed necessary to clarify the benefits of ACEi and ABR use in ED.

5.4 ACE2/Ang-(1–7)/Mas Receptor Axis on Erectile Function

In the last decade, Ang-(1–7) emerged as the main endogenous counter-regulatory effector of Ang II [11, 12, 22]. Acting through the Mas receptor, Ang-(1–7) produces several cardiovascular-protective actions, such as vasodilation, inhibition of oxidative stress, and anti-inflammatory, antithrombotic, antiproliferative, and antifibrotic actions [3, 11, 12, 22]. Likewise, Ang-(1–7) facilitates penile erection and preserves penile structure against pathological alterations [8].

Exogenous administration of Ang-(1–7) was able to produce concentration-dependent relaxation in isolated rabbit corpus cavernosum [43]. Also, its intracavernosal injection potentiated the erectile response induced by electrical stimulation of the major pelvic ganglion of rats and mice [13]. Nevertheless, evidence suggests that endogenous Ang-(1–7) possesses an essential role on penile physiological erection. Intracavernosal administration of A-779, a Mas receptor antagonist, was able to singly reduce erectile response [8, 13]. Moreover, rabbit corpus cavernosum contraction induced by Ang II was enlarged by coadministration of A-779 [43]. Supporting this finding, Mas receptor gene-deleted mice showed a marked reduction in erectile response [13].

Based on the protective role of Ang-(1–7)/Mas axis in erectile function, investigations have been conducted targeting and exploring the contribution of this axis in ED. Indeed, Ang-(1–7)/Mas axis activation may ameliorate or even reverse vasculogenic ED, as was demonstrated by the restoration of impaired erections in DOCA-salt hypertensive rats by acute administration of Ang-(1–7) [13]. Accordingly, treatment with an oral formulation of Ang-(1–7) [Ang-(1–7)-CyD] produced several beneficial effects against hypercholesterolemic-induced corpus cavernosum damage [58]. In particular, Ang-(1–7)-CyD chronic treatment reduced corpus cavernosum fibrosis, which is associated with an attenuation of oxidative stress. Additionally, Ang-(1–7)-CyD improved the cavernosal endothelial function and NO bioavailability [58]. Supporting these observations, Ang-(1–7) treatment was also demonstrated to prevent corpus cavernosum smooth muscle degeneration and oxidative DNA damage in a rat model of diabetic ED [59].

The mechanisms underlying the protective actions of Ang-(1–7) in erectile tissues are still poorly understood. It appears the Ang-(1–7) facilitates erection mainly by increasing the NO bioavailability within the corpus cavernosum [8, 13, 60]. In endothelial cells, the activation of Mas receptor by Ang-(1–7) leads to the activation of the Akt/PKI3 pathways, culminating in the phosphorylation and dephosphorylation of Scr1177 and Thr495 residues, respectively (the stimulatory and inhibitor site of eNOS, respectively), consequently inducing NO production [24]. Accordingly, the in vitro and in vivo actions of Ang-(1–7) on the corpus cavernosum were blocked by the nitric oxide synthase inhibitor, Nω-nitro-L-arginine methyl (L-NAME) [13, 43]. A similar effect was observed with A-779, a synthetic Mas agonist [60]. Using a fluorescent probe to directly measure NO production, rat and mouse corpus cavernosum strips incubated with Ang-(1–7) markedly increased NO production, whereas electrically stimulated release of NO (neuronal-derived) in the rat corpus cavernosum was potentiated by Ang-(1–7) [13]. Consistent with this, chronic treatment with Ang-(1–7)-CyD [an oral formulation of Ang-(1–7)] increased the protein expression of the endothelial and neuronal nitric oxide synthase isoforms in a mouse model of ED [58]. Therefore, it is evident that NO is a crucial factor contributing to the Ang-(1–7)/Mas axis-mediated pro-erectile function. However, it still remains unclear as to the main source of NO, whether neuronal derived or endothelial derived, that participates in Ang-(1–7)/Mas action [8].

In addition to the acute effect of Ang-(1–7)/Mas receptor on erection, this axis produces profound protective actions on penile structure [8]. Chronic treatment with Ang-(1–7) markedly inhibits the penile fibrosis in a hypercholesterolemic-induced ED mouse model [58]. Moreover, Mas receptor gene-deleted mice showed a robust increase of collagen deposition within the corpus cavernosum [13]. It appears that different pathways are involved in the antifibrotic effect of Ang-(1–7)/Mas, such as attenuation of cytokine signaling cascades [61], modulation of MMP activity [62], inhibition of MAPK signaling cascades [63, 64], and oxidative stress reduction [26, 58]. Nevertheless, the direct mechanism by which Ang-(1–7) inhibits penile fibrosis remains unknown.

5.5 Future Directions

The RAS plays a fundamental role in erection physiology, while its unbalance state is associated with ED [8]. Consequently, it is rational to consider RAS as a putative target to treat vasculogenic ED. ACEi and ARBs are potentially effective treatment options for ED; however, more investigation is necessary to elucidate its relevance in clinical practice. Most clinical studies evaluating the effect these drugs on sexual activity present several limitations, such as narrow cohort or lack of proper control. Therefore, large and well-controlled clinical trials are needed to clarify the advantages of the actual RAS blockers against ED.

In addition to Ang II/AT1 axis blockage, the activation of the Ang-(1–7)/Mas receptor axis has emerged as potential target to treat ED. Many studies showed the beneficial actions of this axis on penile erection and structure [8]. Presently, there are no drugs available on the market that activate the Ang-(1–7)/Mas axis. However, several investigations are currently devoted to develop such pharmacological tools [12]. Indeed, some initiatives appear to be promising, including a formulation of Ang-(1–7), based on the inclusion of this peptide in cyclodextrin that allows for the oral administration of Ang-(1–7) [12, 65]. Because of its peptidic nature, the clinical use of Ang-(1–7) is hampered by their rapid proteolytic degradation. The formulation is able to avoid Ang-(1–7) degradation into the gastrointestinal tract, enhancing its stability and absorption across biological barriers. Additionally, synthetic Mas receptor agonists have been developed and are also potential candidates to manage vasculogenic ED [12, 60].

Despite of the described protective action of Ang-(1–7)/Mas receptor axis against ED, the relevance of this axis on human erectile function still remain uncertain. Further preclinical and clinical studies are essential to establish the potential of drugs activating Ang-(1–7)/Mas axis against ED.

References

1. Ma TK et al (2010) Renin-angiotensin-aldosterone system blockade for cardiovascular diseases: current status. Br J Pharmacol 160(6):1273–1292

2. Schiffrin EL (2002) Vascular and cardiac benefits of angiotensin receptor blockers. Am J Med 113(5):409–418
3. Bader M (2010) Tissue renin-angiotensin-aldosterone systems: targets for pharmacological therapy. Annu Rev Pharmacol Toxicol 50:439–465
4. Dzau VJ (1988) Circulating versus local renin-angiotensin system in cardiovascular homeostasis. Circulation 77(6 Pt 2):I4–I13
5. Dostal DE, Baker KM (1999) The cardiac renin-angiotensin system: conceptual, or a regulator of cardiac function? Circ Res 85(7):643–650
6. Paul M, Poyan Mehr A, Kreutz R (2006) Physiology of local renin-angiotensin systems. Physiol Rev 86(3):747–803
7. Bader M, Ganten D (2008) Update on tissue renin-angiotensin systems. J Mol Med (Berl) 86(6):615–621
8. Fraga-Silva RA et al (2013) Pathophysiological role of the renin-angiotensin system on erectile dysfunction. Eur J Clin Invest 43(9):978–985
9. Becker AJ et al (2001) Possible role of bradykinin and angiotensin II in the regulation of penile erection and detumescence. Urology 57(1):193–198
10. Becker AJ et al (2001) Plasma levels of angiotensin II during different penile conditions in the cavernous and systemic blood of healthy men and patients with erectile dysfunction. Urology 58(5):805–810
11. Ferreira AJ et al (2010) Therapeutic implications of the vasoprotective axis of the renin-angiotensin system in cardiovascular diseases. Hypertension 55(2):207–213
12. Fraga-Silva RA, Ferreira AJ, Dos Santos RA (2013) Opportunities for targeting the angiotensin-converting enzyme 2/angiotensin-(1–7)/mas receptor pathway in hypertension. Curr Hypertens Rep 15(1):31–38
13. da Costa Goncalves AC et al (2007) Evidence that the vasodilator angiotensin-(1–7)-Mas axis plays an important role in erectile function. Am J Physiol Heart Circ Physiol 293(4): H2588–H2596
14. Kokubu T et al (1979) Purification and properties of angiotensin I-converting enzyme in human lung and its role on the metabolism of vasoactive peptides in pulmonary circulation. Adv Exp Med Biol 120B:467–475
15. Unger T (2002) The role of the renin-angiotensin system in the development of cardiovascular disease. Am J Cardiol 89(2A):3A–9A; discussion 10A
16. Levy BI (2005) How to explain the differences between renin angiotensin system modulators. Am J Hypertens 18(9 Pt 2):134S–141S
17. Widdop RE et al (2002) AT2 receptor-mediated relaxation is preserved after long-term AT1 receptor blockade. Hypertension 40(4):516–520
18. Savoia C et al (2011) Angiotensin type 2 receptor in hypertensive cardiovascular disease. Curr Opin Nephrol Hypertens 20(2):125–132
19. Steckelings UM et al (2011) Non-peptide AT2-receptor agonists. Curr Opin Pharmacol 11(2):187–192
20. Vickers C et al (2002) Hydrolysis of biological peptides by human angiotensin-converting enzyme-related carboxypeptidase. J Biol Chem 277(17):14838–14843
21. Zisman LS et al (2003) Angiotensin-(1–7) formation in the intact human heart: in vivo dependence on angiotensin II as substrate. Circulation 108(14):1679–1681
22. Ferrario CM et al (1997) Counterregulatory actions of angiotensin-(1–7). Hypertension 30 (3 Pt 2):535–541
23. Santos RA et al (2003) Angiotensin-(1–7) is an endogenous ligand for the G protein-coupled receptor Mas. Proc Natl Acad Sci U S A 100(14):8258–8263
24. Sampaio WO et al (2007) Angiotensin-(1–7) through receptor Mas mediates endothelial nitric oxide synthase activation via Akt-dependent pathways. Hypertension 49(1):185–192
25. Langeveld B et al (2005) Angiotensin-(1–7) attenuates neointimal formation after stent implantation in the rat. Hypertension 45(1):138–141
26. Katovich MJ, Grobe JL, Raizada MK (2008) Angiotensin-(1–7) as an antihypertensive, antifibrotic target. Curr Hypertens Rep 10(3):227–232

27. da Silveira KD et al (2010) Anti-inflammatory effects of the activation of the angiotensin-(1–7) receptor, MAS, in experimental models of arthritis. J Immunol 185(9):5569–5576
28. Rice GI et al (2004) Evaluation of angiotensin-converting enzyme (ACE), its homologue ACE2 and neprilysin in angiotensin peptide metabolism. Biochem J 383(Pt 1):45–51
29. Stanziola L, Greene LJ, Santos RA (1999) Effect of chronic angiotensin converting enzyme inhibition on angiotensin I and bradykinin metabolism in rats. Am J Hypertens 12(10 Pt 1):1021–1029
30. Park JK et al (1997) Renin angiotensin system in rabbit corpus cavernosum: functional characterization of angiotensin II receptors. J Urol 158(2):653–658
31. Jin LM (2009) Angiotensin II signaling and its implication in erectile dysfunction. J Sex Med 6(Suppl 3):302–310
32. Kifor I et al (1997) Tissue angiotensin II as a modulator of erectile function. I. Angiotensin peptide content, secretion and effects in the corpus cavernosum. J Urol 157(5):1920–1925
33. Iwamoto Y et al (2001) Multiple pathways of angiotensin I conversion and their functional role in the canine penile corpus cavernosum. J Pharmacol Exp Ther 298(1):43–48
34. Touyz RM, Berry C (2002) Recent advances in angiotensin II signaling. Braz J Med Biol Res 35(9):1001–1015
35. Wynne BM, Chiao CW, Webb RC (2009) Vascular smooth muscle cell signaling mechanisms for contraction to angiotensin II and endothelin-1. J Am Soc Hypertens 3(2):84–95
36. Ying Z et al (2006) Angiotensin II up-regulates the leukemia-associated Rho guanine nucleotide exchange factor (RhoGEF), a regulator of G protein signaling domain-containing RhoGEF, in vascular smooth muscle cells. Mol Pharmacol 69(3):932–940
37. Bivalacqua TJ et al (2003) Endothelial dysfunction in erectile dysfunction: role of the endothelium in erectile physiology and disease. J Androl 24(6 Suppl):S17–S37
38. Jin L et al (2008) NADPH oxidase activation: a mechanism of hypertension-associated erectile dysfunction. J Sex Med 5(3):544–551
39. Horiuchi M, Iwanami J, Mogi M (2012) Regulation of angiotensin II receptors beyond the classical pathway. Clin Sci (Lond) 123(4):193–203
40. Nguyen Dinh Cat A, Touyz RM (2011) Cell signaling of angiotensin II on vascular tone: novel mechanisms. Curr Hypertens Rep 13(2):122–128
41. Unger T (1999) The angiotensin type 2 receptor: variations on an enigmatic theme. J Hypertens 17(12 Pt 2):1775–1786
42. Lin CS et al (2001) Gene expression profiling of an arteriogenic impotence model. Biochem Biophys Res Commun 285(2):565–569
43. Yousif MH, Kehinde EO, Benter IF (2007) Different responses to angiotensin-(1–7) in young, aged and diabetic rabbit corpus cavernosum. Pharmacol Res 56(3):209–216
44. Li SX, Dai YT (2005) Effects of angiotensin II on male rats with diabetic erectile dysfunction. Zhonghua Nan Ke Xue 11(5):346–349
45. Chen Y et al (2012) Losartan improves erectile dysfunction in diabetic patients: a clinical trial. Int J Impot Res 24(6):217–220
46. Dorrance AM, Lewis RW, Mills TM (2002) Captopril treatment reverses erectile dysfunction in male stroke prone spontaneously hypertensive rats. Int J Impot Res 14(6):494–497
47. Yang R et al (2009) Losartan, an Angiotensin type I receptor, restores erectile function by downregulation of cavernous renin-angiotensin system in streptozocin-induced diabetic rats. J Sex Med 6(3):696–707
48. Schlimmer N et al (2011) Telmisartan, ramipril and their combination improve endothelial function in different tissues in a murine model of cholesterol-induced atherosclerosis. Br J Pharmacol 163(4):804–814
49. Kloner RA et al (2003) Erectile dysfunction in the cardiac patient: how common and should we treat? J Urol 170(2 Pt 2):S46–S50; discussion S50
50. Fogari R et al (2001) Sexual activity in hypertensive men treated with valsartan or carvedilol: a crossover study. Am J Hypertens 14(1):27–31

51. Llisterri JL et al (2001) Sexual dysfunction in hypertensive patients treated with losartan. Am J Med Sci 321(5):336–341
52. Della Chiesa A et al (2003) Sexual activity in hypertensive men. J Hum Hypertens 17(8):515–521
53. Dusing R (2005) Sexual dysfunction in male patients with hypertension: influence of antihypertensive drugs. Drugs 65(6):773–786
54. Suzuki H et al (1988) Effects of first-line antihypertensive agents on sexual function and sex hormones. J Hypertens Suppl 6(4):S649–S651
55. Fogari R et al (1998) Sexual function in hypertensive males treated with lisinopril or atenolol: a cross-over study. Am J Hypertens 11(10):1244–1247
56. Segal RL, Bivalacqua TJ, Burnett AL (2012) Irbesartan promotes erection recovery after nerve-sparing radical retropubic prostatectomy: a retrospective long-term analysis. BJU Int 110(11):1782–1786
57. Ekman E et al (2010) Antihypertensive drugs and erectile dysfunction as seen in spontaneous reports, with focus on angiotensin II type 1 receptor blockers. Drug Healthc Patient Saf 2:21–25
58. Fraga-Silva RA et al (2013) An oral formulation of angiotensin-(1–7) reverses corpus cavernosum damages induced by hypercholesterolemia. J Sex Med 10(10):2430–2442
59. Kilarkaje N et al (2013) Role of angiotensin II and angiotensin-(1–7) in diabetes-induced oxidative DNA damage in the corpus cavernosum. Fertil Steril 100(1):226–233
60. da Costa Goncalves AC et al (2013) AVE 0991, a non-peptide Mas-receptor agonist, facilitates penile erection. Exp Physiol 98(3):850–855
61. Shenoy V et al (2010) The angiotensin-converting enzyme 2/angiogenesis-(1–7)/Mas axis confers cardiopulmonary protection against lung fibrosis and pulmonary hypertension. Am J Respir Crit Care Med 182(8):1065–1072
62. Pei Z et al (2010) Angiotensin-(1–7) ameliorates myocardial remodeling and interstitial fibrosis in spontaneous hypertension: role of MMPs/TIMPs. Toxicol Lett 199(2):173–181
63. Ferreira AJ et al (2011) Angiotensin-converting enzyme 2 activation protects against hypertension-induced cardiac fibrosis involving extracellular signal-regulated kinases. Exp Physiol 96(3):287–294
64. McCollum LT, Gallagher PE, Ann Tallant E (2012) Angiotensin-(1–7) attenuates angiotensin II-induced cardiac remodeling associated with upregulation of dual-specificity phosphatase 1. Am J Physiol Heart Circ Physiol 302(3):H801–H810
65. Lula I et al (2007) Study of angiotensin-(1–7) vasoactive peptide and its beta-cyclodextrin inclusion complexes: complete sequence-specific NMR assignments and structural studies. Peptides 28(11):2199–2210

Erectile Dysfunction and Target Organ Damage

Nikolaos Ioakeimidis

6.1 Target Organ Damage in Hypertension

Several arguments support the investigation for target organ damage (TOD) in hypertensive patients to quantify total cardiovascular (CV) risk before deciding the treatment strategy [1]. Subclinical (or asymptomatic) organ damage involving the structure and/or function of the heart, brain, kidney, or vessels predicts CV death independently of Systematic Coronary Risk Evaluation Project (SCORE), and a combination of both may improve risk prediction, particularly in individuals at low and moderate risk (SCORE 1–4 %) [2]. This has important implications for treatment because therapeutic strategies differ in high- vs moderate-, or low-risk hypertensive patients [3]. Therefore, Guidelines of the European Society of Hypertension and the European Society of Cardiology recommend assessment of asymptomatic organ damage in the diagnostic workup of hypertensive patients [3] (Table 6.1). Furthermore, looking for damage in different organs is meaningful because the risk increases with the increase in the number of organs affected, while evidence exists that this happens even with different measures of damage within the same organ. In the kidney, for example, microalbuminuria and reduced estimated glomerular filtration rate are associated with a greater risk of renal and CV events than either abnormality alone [4].

N. Ioakeimidis
1st Cardiology Department, Athens Medical School,
Hippokration Hospital, 114 Vas Sofias, Athens 11528, Greece
e-mail: nioakim@gmail.com

Table 6.1 Asymptomatic organ damage

Pulse pressure (in the elderly) ≥60 mmHg
Electrocardiographic LVH (Sokolow–Lyon index >3.5 mV; RaVL >1.1 mV; Cornell voltage duration product >244 mV*ms), or
Echocardiographic LVH [LVM index: men >115 g/m^2; women >95 g/m^2 (BSA)]
Carotid wall thickening (IMT >0.9 mm) or plaque
Carotid–femoral PWV >10 m/s
Ankle-brachial index <0.9
CKD with eGFR 30–60 mL/min/1.73 m^2 (BSA)
Microalbuminuria (30–300 mg/24 h), or albumin–creatinine ratio (30–300 mg/g; 3.4–34 mg/mmol) (preferentially on morning spot urine)

CKD chronic kidney disease, *eGFR* estimated glomerular filtration rate, *IMT* intima media thickness, *LVH* left ventricular hypertension

Table 6.2 Association with erectile dysfunction, availability, response to treatment, prognostic value and cost of markers of asymptomatic organ damage in men with hypertension (scored from 0 to 4+)

Target organ damage	Association with vasculogenic ED	Overall CVD predictive value	CVD predictive value in ED[a]	Availability	Cost
LVH (ECG/Echo)	–/+	+++	–	++	++
Aortic PWV	++	+++	+	++	++
IMT	+++	+++	–	++	++
ABI	++	+++	–	+++	+
eGFR	–/+	+++	–	++++	+
Microalbuminuria	+	+++	+	++++	+

ABI Ankle-brachial index, *eGFR* estimated glomerular filtration rate, *IMT* intima media thickness *LVH* left ventricular hypertension, *PWV* pulse wave velocity
[a]Data available from studies in the ED population

6.2 Target Organ Damage in Patients with Hypertension and Erectile Dysfunction (Table 6.2)

Vasculogenic erectile dysfunction (ED) is considered an early manifestation of generalized arterial disease. ED is frequent in patients with established coronary artery disease (CAD) [5], it co-exists with occult CAD [6], and it is an independent predictor of CV outcomes [7]. In hypertensive patients, it is currently unknown whether ED is related to any additional risk on top of hypertension. Furthermore, data regarding the extent of hypertension-related TOD in hypertensive men with ED are scarce.

Ultrasound examination of the carotid arteries with measurement of *intima-media thickness* (*IMT*) or identification of the presence of *plaques* is a reliable surrogate of systemic atherosclerosis, including CAD [8]. The presence but not the severity of ED (as quantified by the International Index of Erectile

Function-IIEFquestionnaire) has been associated with increased carotid IMT specifically in hypertensive patients [9]. Other studies have shown a trend towards a more severe impairment of vascular function and structure at penile arteries (by measurement of dynamic penile peak systolic velocity and IMT) in ED patients with higher carotid IMT [10, 11].

Measurement of *carotid-femoral pulse wave velocity* (*PWV*) provides a comprehensive non-invasive assessment of aortic stiffness [12, 13]. Aortic stiffness has been associated with the presence and severity of penile vascular disease as measured by penile Doppler in hypertensive (treated and never treated) individuals [9]. In men without hypertension or other traditional risk factors (as well as in individuals with early stage high blood pressure) aortic PWV level was similar between the ED patients and men with normal erectile function [14, 15].

Left ventricular hypertrophy (*LVH*) is highly prevalent among hypertensive patients. The association of LVH and increased CV morbidity and mortality has been convincingly documented [16]. Left ventricular diastolic function is impaired in ED patients with hypertension but without overt cardiovascular disease compared to men with normal erectile function [17], however, differences in LV structure are not evident between ED patients and non-ED subjects, at least in the early stages of hypertension [15].

A *low ankle-brachial blood pressure index* (*ABI*) signals peripheral artery disease (PAD) and, in general, advanced atherosclerosis, and relates to further development of CV morbidity and mortality [18]. In a study evaluating the relationship between ED and PAD, Polonsky et al. showed that ABI successfully identified PAD in men with ED and suggested that men with ED be targeted for ABI examination [19]. The association of ABI with ED in the context of hypertension has not been studied yet.

The finding of an impaired renal function in a hypertensive patient, expressed as *increased urinary protein excretion* and/or a *reduced estimated glomerular filtration rate*, constitutes a very potent predictor of future CV events and death [20]. The association of ED with glomerular filtration rate and albuminuria, particularly in men with hypertension has not been adequately addressed. Although albuminuria has been associated with ED in type 2 diabetes patients [21], data on the impact of ED in treated and untreated essential hypertensive patients are not yet available [22].

6.3 Target Organ Damage and CV Prediction Within ED

As there are no data on the predictive value of TOD specifically for hypertensive patients with ED, we rely on the evidence available from studies in patients either with hypertension or with ED. It should be noted, however, that patients in ED studies were to a large percentage hypertensives [7] (Table 6.2). Recent data show an independent predictive ability of *aortic PWV* for future cardiovascular events specifically in ED patients without established cardiovascular disease (Vlachopoulos et al. submitted). Subjects in the highest PWV tertile (>8.8 m/s) had a fourfold higher risk of MACE compared to those in the lowest PWV tertile (<7.6 m/s). When added to standard risk models, such as the Framingham Risk Score, aortic PWV reclassifies correctly a considerable percentage (27.6 %) of patients to a higher or lower risk category in the whole population. In addition, *pulse pressure*, a crude index of arterial stiffness, has also been shown to predict outcome in ED patients: the risk of cardiac events is increased by 60 % for each 10 mmHg increment in pulse pressure [23]. *Microalbuminuria*, as defined by albumin/creatinine ratio 3.4–34 mg/mmol and albumin excretion ratio 30–300 mg/day, is an easily measured non-circulating marker of microvascular injury. Microalbuminuria has been shown to predict CV events specifically in a population of diabetic ED patients with angiographically proven CAD; in this studied population, hypertension was highly prevalent [24].

Further to the identification of organs that can serve as risk predictors, it would be important to assess whether TOD regression predicts risk reduction. Such evidence, documented in hypertensive patients [3, 25], offers valuable information on whether specific treatment confers additional therapeutic benefit. Currently there are no data in the ED population to document the impact of antihypertensive drugs (with neutral or even a positive effect on erectile function) on TOD regression. Likewise, whether treatment-induced reduction in TOD affects incidence of adverse CV events is also an interesting, yet unexplored, field.

6.4   Is Erectile Dysfunction a Target Organ Damage Per Se?

The frequent co-existence of hypertension and ED and the impact of antihypertensive drugs on sexual function raise the question whether ED is the result of hypertension per se, an adverse event of antihypertensive treatment, or a combination of both [26]. Several lines of evidence indicate that drugs used in the treatment of hypertension can indeed deteriorate sexual function, but such an effect appears mainly with older generation drugs (older beta blockers, diuretics), while newer agents (nebivolol, renin-angiotensin-aldosterone system blockers) might even improve sexual function [27]. On the other hand, hypertension appears to cause ED per se, through a multitude of mechanisms that include prolonged exposure to elevated levels of systemic blood pressure, endothelial dysfunction and circulation of vasoactive substances (with a pivotal role of angiotensin II) that lead to structural and functional alterations in the penile arteries [28]. Penile doppler studies have shown that the presence of hypertension is associated with a approximately twofold increase in the likelihood of having an abnormal penile blood flow [29]. Specifically, patients with hypertension exhibit a significantly low penile blood inflow and venous leakage as expressed by reduced penile peak systolic velocity (PSV) and increased end-diastolic velocity (EDV) respectively, compared to men without vascular risk factors.

Screening for vasculogenic ED as a TOD per se could be incorporated in diagnostic algorithms for the management and treatment of arterial hypertension

[30] in men for three reasons: First, ED is easy to recognize and it gravely affects a man's quality of life. Second, the presence of ED per se increases the risk for future CV events [7]. The predictive ability of ED is higher in young subjects and in subjects with intermediate baseline CV risk [7]. Third, testosterone deficiency, which is frequent in aged males who suffer from vasculogenic ED [31], is associated with subclinical organ damage (LVH, IMT, aortic stiffness, ABI) [31–33], and it is an important predictor of future CV events in men with hypertension [34].

6.5 Screening for Target Organ Damage in Hypertensive ED Patients

ED as a TOD: The use of the Sexual Health Inventory for Men (SHIM) validated questionnaire for diagnosis and evaluation of ED as a TOD should be incorporated in the investigation of all hypertensive patients [35, 36]. Importantly, according to recent evidence validated questionnaires correlate with the vascular markers of TOD [9, 19, 37] (aortic PWV, carotid IMT, ABI) and improve the predictive value of ED for total CV events compared with a single question [7]. Evaluation of penile vasculature by dynamic color Doppler ultrasound (with intracavernous injection of alprostadil) still remains the cornerstone of the diagnostic workup of the patients with vasculogenic ED, by differentiating psychogenic and vasculogenic causes of ED [38, 39]. Penile doppler indices strongly correlate with atherosclerotic lesions in other vascular beds and major adverse CV events [40].

Screening for TOD in ED (Table 6.3): Within the context of ED and hypertension combined, tests to reveal TOD that appear appealing include those that assess vascular function and structure, ventricular hypertrophy and function, and renal function. As such, a resting electrocardiogram, estimation of glomerular filtration rate, conventional echocardiography, carotid ultrasonography (for measurement of IMT and identification of plaques), aortic PWV, ABI, and detection of microalbuminuria are principal screening tests to identify TOD. Although many of these tests have not yet been evaluated in hypertensive ED patients, as stated earlier, their use is progressively being extended from the research to the clinical field [36, 41, 42].

Table 6.3 Searching for asymptomatic organ damage in hypertensive patients with ED

Screening test	Necessity
Electrocardiography	Necessary
Estimation of GFR	
Echocardiography	Recommended
Aortic PWV	
Carotid IMT and plaques	
ABI	
Microalbuminuria	

Conclusions

ED is considered to be an independent CV risk factor and an early diagnostic indicator for asymptomatic or clinical organ damage. Although the links between hypertension and ED are increasingly recognized, data regarding the presence of TOD and their prognostic role within the context of ED and hypertension are not ample. Assessment of target organ damage allows better prediction of CV risk compared with conventional risk assessment, and identifies high-risk individuals in whom a more intense treatment is needed. Cardiac echocardiography, carotid ultrasound, aortic PWV, ABI and microalbuminuria should be considered as recommended tests in hypertensive ED patients. ED per se can also be perceived as organ damage in hypertension due to its prognostic ability. Increased recognition of the potential for TOD in hypertensive men with ED, followed by appropriate preventive action, can improve sexual function and may affect incidence of adverse CV events. We recommend that inquiry of ED is part of recommended cardiovascular risk assessment in all hypertensive males.

References

1. Mancia G, Laurent S, Agabiti-Rosei E et al (2009) Reappraisal of European guidelines on hypertension management: a European Society of Hypertension Task Force document. J Hypertens 27:2121–2158
2. Perk J, DeBaker G, Gohlke H et al (2012) European guidelines on cardiovascular disease prevention in clinical practice (version 2012). The fifth joint task force of the European Society of Cardiology and other societies on cardiovascular disease prevention in clinical practice (constituted by representatives of nine societies and by invited experts). Developed with the special contribution of the European Association for Cardiovascular Prevention & Rehabilitation (EACPR). Eur Heart J33:1635–1701
3. Mancia G, Fagard R, Narkiewicz K et al (2013) 2013 ESH/ESCguidelines for the management of arterial hypertension: the task force for the management of arterial hypertension of the European Society of Hypertension (ESH) and of the European Society of Cardiology (ESC). Eur Heart J 34(28):2159–2219
4. Patel A, MacMahon S, Chalmers J et al (2007) Effects of a fixed combination of perindopril and indapamide on macrovascular and microvascular outcomes in patients with type 2 diabetes mellitus (the ADVANCE trial): a randomised controlled trial. Lancet 370:829–840
5. Montorsi P, Ravagnani PM, Galli S et al (2006) Association between erectile dysfunction and coronary artery disease. Role of coronary clinical presentation and extent of coronary vessels involvement: the COBRA trial. Eur Heart J 22:2632–2639
6. Vlachopoulos C, Rokkas K, Ioakeimidis N et al (2005) Prevalence of asymptomatic coronary artery disease in men with vasculogenic erectile dysfunction: a prospective angiographic study. Eur Urol 48:996–1002
7. Vlachopoulos CV, Terentes-Printzios DG, Ioakeimidis NK et al (2013) Prediction of cardiovascular events and all-cause mortality with erectile dysfunction: a systematic review and meta-analysis of cohort studies. Circ Cardiovasc Qual Outcome 6:99–109
8. Nambi V, Chambless L, Folsom AR et al (2010) Carotid intima-media thickness and presence or absence of plaque improves prediction of coronary heart disease risk: the ARIC (Atherosclerosis Risk In Communities) study. J Am Coll Cardiol 55:1600–1607
9. Vlachopoulos C, Aznaouridis K, Ioakeimidis N et al (2008) Arterial function and intima-media thickness in hypertensive patients with erectile dysfunction. J Hypertens 26:1829–1836

10. Bocchio M, Scarpelli P, Necozione S et al (2006) Penile duplex pharmaco-ultrasonography of cavernous arteries in men with erectile dysfunction and generalized atherosclerosis. Int J Androl 29:496–501
11. Caretta N, Palego P, Roverato A et al (2006) Age-matched cavernous peak systolic velocity: a highly sensitive parameter in the diagnosis of arteriogenic erectile dysfunction. Int J Impot Res 18(3):306–310
12. Vlachopoulos C, Aznaouridis K, Stefanadis C (2014) Aortic stiffness for cardiovascular risk prediction: just measure it, just do it! J Am Coll Cardiol 63:647–649
13. Vlachopoulos C, Aznaouridis K, Stefanadis C (2010) Prediction of cardiovascular events and all-cause mortality with arterial stiffness: a systematic review and meta-analysis. J Am Coll Cardiol 55:1318–1327
14. Kaiser DR, Billups K, Mason C et al (2004) Impaired brachial artery endothelium-dependent and -independent vasodilation in men with erectile dysfunction and no other clinical cardiovascular disease. J Am Coll Cardiol 43:179–184
15. Kakkavas A, Tsioufis C, Tsiachris D et al (2013) Erectile dysfunction and target organ damage in the early stages of hypertension. J Clin Hypertens (Greenwich) 15:644–649
16. Armstrong AC, Gidding S, Gjesdal O et al (2012) LV mass assessed by echocardiography and CMR, cardiovascular outcomes, and medical practice. JACC Cardiovasc Imaging 5:837–848
17. Uslu N, Eren M, Gorgulu S et al (2006) Left ventricular diastolic function and endothelial function in patients with erectile dysfunction. Am J Cardiol 97:1785–1788
18. Ankle Brachial Index Collaboration, Fowkes FG, Murray GD, Butcher I et al (2008) Ankle brachial index combined with Framingham risk score to predict cardiovascular events and mortality: a meta-analysis. JAMA 300:197–208
19. Polonsky TS, Taillon LA, Sheth H et al (2009) The association between erectile dysfunction and peripheral arterial disease as determined by screening ankle-brachial index testing. Atherosclerosis 207:440–444
20. Perkovic V, Verdon C, Ninomiya T et al (2008) The relationship between proteinuria and coronary risk: a systematic review and meta-analysis. PLoS Med 5:e207
21. Chuang YC, Chung MS, Wang PW et al (2012) Albuminuria is an independent risk factor of erectile dysfunction in men with type 2 diabetes. J Sex Med 9:1055–1064
22. Busari OA, Opadijo OG, Olarewaju TO et al (2013) Male erectile dysfunction and microalbuminuria in adult Nigerians with essential hypertension. N Am J Med Sci 5:32–36
23. Corona G, Monami M, Boddi V et al (2011) Pulse pressure independently predicts major cardiovascular events in younger but not in older subjects with erectile dysfunction. J Sex Med 8:247–254
24. Gazzaruso C, Solerte SB, Pujia A et al (2008) Erectile dysfunction as a predictor of cardiovascular events and death in diabetic patients with angiographically proven asymptomatic coronary artery disease: a potential protective role for statins and 5-phosphodiesterase inhibitors. J Am Coll Cardiol 51:2040–2044
25. Fagard RH, Celis H, Thijs L et al (2009) Regression of left ventricular mass by antihypertensive treatment: a meta-analysis of randomized comparative studies. Hypertension 54:1084–1091
26. Manolis A, Doumas M (2012) Antihypertensive treatment and sexual dysfunction. Curr Hypertens Rep 14:285–292
27. Doumas M, Douma S (2006) The effect of antihypertensive drugs on erectile function: a proposed management algorithm. J Clin Hypertens (Greenwich) 8:359–364
28. Nunes KP, Labazi H, Webb RC (2012) New insights into hypertension-associated erectile dysfunction. Curr Opin Nephrol Hypertens 21:163–170
29. Kendirci M, Trost L, Sikka SC et al (2007) The effect of vascular risk factors on penile vascular status in men with erectile dysfunction. J Urol 178:2516–2520
30. Viigimaa M, Doumas M, Vlachopoulos C et al (2011) European Society of Hypertension working group on sexual dysfunction. Hypertension and sexual dysfunction: time to act. J Hypertens 29:403–407

31. Fogari R, Zoppi A, Preti P et al (2002) Sexual activity and plasma testosterone levels in hypertensive males. Am J Hypertens 15:217–221
32. Vlachopoulos C, Ioakeimidis N, Miner M et al (2014) Testosterone deficiency: a determinant of aortic stiffness in men. Atherosclerosis 233:278–283
33. Muller M, van den Beld AW, Bots ML et al (2004) Endogenous sex hormones and progression of carotid atherosclerosis in elderly men. Circulation 109:2074–2079
34. Vlachopoulos C, Ioakeimidis N, Terentes-Printzios D et al (2013) Plasma total testosterone and incident cardiovascular events in hypertensive patients. Am J Hypertens 26:373–378
35. Cappelleri JC, Rosen RC (2005) The Sexual Health Inventory for Men (SHIM): a 5-year review of research and clinical experience. Int J Impot Res 17:307–319
36. Vlachopoulos C, Jackson G, Stefanadis C et al (2013) Erectile dysfunction in the cardiovascular patient. Eur Heart J34:2034–2046
37. Caretta N, Pallego P, Ferlin A et al (2006) Resumption of spontaneous erections in selected patients affected by erectile dysfunction and various degrees of carotid wall alteration: role of tadalafil. Eur Urol 48:326–331
38. Aversa A, Sarteschi LM (2007) The role of penile color-duplex ultrasound for the evaluation of erectile dysfunction. J Sex Med 4:1437–1447
39. Ioakeimidis N, Vlachopoulos C, Rokkas K et al (2011) Relationship of asymmetric dimethylarginine with penile Doppler ultrasound parameters in men with vasculogenic erectile dysfunction. Eur Urol 59:948–955
40. Corona G, Monami M, Boddi V et al (2010) Male sexuality and cardiovascular risk. A cohort study in patients with erectile dysfunction. J Sex Med 7:1918–1927
41. Nehra A, Jackson G, Miner M et al (2012) The Princeton III consensus recommendations for the management of erectile dysfunction and cardiovascular disease. Mayo Clin Proc 87:766–778
42. Miner M, Seftel AD, Nehra A et al (2012) Prognostic utility of erectile dysfunction for cardiovascular disease in younger men and those with diabetes. Am Heart J 164:21–28

Erectile Dysfunction in Coronary Artery Disease and Heart Failure

Giorgio Gandaglia, Alberto Briganti, Piero Montorsi, Francesco Montorsi, and Charalambos Vlachopoulos

7.1 Introduction

Erectile dysfunction (ED), coronary artery disease (CAD), and heart failure (HF) represent highly prevalent conditions, especially in the aging population. These complex conditions share many common risk factors and pathophysiological mechanisms. As a consequence, several authors proposed that they might be considered as different manifestations of the same systemic disorder; in this context, ED would precede cardiovascular events in the majority of cases. Additionally, ED could also become clinically evident in patients with HF as a consequence of a global cardiovascular impairment that involves both the heart and the arteries. In this chapter, we analyze the complex relationship between ED, CAD, and HF. Particularly, we focus on the clinical implications for the cardiologist and urologist.

G. Gandaglia (✉)
Department of Oncology, Unit of Urology, IRCCS San Raffaele Hospital,
Via Olgettina 58, Milan 20132, Italy

Division of Oncology/Unit of Urology; URI, IRCCS Ospedale San Raffaele, Milan, Italy
e-mail: gandaglia.giorgio@hsr.it

A. Briganti • F. Montorsi
Division of Oncology/Unit of Urology; URI,
IRCCS Ospedale San Raffaele, Milan, Italy
e-mail: briganti.alberto@hsr.it; Montorsi.francesco@hsr.it

P. Montorsi
Centro Cardiologico Monzino, Institute of Cardiology,
University of Milan, Milan 20132, Italy
e-mail: piero.montorsi@unimi.it

C. Vlachopoulos
1st Department of Cardiology, Athens Medical School,
Profiti Elia 24, Athens 14575, Greece
e-mail: cvlachop@otenet.gr

7.2 Erectile Dysfunction and Coronary Artery Disease

7.2.1 Common Risk Factors Between Erectile Dysfunction and Coronary Artery Disease

Erectile dysfunction is considered a primarily vascular disease in the majority of the cases. Numerous risk factors that contribute to the development and onset of ED are principal for the development of CAD [1–3]. These risk factors may be classified as modifiable and non-modifiable. While the former principally include aging and genetic susceptibility [4], the latter are mainly related to lifestyle habits [3]. Hypertension, smoking, diabetes, dyslipidemia, hypertriglyceridemia, obesity, and metabolic syndrome are well-known modifiable risk factors for both ED and cardiac diseases [2]. In this context, a prospective study comprehensively demonstrated that age, increased BMI, cholesterol and triglycerides, as well as cigarette smoking were significantly associated with an increased risk of ED at a 25-year follow-up [2, 5]. Therefore, it should be emphasized that improving cardiac risk factor profile would result not only in reduced risk of cardiac events over time, but it would also help patients to maintain adequate sexual activity [2, 5–7].

Although endothelial dysfunction and penile atherosclerosis have been proposed as the common denominators between ED and cardiac conditions, the relationship between these disorders is complex and might involve other pathophysiological mechanisms [8, 9].

7.2.2 Pathophysiological Mechanisms Explaining the Association Between Erectile Dysfunction and Coronary Artery Disease

The Artery-Size Hypothesis
The empirical knowledge derived by the effectiveness of the administration of phosphodiesterase type-5 inhibitors in patients with ED was comprehensively founded by Ganz et al. in 2005 who described that NO activation pathway leads to the vasodilatation necessary for achievement of erections [10]. Accordingly, although normal erectile function is a neurovascular event modulated also by hormonal and psychological factors, endothelial integrity plays a major role in the physiology of erections [6, 7, 11–13].

The initial impairment in endothelial-dependent vasodilatation might lead to a number of structural vascular abnormalities, resulting in penile artery atherosclerosis and flow-limiting stenosis [14–16]. The observation that ED usually precedes CAD raised the hypothesis that ED and CAD might be two different manifestations of the same systemic disorder and that their onset might be related to the size of the arteries supplying the different districts [6, 7, 17, 18]. Under this perspective, the pioneering study by Montorsi et al. [17] proposed the so-called artery-size hypothesis. According to this concept, all vascular beds would be affected to the same extent by endothelial dysfunction and atherosclerosis, given their systemic nature

[15, 18, 19]. However, the reason why ED and CAD do not become clinically manifest simultaneously can be explained according to differences in the artery size of the penile and cardiac territories. Indeed, larger vessels better tolerate the same amount of endothelial dysfunction and atherosclerosis compared to the smaller ones. Since the size of penile arteries is smaller (1–2 mm) compared to that of coronary arteries (3–4 mm), the same level of endothelial dysfunction and atherosclerosis may lead to a more significant reduction of blood flow in erectile tissues compared to that in coronary arteries [15]. This, in turn, would result into an earlier onset of ED compared to CAD.

Although this concept is, at least, intriguing, studies reported contrasting results according to which not all patients affected by CAD have hemodynamically relevant penile artery lesions [18, 20–22]. Consequently, it was hypothesized that other pathophysiological mechanisms might be involved in the complex relationship between ED and CAD.

Hormonal Alterations

The detection of low androgen levels has been proposed as a common denominator in the pathogenesis of ED, diabetes, and CAD [23–26]. Besides the well-known association between testosterone and erectile function (and dysfunction), androgen levels have been shown to be associated with the risk of cardiac events. Particularly, patients with low testosterone are considered at higher risk of CAD and cardiac mortality compared to their counterparts with normal androgen levels [24, 26, 27]. Of note, androgens act on arterial tissues and vascular remodeling both directly, allowing the preservation of smooth muscle homeostasis, and indirectly. For example, low androgen levels might have proinflammatory and proapoptotic effects on endothelial cells [23, 28]. Thus, testosterone plays a crucial role in the homeostasis of vascular tissues and the presence of low androgens might in part explain the association between ED and CAD.

Chronic Inflammation

The development of ED has been shown to be associated with an increased expression of markers of inflammation and endothelial dysfunction, as well as prothrombotic factors [28–31]. Similarly, increased expression of proinflammatory factors has been found in patients with metabolic syndrome and diabetes [7, 30, 32]. Previous studies investigating the role of chronic inflammation in patients with ED and CAD showed that patients with ED alone have similar expression of proinflammatory markers as compared to their counterparts with CAD alone [28]. Thus, these two pathological conditions are characterized by a similar proinflammatory and prothrombotic environment. This might predispose to the rupture of unstable coronary plaques, thus increasing the risk of CAD in patients with ED. On the other hand, this might also favor endothelial dysfunction at the penile circulation level in patients with CAD, predisposing to the development of ED.

Taken together, these three pathological mechanisms (i.e., "the artery-size hypothesis," low androgen levels, and chronic inflammation) might be responsible for the complex relationship between ED and CAD.

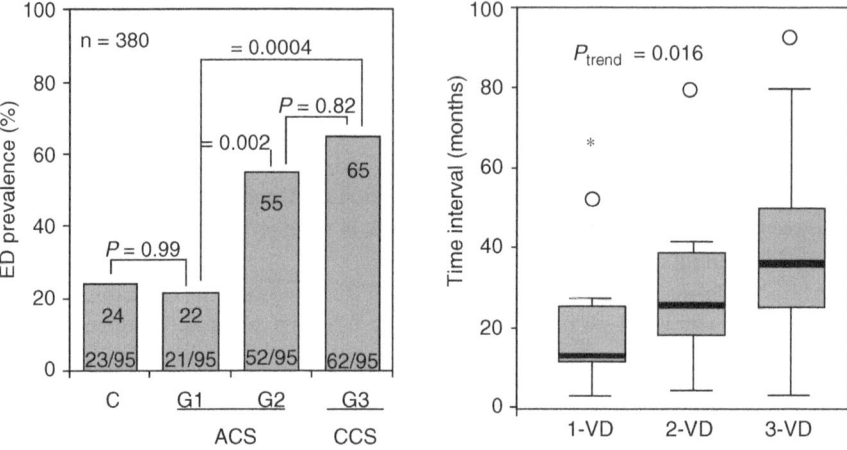

Fig. 7.1 Relation between erectile dysfunction prevalence and type of coronary syndrome (**a**). Time interval (months) between erectile dysfunction and coronary artery disease symptom onset in chronic coronary syndrome according to the number of vessels involved (**b**). *ACS* acute coronary syndrome, *CCS* chronic coronary syndrome, *G1* ACS and 1-VD, *G2* ACS and 2-,3-VD, *G3* CCS, *VD* vessel disease, *C* the control group with normal coronary angiography (With permission from Montorsi et al. The COBRA trial [20])

7.2.3 Clinical Evidence for the Association Between ED and CAD

The first evidence of an association between ED and CAD comes from the study by Montorsi et al. [18] in 2003. By evaluating 300 consecutive patients with acute chest pain and angiographically documented CAD, the authors showed that 49 % of them had a history of ED. Of note, ED symptoms became clinically evident before cardiac disorders in 70 % of the patients, and the mean time interval between ED onset and CAD was approximately 3 years. Similarly, the COBRA trial showed that ED prevalence differs across subsets of patients with CAD (i.e., patients with acute coronary syndrome vs. those with chronic coronary syndrome) and might be related to coronary clinical presentation and extent of CAD (Fig. 7.1). Indeed, in patients with chronic coronary syndrome, ED became clinically manifest before CAD in the vast majority of cases by an average of 2 up to 3 years [20]. Based on these results, the authors concluded that ED might be considered as a predictor of CAD [18, 20]. Other retrospective studies confirmed successively these findings [33–35].

It is also important to stress that ED severity might impact on the risk of CAD events and extent of CAD [20, 36–40]. In this context, the erectile function domain of the International Index of Erectile Function (IIEF), a validated 15-item self-administered questionnaire used to assess the degree of erectile dysfunction, has been shown to be correlated to the plaque burden calculated according to the Gensini's score [20, 37, 39].

These mounting pieces of evidence coming from retrospective studies led to an increased attention to the relationship between ED and CAD. This ultimately resulted in the planning and execution of prospective studies that tried to better characterize the role of ED in patients with CVD. Large investigations that included elderly patients as well found a strong association between sexual dysfunction and the subsequent risk of cardiovascular events: individuals complaining of ED had roughly 1.5–2-fold higher risk of experiencing CAD during follow-up compared to their counterparts with satisfactory erectile function [38, 41]. Of note, this held true even when considering patients at increased risk of CAD, such as diabetic individuals [42–45]. On the other hand, conflicting results have been reported by other smaller prospective studies [46, 47]. However, the validity of these observations is undermined by the inclusion of relatively young patients at lower risk of CAD with an inadequate follow-up period.

Recently, two meta-analyses provided additional evidence in favor to the association between ED and the risk of CAD [48, 49]. The most recent one included more than 90,000 patients from 14 studies and showed that, after a mean follow-up of 6.1 years, patients with ED had a risk of cardiovascular events, myocardial infarction, and overall mortality by 44, 62, and 25 %, respectively [48].

7.3 Erectile Dysfunction and Heart Failure

Erectile dysfunction is a highly prevalent condition among patients with HF, where up to 90 % of these individuals complain of decrease in sexual interest or varying degrees of cessation of sexual activity altogether [3, 50, 51]. Although ED and HF might share many risk factors and pathophysiological conditions, this relationship might be more complex than what observed in patients with CAD. Indeed, HF itself might profoundly affect patients' sexual activity, eventually causing ED [3, 50, 51].

7.3.1 Association Between Erectile Dysfunction and Heart Failure

Endothelial Dysfunction
As previously discussed, endothelial dysfunction is a key factor in the pathogenesis and development of ED [6, 7]. Similarly, it plays a major role in HF progression and impairment of the patient's general health status. Indeed, HF is a complex syndrome associated with several metabolic alterations, which include impairment of nitric oxide synthase activity and vascular relaxation [3]. This, in turn, leads to the production of free oxygen radical products and ultimately to a decrease in peripheral oxygen supply [52–54].

Cardiac Drugs in HF Patients and ED
The administration of many drugs used in patients with HF is known to be associated with an increased risk of ED. This is mainly related to their multiple metabolic, vascular, and neural activities.

Diuretics are one of the most commonly implicated drugs in the pathogenesis of ED in HF patients. Sexual dysfunction is a well-known side effect in patients treated with thiazide diuretics, such as hydrochlorothiazide, chlorthalidone, and bendroflumethiazide [55]. Despite their beneficial effect in treating hypertension, these agents have been shown to cause endothelial dysfunction, increased oxidative stress, stimulation of the sympathetic nervous system, hyperlipidemia, and insulin resistance [3, 56–58]. As a consequence, ED may ensue in the long term [56]. Similarly, spironolactone, an effective anti-aldosterone agent, has been associated with breast tenderness, gynecomastia, and ED [59].

The administration of beta-blockers is also associated with an impairment of sexual function in patients with HF. First- and second-generation beta-blockers might act both on the central nervous system and peripherally, finally resulting in an increased risk of ED [55, 60]. Particularly, these drugs might induce sexual dysfunction through the inhibition of the sympathetic nervous system, which is involved in the control of erection and ejaculation [55, 61]. On the other hand, it should be emphasized that nebivolol, a novel third-generation beta-1 blocker, appears to be associated with neutral or beneficial effects in hypertensive patients [55, 61, 62].

When considering lipid-lowering medications, results are conflicting regarding the role of these drugs on sexual function [3, 55]. While some authors proposed a protective effect of statins on erectile function [63–65], other studies demonstrated an increased risk of ED in patients using statins and fibrates [3, 55]. Finally, digoxin use has been shown to be associated with an increased risk of experiencing ED [66]. However, the underlying mechanism has not been completely understood yet.

Despite the fact that the abovementioned medications might be associated with an increased risk of ED, other classes of drugs, such as ACE inhibitors, angiotensin II receptor antagonists, and calcium channel antagonists, have been shown to be safe in terms of sexual side effects [55]. Additionally, recent studies suggest that these agents might include improved erectile function in their array of actions [55, 67, 68].

Psychological Factors

The impact of psychological factors on the subsequent risk of sexual dysfunctions in patients with HF should not be underestimated. Indeed, HF patients often suffer from depression, which might result in decreased libido and impaired erectile function [3, 69]. Additionally, these individuals might be afraid of triggering new cardiovascular events during sexual activity [3]. On the other hand, moderate physical exercise is not contraindicated in patients with stable HF, but it is beneficial for their general health status. In this context, accurate individual risk assessment and detailed counseling is mandatory in HF patients interested in sexual activity [70].

7.3.2 Sexual Activity in Patients with ED and HF

Sexual intercourse requires a modest exertion. It is equivalent to walking 1 mile on the flat in 20 min or briskly climbing two flights of stairs in 10 s. Sexual intercourse averages 2–3 metabolic equivalents (METs) in the pre-orgasm phase and 3–4 METs in the orgasm phase [3]. Consequently, sexual activity leads to a modest increase in myocardial oxygen demand with a peak lasting only for a short time period.

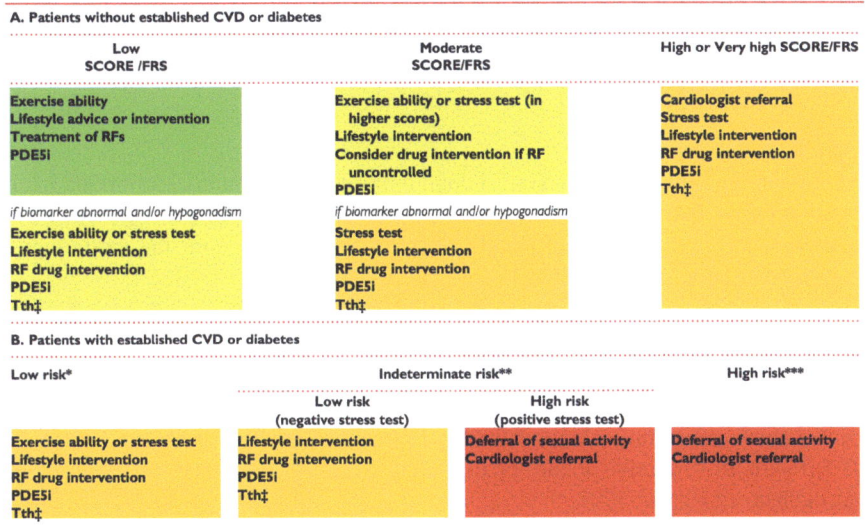

Fig. 7.2 Management of a patient with CVD (**a**) or without known CVD (**b**) (With permission from Vlachopoulos et al. [51]). *Low-risk patients include those with complete revascularization (e.g., via coronary artery bypass grafting, stenting, or angioplasty), patients with asymptomatic controlled hypertension, those with mild valvular disease, and patients with left ventricular dysfunction/heart failure (NYHA classes I and II) who achieved five metabolic equivalents of the task (*METS*) without ischemia on recent exercise testing. **Indeterminate risk patients include diabetics, those with mild or moderate stable angina pectoris, past myocardial infarction (2–8 weeks) without intervention awaiting exercise electrocardiography, congestive heart failure (NYHA class III), and noncardiac sequelae of atherosclerotic disease (e.g., peripheral artery disease and a history of stroke or transient ischemic attack); this patient with ED may require assessment for additional vascular disease using carotid intima-media thickness or ankle-brachial index and subsequent reclassification to low or high risk. ***High-risk patients include those with unstable or refractory angina pectoris, uncontrolled hypertension, congestive heart failure (NYHA class IV), recent myocardial infarction without intervention (2 weeks), high-risk arrhythmia (exercise-induced ventricular tachycardia, implanted internal cardioverter defibrillator with frequent shocks, and poorly controlled atrial fibrillation), obstructive hypertrophic cardiomyopathy with severe symptoms, and moderate to severe valve disease, particularly aortic stenosis. ‡Where appropriate *CVD* cardiovascular disease, *FRS* Framingham risk score, *PDE5i* phosphodiesterase type 5 inhibitors, *RF* risk factor, *Tth* testosterone therapy; *NYHA* New York Heart Association

In 2012, the Third Princeton Consensus Conference developed a novel algorithm for the management of patients with ED [70]. The objective of this tool was to estimate the risk associated with sexual activity in patients with ED and known CVD (Fig. 7.2). These recommendations are based on the most widely used clinical classification of HF, which is the New York Heart Association (NYHA) classification.

Low-Risk Patients

In patients included in the low-risk group (i.e., NYHA I and II or individuals who achieved 5 METs without ischemia on exercise testing should be included in this category), sexual activity does not represent a significant cardiac risk [70]. These patients can safely perform sexual activity without further testing or evaluation. Additionally, they might benefit from the administration of pharmacological treatments for ED, such as phosphodiesterase type-5 inhibitors [6].

High-Risk Patients
These individuals have CVD severe enough to pose a significant risk of events with sexual activity. Patients in the NYHA IV class are included in this group [70]. Patients in the high-risk group should defer sexual activity until the cardiologic condition has been stabilized [6].

Intermediate-Risk Patients
The intermediate-risk group includes patients with NYHA III. These men should receive exercise stress test in order to be reassigned to low- or high-risk groups [6, 70]. Of note, completing 4 min of the Bruce treadmill protocol (equivalent to 5–6 METs) without symptoms identifies the safety of sexual activity in patients in the intermediate-risk group [70].

7.3.3 Use of Phosphodiesterase Type-5 Inhibitors in Patients with HF

Phosphodiesterase type-5 inhibitors represent a safe treatment for ED in patients with CVD. Additionally, (PDE-5) the well-known pathophysiological association between ED and CVD led to the hypothesis that patients with CVD and HF might benefit from the administration of PDE-5 inhibitors not only in terms of improved erectile function but also to improve HF [52]. Studies have evaluated the effect of PDE-5 inhibitors on HF both at short- and long-term follow-up. For example, the acute administration of sildenafil decreased heart rate during exercise, leading to a reduction of oxygen demand and risk of ischemia [71]. This drug significantly decreases resting mean pulmonary artery pressure and pulmonary and systemic vascular resistance and increases cardiac index [72–75].

Regarding the chronic effects, PDE-5 inhibitors' administration in HF patients has shown that these drugs may lead to NO-mediated vasodilatation, improved exercise capacity, reduced pulmonary hypertension, and improved ventilatory performance [76–79]. The beneficial effects of PDE-5 inhibitors might be attributed to increased production of cAMP which, in turn, activates protein kinase A, leading ultimately to an increase in intracellular calcium concentration and improvement of myocardial contractility [80]. Moreover, other mechanisms that decrease fibrosis, apoptosis, and hypertrophy, and prevent cardiovascular remodeling may also be responsible [78, 79].

In patients with preserved ejection fraction, results are neutral. Administration of sildenafil for 24 weeks, compared with placebo, did not result in significant improvement in exercise capacity or clinical status [81].

Importantly, when considering the use of PDE-5 inhibitors in HF patients, some clinically relevant issues warrant discussion. Indeed, the concomitant use of nitrates represents one of the main contraindications for the administration of these agents. A time interval of at least 24 h is recommended between the administration of nitrates and PDE-5 inhibitors (24 for sildenafil and vardenafil and 36 for tadalafil) [82].

Finally, it should be noted that other substances, such as L-arginine or capsaicin, might be beneficial in terms of improved erectile and cardiac function in HF patients since they act through an improvement of endothelial function [83–85]. However, clinical evidence regarding the efficacy of these agents is still poor and further well-designed prospective studies are needed.

References

1. Feldman HA, Johannes CB, Derby CA et al (2000) Erectile dysfunction and coronary risk factors: prospective results from the Massachusetts male aging study. Prev Med 30(4): 328–338
2. Fung MM, Bettencourt R, Barrett-Connor E (2004) Heart disease risk factors predict erectile dysfunction 25 years later: the Rancho Bernardo study. J Am Coll Cardiol 43(8):1405–1411
3. Alberti L, Torlasco C, Lauretta L et al (2013) Erectile dysfunction in heart failure patients: a critical reappraisal. Andrology 1(2):177–191
4. Ianni M, Callegari S, Rizzo A et al (2012) Pro-inflammatory genetic profile and familiarity of acute myocardial infarction. Immun Ageing Immun Ageing 9(1):14
5. Wu C, Zhang H, Gao Y et al (2012) The association of smoking and erectile dysfunction: results from the Fangchenggang Area Male Health and Examination Survey (FAMHES). J Androl 33(1):59–65
6. Gandaglia G, Briganti A, Jackson G et al (2014) A systematic review of the association between erectile dysfunction and cardiovascular disease. Eur Urol 65(5):968–978
7. Gandaglia G, Salonia A, Passoni N, Montorsi P, Briganti A, Montorsi F (2013) Erectile dysfunction as a cardiovascular risk factor in patients with diabetes. Endocrine 43(2):285–292
8. Shamloul R, Ghanem H (2013) Erectile dysfunction. Lancet 381(9861):153–165
9. Ryan JG, Gajraj J (2012) Erectile dysfunction and its association with metabolic syndrome and endothelial function among patients with type 2 diabetes mellitus. J Diabetes Complications 26(2):141–147
10. Ganz P (2005) Erectile dysfunction: pathophysiologic mechanisms pointing to underlying cardiovascular disease. Am J Cardiol 96(12B):8M–12M
11. Gratzke C, Angulo J, Chitaley K et al (2010) Anatomy, physiology, and pathophysiology of erectile dysfunction. J Sex Med 7(1 Pt 2):445–475
12. Billups KL, Bank AJ, Padma-Nathan H, Katz SD, Williams RA (2008) Erectile dysfunction as a harbinger for increased cardiometabolic risk. Int J Impot Res 20(3):236–242
13. Jackson G, Montorsi P, Adams MA et al (2010) Cardiovascular aspects of sexual medicine. J Sex Med 7(4 Pt 2):1608–1626, Epub 2010/04/15
14. Solomon H, Man JW, Jackson G (2003) Erectile dysfunction and the cardiovascular patient: endothelial dysfunction is the common denominator. Heart 89(3):251–253, Epub 2003/02/20
15. Montorsi P, Ravagnani PM, Galli S et al (2006) Association between erectile dysfunction and coronary artery disease: matching the right target with the right test in the right patient. Eur Urol 50(4):721–731, Epub 2006/08/12
16. Montorsi P, Ravagnani PM, Galli S et al (2004) Common grounds for erectile dysfunction and coronary artery disease. Curr Opin Urol 14(6):361–365, Epub 2005/01/01
17. Montorsi P, Montorsi F, Schulman CC (2003) Is erectile dysfunction the "tip of the iceberg" of a systemic vascular disorder? Eur Urol 44(3):352–354

18. Montorsi F, Briganti A, Salonia A et al (2003) Erectile dysfunction prevalence, time of onset and association with risk factors in 300 consecutive patients with acute chest pain and angiographically documented coronary artery disease. Eur Urol 44(3):360–364; discussion 4–5; Epub 2003/08/23
19. Kirby M, Jackson G, Betteridge J, Friedli K (2001) Is erectile dysfunction a marker for cardiovascular disease? Int J Clin Pract 55(9):614–618
20. Montorsi P, Ravagnani PM, Galli S et al (2006) Association between erectile dysfunction and coronary artery disease. Role of coronary clinical presentation and extent of coronary vessels involvement: the COBRA trial. Eur Heart J 27(22):2632–2639, Epub 2006/07/21
21. Chang ST, Chu CM, Hsiao JF et al (2010) Coronary phenotypes in patients with erectile dysfunction and silent ischemic heart disease: a pilot study. J Sex Med 7(8):2798–2804, Epub 2010/06/22
22. Ponholzer A, Stopfer J, Bayer G et al (2012) Is penile atherosclerosis the link between erectile dysfunction and cardiovascular risk? An autopsy study. Int J Impot Res 24(4):137–140, Epub 2012/03/23
23. Mirone V, Imbimbo C, Fusco F, Verze P, Creta M, Tajana G (2009) Androgens and morphologic remodeling at penile and cardiovascular levels: a common piece in complicated puzzles? Eur Urol 56(2):309–316, Epub 2009/01/17
24. Khaw KT, Dowsett M, Folkerd E et al (2007) Endogenous testosterone and mortality due to all causes, cardiovascular disease, and cancer in men: European prospective investigation into cancer in Norfolk (EPIC-Norfolk) prospective population study. Circulation 116(23): 2694–2701, Epub 2007/11/28
25. Traish AM, Goldstein I, Kim NN (2007) Testosterone and erectile function: from basic research to a new clinical paradigm for managing men with androgen insufficiency and erectile dysfunction. Eur Urol 52(1):54–70, Epub 2007/03/03
26. Corona G, Rastrelli G, Monami M et al (2011) Hypogonadism as a risk factor for cardiovascular mortality in men: a meta-analytic study. Eur J Endocrinol 165(5):687–701, Epub 2011/08/20
27. Vlachopoulos C, Ioakeimidis N, Terentes-Printzios D et al (2013) Plasma total testosterone and incident cardiovascular events in hypertensive patients. Am J Hypertens 26(3):373–381
28. Vlachopoulos C, Aznaouridis K, Ioakeimidis N et al (2006) Unfavourable endothelial and inflammatory state in erectile dysfunction patients with or without coronary artery disease. Eur Heart J 27(22):2640–2648, Epub 2006/10/24
29. Chiurlia E, D'Amico R, Ratti C, Granata AR, Romagnoli R, Modena MG (2005) Subclinical coronary artery atherosclerosis in patients with erectile dysfunction. J Am Coll Cardiol 46(8): 1503–1506
30. Arana Rosainz Mde J, Ojeda MO, Acosta JR et al (2011) Imbalanced low-grade inflammation and endothelial activation in patients with type 2 diabetes mellitus and erectile dysfunction. J Sex Med 8(7):2017–2030
31. Bocchio M, Desideri G, Scarpelli P et al (2004) Endothelial cell activation in men with erectile dysfunction without cardiovascular risk factors and overt vascular damage. J Urol 171(4): 1601–1604
32. Vlachopoulos C, Rokkas K, Ioakeimidis N, Stefanadis C (2007) Inflammation, metabolic syndrome, erectile dysfunction, and coronary artery disease: common links. Eur Urol 52(6):1590–1600
33. Vlachopoulos C, Rokkas K, Ioakeimidis N et al (2005) Prevalence of asymptomatic coronary artery disease in men with vasculogenic erectile dysfunction: a prospective angiographic study. Eur Urol 48(6):996–1002
34. Ponholzer A, Temml C, Obermayr R, Wehrberger C, Madersbacher S (2005) Is erectile dysfunction an indicator for increased risk of coronary heart disease and stroke? Eur Urol 48(3):512–518
35. Ponholzer A, Temml C, Mock K, Marszalek M, Obermayr R, Madersbacher S (2005) Prevalence and risk factors for erectile dysfunction in 2869 men using a validated questionnaire. Eur Urol 47(1):80–85
36. Greenstein A, Chen J, Miller H, Matzkin H, Villa Y, Braf Z (1997) Does severity of ischemic coronary disease correlate with erectile function? Int J Impot Res 9(3):123–126

37. Solomon H, Man JW, Wierzbicki AS, Jackson G (2003) Relation of erectile dysfunction to angiographic coronary artery disease. Am J Cardiol 91(2):230–231
38. Banks E, Joshy G, Abhayaratna WP et al (2013) Erectile dysfunction severity as a risk marker for cardiovascular disease hospitalisation and all-cause mortality: a prospective cohort study. PLoS Med 10(1):e1001372
39. Yaman O, Gulpinar O, Hasan T, Ozdol C, Ertas FS, Ozgenci E (2008) Erectile dysfunction may predict coronary artery disease: relationship between coronary artery calcium scoring and erectile dysfunction severity. Int Urol Nephrol 40(1):117–123
40. Schouten BW, Bohnen AM, Bosch JL et al (2008) Erectile dysfunction prospectively associated with cardiovascular disease in the Dutch general population: results from the Krimpen study. Int J Impot Res 20(1):92–99
41. Thompson IM, Tangen CM, Goodman PJ, Probstfield JL, Moinpour CM, Coltman CA (2005) Erectile dysfunction and subsequent cardiovascular disease. JAMA 294(23): 2996–3002
42. Bohm M, Baumhakel M, Teo K et al (2010) Erectile dysfunction predicts cardiovascular events in high-risk patients receiving telmisartan, ramipril, or both: the ONgoing Telmisartan Alone and in combination with Ramipril Global Endpoint Trial/Telmisartan Randomized AssessmeNt Study in ACE iNtolerant subjects with cardiovascular Disease (ONTARGET/TRANSCEND) trials. Circulation 121(12):1439–1446
43. Batty GD, Li Q, Czernichow S et al (2010) Erectile dysfunction and later cardiovascular disease in men with type 2 diabetes: prospective cohort study based on the ADVANCE (Action in Diabetes and Vascular Disease: Preterax and Diamicron Modified-Release Controlled Evaluation) trial. J Am Coll Cardiol 56(23):1908–1913
44. Gazzaruso C, Solerte SB, Pujia A et al (2008) Erectile dysfunction as a predictor of cardiovascular events and death in diabetic patients with angiographically proven asymptomatic coronary artery disease: a potential protective role for statins and 5-phosphodiesterase inhibitors. J Am Coll Cardiol 51(21):2040–2044
45. Ma RC, So WY, Yang X et al (2008) Erectile dysfunction predicts coronary heart disease in type 2 diabetes. J Am Coll Cardiol 51(21):2045–2050
46. Ponholzer A, Gutjahr G, Temml C, Madersbacher S (2010) Is erectile dysfunction a predictor of cardiovascular events or stroke? A prospective study using a validated questionnaire. Int J Impot Res 22(1):25–29
47. Hotaling JM, Walsh TJ, Macleod LC et al (2012) Erectile dysfunction is not independently associated with cardiovascular death: data from the vitamins and lifestyle (VITAL) study. J Sex Med 9(8):2104–2110
48. Vlachopoulos CV, Terentes-Printzios DG, Ioakeimidis NK, Aznaouridis KA, Stefanadis CI (2013) Prediction of cardiovascular events and all-cause mortality with erectile dysfunction: a systematic review and meta-analysis of cohort studies. Circ Cardiovasc Qual Outcomes 6(1):99–109
49. Dong JY, Zhang YH, Qin LQ (2011) Erectile dysfunction and risk of cardiovascular disease: meta-analysis of prospective cohort studies. J Am Coll Cardiol 58(13):1378–1385
50. Apostolo A, Vignati C, Brusoni D et al (2009) Erectile dysfunction in heart failure: correlation with severity, exercise performance, comorbidities, and heart failure treatment. J Sex Med 6(10):2795–2805
51. Vlachopoulos C, Jackson G, Stefanadis C, Montorsi P (2013) Erectile dysfunction in the cardiovascular patient. Eur Heart J 34(27):2034–2046
52. Al-Ameri H, Kloner RA (2009) Erectile dysfunction and heart failure: the role of phosphodiesterase type 5 inhibitors. Int J Impot Res 21(3):149–157
53. Torre-Amione G, Kapadia S, Lee J et al (1996) Tumor necrosis factor-alpha and tumor necrosis factor receptors in the failing human heart. Circulation 93(4):704–711
54. Tostes RC, Carneiro FS, Lee AJ et al (2008) Cigarette smoking and erectile dysfunction: focus on NO bioavailability and ROS generation. J Sex Med 5(6):1284–1295
55. Nicolai MP, Liem SS, Both S et al (2014) A review of the positive and negative effects of cardiovascular drugs on sexual function: a proposed table for use in clinical practice. Neth Heart J Mon J Neth Soc Cardiol Neth Heart Found 22(1):11–19

56. Zhou MS, Schulman IH, Jaimes EA, Raij L (2008) Thiazide diuretics, endothelial function, and vascular oxidative stress. J Hypertens 26(3):494–500
57. Grassi G, Seravalle G, Dell'Oro R et al (2003) Comparative effects of candesartan and hydrochlorothiazide on blood pressure, insulin sensitivity, and sympathetic drive in obese hypertensive individuals: results of the CROSS study. J Hypertens 21(9):1761–1769
58. Eriksson JW, Jansson PA, Carlberg B et al (2008) Hydrochlorothiazide, but not Candesartan, aggravates insulin resistance and causes visceral and hepatic fat accumulation: the mechanisms for the diabetes preventing effect of Candesartan (MEDICA) study. Hypertension 52(6):1030–1037
59. Epstein M, Calhoun DA (2011) Aldosterone blockers (mineralocorticoid receptor antagonism) and potassium-sparing diuretics. J Clin Hypertens 13(9):644–648
60. Ko DT, Hebert PR, Coffey CS, Sedrakyan A, Curtis JP, Krumholz HM (2002) Beta-blocker therapy and symptoms of depression, fatigue, and sexual dysfunction. JAMA 288(3): 351–357
61. Barksdale JD, Gardner SF (1999) The impact of first-line antihypertensive drugs on erectile dysfunction. Pharmacotherapy 19(5):573–581
62. Brixius K, Middeke M, Lichtenthal A, Jahn E, Schwinger RH (2007) Nitric oxide, erectile dysfunction and beta-blocker treatment (MR NOED study): benefit of nebivolol versus metoprolol in hypertensive men. Clin Exp Pharmacol Physiol 34(4):327–331
63. Saltzman EA, Guay AT, Jacobson J (2004) Improvement in erectile function in men with organic erectile dysfunction by correction of elevated cholesterol levels: a clinical observation. J Urol 172(1):255–258
64. Dogru MT, Basar MM, Simsek A et al (2008) Effects of statin treatment on serum sex steroids levels and autonomic and erectile function. Urology 71(4):703–707
65. Trivedi D, Kirby M, Wellsted DM et al (2013) Can simvastatin improve erectile function and health-related quality of life in men aged >/=40 years with erectile dysfunction? Results of the erectile dysfunction and statins trial [ISRCTN66772971]. BJU Int 111(2):324–333
66. Gupta S, Salimpour P, Saenz de Tejada I et al (1998) A possible mechanism for alteration of human erectile function by digoxin: inhibition of corpus cavernosum sodium/potassium adenosine triphosphatase activity. J Urol 159(5):1529–1536
67. Baumhakel M, Schlimmer N, Bohm M, Investigators D-I (2008) Effect of irbesartan on erectile function in patients with hypertension and metabolic syndrome. Int J Impot Res 20(5):493–500
68. Rastogi S, Rodriguez JJ, Kapur V, Schwarz ER (2005) Why do patients with heart failure suffer from erectile dysfunction? A critical review and suggestions on how to approach this problem. Int J Impot Res 17(Suppl 1):S25–S36
69. Huang SS, Lin CH, Chan CH, el Loh W, Lan TH (2013) Newly diagnosed major depressive disorder and the risk of erectile dysfunction: a population-based cohort study in Taiwan. Psychiatry Res 210(2):601–606
70. Nehra A, Jackson G, Miner M et al (2012) The Princeton III Consensus recommendations for the management of erectile dysfunction and cardiovascular disease. Mayo Clin Proc 87(8):766–778
71. Bocchi EA, Guimaraes G, Mocelin A, Bacal F, Bellotti G, Ramires JF (2002) Sildenafil effects on exercise, neurohormonal activation, and erectile dysfunction in congestive heart failure: a double-blind, placebo-controlled, randomized study followed by a prospective treatment for erectile dysfunction. Circulation 106(9):1097–1103
72. Lewis GD, Lachmann J, Camuso J et al (2007) Sildenafil improves exercise hemodynamics and oxygen uptake in patients with systolic heart failure. Circulation 115(1):59–66
73. Katz SD, Balidemaj K, Homma S, Wu H, Wang J, Maybaum S (2000) Acute type 5 phosphodiesterase inhibition with sildenafil enhances flow-mediated vasodilation in patients with chronic heart failure. J Am Coll Cardiol 36(3):845–851
74. Hirata K, Adji A, Vlachopoulos C, O'Rourke MF (2005) Effect of sildenafil on cardiac performance in patients with heart failure. Am J Cardiol 96(10):1436–1440

75. Al-Hesayen A, Floras JS, Parker JD (2006) The effects of intravenous sildenafil on hemodynamics and cardiac sympathetic activity in chronic human heart failure. Eur J Heart Fail 8(8):864–868
76. Chau VQ, Salloum FN, Hoke NN, Abbate A, Kukreja RC (2011) Mitigation of the progression of heart failure with sildenafil involves inhibition of RhoA/Rho-kinase pathway. Am J Physiol Heart Circ Physiol 300(6):H2272–H2279
77. Cvelich RG, Roberts SC, Brown JN (2011) Phosphodiesterase type 5 inhibitors as adjunctive therapy in the management of systolic heart failure. Ann Pharmacother 45(12):1551–1558
78. Chrysant SG (2013) Effectiveness and safety of phosphodiesterase 5 inhibitors in patients with cardiovascular disease and hypertension. Curr Hypertens Rep 15(5):475–483
79. Ioakeimidis N, Kostis JB (2014) Pharmacologic therapy for erectile dysfunction and its interaction with the cardiovascular system. J Cardiovasc Pharmacol Ther 19(1):53–64
80. Westermann D, Becher PM, Lindner D et al (2012) Selective PDE5A inhibition with sildenafil rescues left ventricular dysfunction, inflammatory immune response and cardiac remodeling in angiotensin II-induced heart failure in vivo. Basic Res Cardiol 107(6):308
81. Redfield MM, Chen HH, Borlaug BA et al (2013) Effect of phosphodiesterase-5 inhibition on exercise capacity and clinical status in heart failure with preserved ejection fraction: a randomized clinical trial. JAMA 309(12):1268–1277
82. Cheitlin MD, Hutter AM Jr, Brindis RG et al (1999) ACC/AHA expert consensus document. Use of sildenafil (Viagra) in patients with cardiovascular disease. American College of Cardiology/American Heart Association. J Am Coll Cardiol 33(1):273–282
83. Hambrecht R, Hilbrich L, Erbs S et al (2000) Correction of endothelial dysfunction in chronic heart failure: additional effects of exercise training and oral L-arginine supplementation. J Am Coll Cardiol 35(3):706–713
84. Gentile V, Antonini G, Antonella Bertozzi M et al (2009) Effect of propionyl-L-carnitine, L-arginine and nicotinic acid on the efficacy of vardenafil in the treatment of erectile dysfunction in diabetes. Curr Med Res Opin 25(9):2223–2228
85. Fragasso G, Palloshi A, Piatti PM et al (2004) Nitric-oxide mediated effects of transdermal capsaicin patches on the ischemic threshold in patients with stable coronary disease. J Cardiovasc Pharmacol 44(3):340–347

Erectile Dysfunction as an 'Early Diagnostic Window' for Asymptomatic Coronary Artery Disease

Graham Jackson

8.1 Introduction

Erectile dysfunction (ED) is common and increases with increasing age [1]. As we are an ageing population, management will become an increasing challenge. In the 1990s, ED and cardiovascular disease (CVD) were first recognised to frequently coexist [2]. However, it was 2001 before angiographic evidence demonstrated ED occurring before coronary artery disease (CAD) was symptomatic [3]. Since then there has been an overwhelming body of evidence linking ED with CAD in particular, in that ED often precedes a cardiovascular event and ED is common in patients with CVD. Unfortunately, ED is not discussed proactively by many cardiologists or general physicians. So the first premise in the management of ED is talking about sex, because giving sexual advice to cardiac patients is an important aspect of their overall management, no matter the cardiovascular disease condition [4]. The 2nd Princeton Guidelines stated that ED and CVD shared the same common denominator, namely, endothelial dysfunction, with the result that the principal problem of ED was vascular. Their conclusion was 'the recognition of ED as a warning sign of silent vascular disease has led to the concept that a man with ED and no cardiac symptoms is a cardiac (or vascular) patient until proven otherwise' [5].

G. Jackson
Department of Cardiac, Guy's and St Thomas' Hospitals NHS Trust, London, UK

Department of Cardiac, London Bridge Hospital, Suite 301 Emblem House,
27 Tooley Street, London SE1 2PR, UK
e-mail: gjcardiol@talk21.com

Table 8.1 Artery size and atherothrombosis. A significant restriction to flow in the penile arteries may be subclinical in larger vessels

Artery	Diameter (mm)	Clinical event
Penile	1–2	ED
Coronary	3–4	Ischaemic heart disease
Carotid	5–7	TIA/stroke
Femoral	6–8	Claudication

TIA transient ischaemic attack

8.2 ED and CVD: Examining the Link

The endothelium is the same throughout arterial tree; it follows that if there is a problem at one part of the circulation (ED), there could be a problem elsewhere which need not be symptomatic (e.g. 'silent' CAD or carotid disease). The artery size hypothesis seeks to explain the differing presentations of the same pathology and why ED could be a marker for silent disease elsewhere [6].

Artery size varies according to location within the vascular system (Table 8.1). For example, the lumen of the penile arteries is considerably smaller (1–2 mm) compared with that of the coronary (3–4 mm), carotid (5–6 mm) and femoral (6–8 mm) arteries. Because of their smaller size and greater surface area, the same level of plaque burden and/or endothelial dysfunction has a greater effect on blood flow through the penile arteries than through the coronary, carotid and femoral arteries. Therefore, the clinical manifestations of penile endothelial dysfunction may become evident before the consequences of coronary or peripheral vascular disease. By the time the lumen of the larger arteries become significantly obstructed (>50 %), the penile blood flow may have already decreased considerably, which explains why so many men with CAD have ED.

Thus, on the basis of the artery size hypothesis, a malfunction in the penile arteries causing ED may be a predictor of silent subclinical CVD. In addition, because an acute coronary syndrome often arises as a result of the rupture of a subclinical plaque, the presence of ED may also be an early warning sign of an acute coronary event including mortality [7].

In support of this concept, a series of 300 patients with acute chest pain and angiographically proven CAD were evaluated with a semi-structured interview to assess their medical and sexual histories prior to presentation [8]. The prevalence of ED among these patients was 49 % ($n=147$). In these 147 men with both ED and CAD, ED was experienced before CAD symptoms in 99 patients (67 %). The mean time interval between the occurrence of ED and the occurrence of CAD was 38.8 months (range 1–168 months). Interestingly, all men with ED and type I diabetes developed sexual dysfunction before the onset of CAD symptoms.

ED is more frequent in diabetic patients with silent CAD than in those without. In a study of men with type II diabetes ($n=260$), the incidence of ED (IIEF questionnaire) was significantly higher in the population with asymptomatic CAD than in the population without CAD (33.8 % vs 4.7 %; $p<0001$) [9]. ED not only predicted CAD independently of other risk factors but also was the strongest predictor of silent CAD in this study.

The large Prostate Cancer Prevention Trial provided the first evidence of a strong association between ED and the subsequent development of clinical cardiovascular events [10]. ED at entry or that developed during follow-up was found to predict significantly any cardiac event with a hazard ratio of 1.45 ($p<0.001$; 95 % confidence interval (CI): 1.25–1.69). The data also showed that the cardiovascular risk associated with incident ED (i.e., developed during follow-up) was at least as great as the risk associated with a family history of myocardial infarction, current smoking or hypercholesterolaemia.

8.3 Case History

A 49-year-old gentleman who was a company director attended my outpatient clinic with his wife. He was a type II diabetic with treated hypertension and a non-smoker. He was treated for hyperlipidaemia with atorvastatin 40 mg daily.

He had suffered from ED for 1 year. I began to advise the patient about the treatment of ED when his wife interrupted the conversation and said she did not want her husband to be treated for ED, she just wanted his heart checked up. She had read in a newspaper that ED may be a marker of silent CAD. She was quite adamant that was the priority, and that was the reason for the consultation with a cardiologist.

Further evaluation followed direct questioning to make sure he was asymptomatic, which he was, and the lack of symptoms had also been documented by the family doctor who referred him.

A 12 lead ECG was normal and an echocardiogram showed good left ventricular function but did demonstrate left ventricular hypertrophy and some impaired left ventricular relaxation. There was no evidence of valvar heart disease.

Because of the risk factor of ED which we knew added to conventional risk factors, he underwent CT angiography. He had a calcium score of 1,598 (normal score 0, >1,000 extensive plaque) and evidence of widespread and significant CAD, and invasive angiography was recommended.

Invasive angiogram (Fig. 8.1) showed that the left anterior descending coronary artery was totally occluded but filled retrogradely from the right system. There was atheromatous disease to about 90 % in the circumflex coronary artery and a 90 % lesion in the right coronary artery which was particularly important as the right coronary artery was filling the left anterior descending retrogradely.

He had severe three-vessel coronary artery disease therefore, and was at risk because he was type II diabetic. The evidence base would support coronary artery bypass grafting rather than attempted angioplasty. Quadruple coronary bypass grafting was therefore performed with three arterial grafts and one vein graft: the left internal mammary was grafted to an occluded heavily diseased left anterior descending and after a long arteriotomy a radial sequential graft was applied to obtuse marginal 1 and 2; a vein graft was applied to the right coronary artery.

The post operative course was uneventful and he was discharged home on the seventh post operative day fully well. He has been seen in the outpatient clinic, and on the statin therapy his cholesterol is 3.6 mmol/L with LDL 1.5. He has been advised about treatment for his ED.

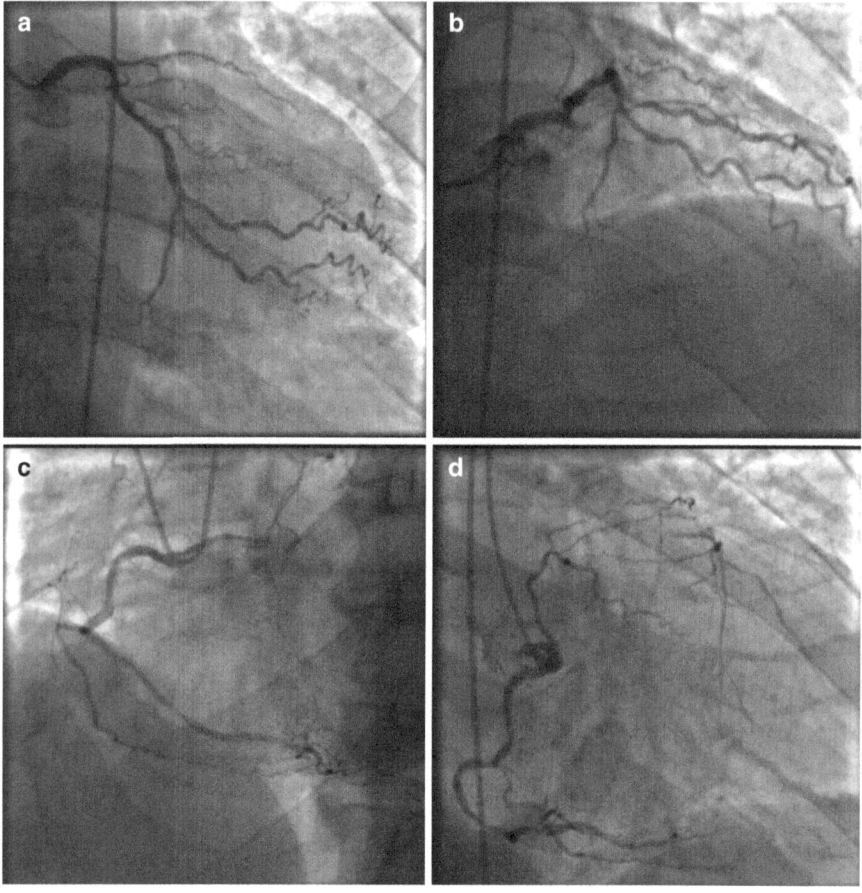

Fig. 8.1 (**a, b**) Show an occluded left anterior descending coronary artery and significant circumflex coronary artery disease. (**c, d**) Pictures demonstrate disease in the right coronary artery which fills the left anterior descending retrogradely

8.4 The Temporal Relationship

Several studies suggest that there is a strong temporal relationship between ED and CAD, with ED preceding a cardiovascular event by at least 2–5 years [11]. This temporal relationship was investigated in a questionnaire-based study that included 207 patients with CVD attending cardiovascular rehabilitation programmes and 165 age-matched controls from general practice in the UK. Patients completed up to four questionnaires including the IIEF. Of the individuals with CVD, 56 % were experiencing symptoms of ED at the time of the study and had done so for a mean of 5 ± 5.3 years. In contrast, 37 % of individuals in the control group had ED symptoms for a mean of 6.6 ± 6.8 years. This interesting finding in the controls reflects the importance of asking about ED routinely.

In the AssoCiation Between eRectile dysfunction and coronary Artery disease (COBRA) trial, 93 % of patients with a chronic coronary syndrome reported ED symptoms before the onset of angina pectoris, with a mean interval of 24 (range 12–36) months [12]. This finding further reinforces the concept of a lead time of at least 2–5 years between the development of ED and symptomatic CAD. The time intervals (range) for patients with one-, two- and three-vessel disease were 12 (9.5–24), 24 (16.5–36) and 33 (21–47) months, respectively. There was a significant relationship between the length of time from ED to CAD onset and the number of vessels involved ($p=0.016$). Importantly, given that men with ED may be at cardiovascular risk, this long lead time provides an early opportunity for cardiovascular risk reduction.

8.5 Prediction of CVD Events and Mortality

Two recent meta-analyses and one systematic review have greatly helped our assessment of the link between ED and the prediction of CVD including mortality [7, 13–15]. Prior to these analyses studies had evaluated the effect of age on the ED link to increased cardiovascular risk, identifying the importance of ED as an especially powerful predictor of CVD events in young- and middle-aged men (ages 30–60 years) where CVD preventative resources should be maximised.

A study of 1,400 men aged 40–75 years with no known CAD was prospectively followed for 10 years [15]. As can be seen from Table 8.2, men in their 40s with ED have a 50-fold increase in CAD events per 1,000 patient years compared with men with normal erectile function, and fivefold in men in their 50s (is there a more powerful risk factor?). In a retrospective study from Western Australia over 10–15 years, men in their 20s and 30s were more than seven times more likely to have a CVD event if they had ED [16], and Riedner and colleagues found in a coronary angiographic study that CAD was 2.3 times higher in men <60 years of age with ED [17]. In all three studies the ED/CAD link became less marked with age over 70 years.

Table 8.2 ED predicts coronary events [15]

Age group	ED at baseline	No baseline ED
1,400 men with no known CAD –10-year follow-up	CAD events per 1,000 pt years with CI intervals	CAD events per 1,000 pt years with CI intervals
40–49	48.52 (1.23–269.26)	0.94 (0.02–5.21)
50–59	27.15 (7.40–69.56)	5.09 (3.38–7.38)
60–69	23.97 (11.49–44.10)	10.72 (7.62–14.66)
70+	29.63 (19.37–43.75)	23.30 (17.18–30.89)

The younger the age group, the increased cardiovascular risk from erectile dysfunction. In men in their 40s who have ED at baseline, cardiovascular risk over a 10-year follow-up is 50-fold greater than men who have normal erections

Table 8.3 Relative risk of increased events and mortality: erectile dysfunction (ED vs no ED [7, 13])

	Meta-analysis [7] ($n=92,757$)	Meta-analysis [13] ($n=36,744$)
Pooled end points	1.44[a]	1.48[a]
Cardiovascular disease mortality	1.19	n/a
Myocardial infarction	1.62[a]	1.46[a]
Stroke	1.39[a]	1.35[a]
All-cause mortality	1.25[a]	1.19

[a]All significant except cardiovascular disease mortality

Dong et al. performed a meta-analysis from 12 prospective studies involving 36,744 men [13]. In Table 8.3, the relative risks for men with ED are seen to be significantly increased for CVD, CAD, stroke and all-cause mortality. Importantly, the ED risk was independent of conventional risk factors and the mortality increase fits in with the rupture of a vulnerable plaque, as previously discussed.

Vlachopoulos and colleagues (Table 8.3) included 14 studies involving 92,757 men with similar findings to the Dong meta-analysis [7]. However, of especial importance is that they found the relative risk to be higher in younger men and intermediate-risk groups (5–20 % 10-year conventional risk).

Both meta-analyses and later a systematic review [14] of the association between ED and CVD confirmed that the presence of ED increases the risk for future CVD events, MI, stroke and all-cause mortality. ED should therefore be incorporated into routine clinical practice as a diagnosis needing treatment as well as a diagnosis which could trigger an aggressive CVD risk-reduction strategy [18].

8.6 Methods of Detection of Silent Coronary Artery Disease

Vlachopoulos and colleagues have extensively studied the role of biomarkers in predicting the unfavourable endothelial and inflammatory state in ED patients with or without coronary artery disease [19]. They have linked the triad of ED to endothelial dysfunction and CVD and concluded that low-grade systemic inflammation could be an important element of the association between ED and CAD and that its individualised assessment could be a valuable tool for ED diagnosis risk assessment and a rationalised therapeutic approach to risk factor reduction in patients with ED with or without CVD symptoms [20]. The importance of risk factor reduction has been emphasised previously in several articles [18]. As ED and CAD share the same risk factors and the penis and the heart share the same endothelium, it is proposed that intensive intervention with lifestyle advice focusing on a healthy diet, weight loss and increased physical activity benefits men with ED, reducing the markers of inflammation and improving endothelial function. Vlachopoulos and colleagues have provided a clinical update on endothelial dysfunction in the cardiovascular patient, and the assessment of vascular risk in men with ED and the role of the cardiologist and general physician have been emphasised, with the recommendation that a question about ED is included in the established assessment of CVD risk in all men and be added to CVD risk assessment guidelines [7, 21].

The 3rd Princeton Consensus Conference identified the link between ED and CVD which may be asymptomatic and may benefit from cardiac risk reduction [22]. The authors went on to conclude that 'all men with vasculogenic ED require a cardiovascular work-up' [23].

8.7 The Role of Computed Tomography Coronary Angiography

Evaluation of chest pain is becoming more anatomical with multidetector cardiac computed tomography (MDCT) being proven the most sensitive way of detecting underlying coronary artery disease. Is this detection rate superior to exercise testing and does it apply to people without chest pain symptoms but with the risk factor of ED? In a study of 65 men with organic ED and no cardiac symptoms, all underwent maximal exercise testing and MDCT in the same 7-day period [24]. The exercise ECG was borderline abnormal in three men and completely normal in 62 with a good functional ability. However, on CT calcium was present in 53 men with the score ranging from 5 to 1,671, and in addition non-calcified plaque was seen in seven men and theoretically this could well be the plaque most vulnerable to rupture. The MDCT angiogram was normal in only 5 (3.25 %). Importantly, as a result of the MDCT, nine men underwent invasive coronary angiography and the severity of the CAD led to five men receiving coronary stents and four men coronary artery bypass surgery (see Case Report Figure).

In this study, most men with ED had subclinical cardiac disease. All were without cardiac symptoms and had been referred prospectively because of their ED and the increasing recognition of the link between ED and CVD.

Depending on location not every man with ED will have access to MDCT. A reasonable approach is to use calcium screening (1–2 mSU X-rays compared with CXR 0.02) in those most at risk, especially men aged 30–60 years, but preferably MDCT (5–20 mSU) to detect soft and/or non-calcified plaque. Alternatively, biomarkers that are abnormal drive a policy of aggressive risk reduction in all identified men with ED (ask routinely), and elective investigation when clinically appropriate could be pursued but this demands detailed and regular follow-up [19]. An ideal algorithm is provided in Fig. 8.2.

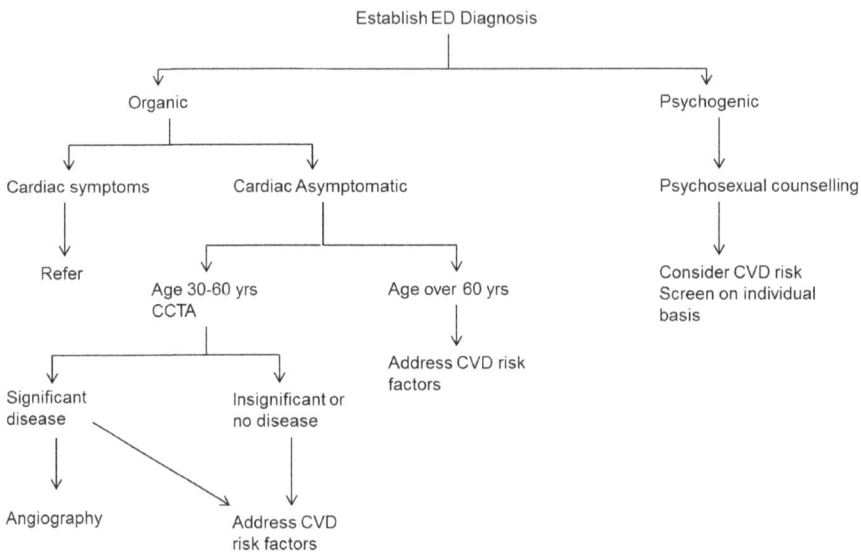

Fig. 8.2 Algorithm

Conclusion

There are several '**ED**s'[1]. There is **E**ndothelial **D**ysfunction which is the common denominator between ED and CVD. There is the importance of **E**arly **D**etection and **ED**ucation, both of the patient and the healthcare professional. Finally, we have the most important **ED** with the time window of opportunity giving us chance to prevent **E**arly **D**eath.

However, there is no point in having windows of opportunity if you do not look through the window and do something about the condition [18]. The window of 2–5 years between ED and CAD events offers us an opportunity for aggressive risk factor reduction. It is time we turned the overwhelming evidence into action, not just recognising the link between ED and CVD but doing something about it.

References

1. Jackson G (2006) Erectile dysfunction: a marker of silent coronary artery disease. Eur Heart J 27:2613–2614
2. Jackson G (1999) Erectile dysfunction and cardiovascular disease. Int J Clin Pract 53:363–368
3. O'Kane PD, Jackson G (2001) Erectile dysfunction: is there silent obstructive coronary artery disease? Int J Clin Pract 55:219–220
4. Jackson G (2013) Let's talk about sex. Clin Res Cardiol 102:327–328
5. Jackson G, Rosen RC, Kloner RA et al (2006) The second Princeton consensus on sexual dysfunction and cardiac risk: new guidelines for sexual medicine. J Sex Med 3:28–36

6. Montorsi P, Montorsi F, Schulman CC (2003) Is erectile dysfunction the "tip of the iceberg" of a systemic vascular disorder? Eur Urol 44:352–354
7. Vlachopoulos CV, Terentes-Printzios DG, Ioakeimidis N et al (2013) Prediction of cardiovascular events and all-cause mortality with erectile dysfunction: a systematic review and meta-analysis of cohort studies. Circ Cardiovasc Qual Outcomes 6:99–109
8. Montorsi F, Briganti A, Salonia A et al (2003) Erectile dysfunction prevalence, time of onset and association with risk factors in 300 consecutive patients with acute chest pain and angiographically documented coronary artery disease. Eur Urol 44:360–364
9. Gazzaruso C, Solerte SB, Pujia A et al (2008) Erectile dysfunction as a predictor of cardiovascular events and death in diabetic patients with angiographically proven asymptomatic coronary artery disease: a potential protective role for statins and 5-phosphodiesterase inhibitors. J Am Coll Cardiol 51:2040–2044
10. Thompson IM, Tangen CM, Goodman PJ et al (2005) Erectile dysfunction and subsequent cardiovascular disease. JAMA 294:2996–3002
11. Hodges LD, Kirby M, Solanki J et al (2007) The temporal relationship between erectile dysfunction and cardiovascular disease. Int J Clin Pract 61:2019–2025
12. Montorsi P, Ravagnani PM, Galli S et al (2006) Association between erectile dysfunction and coronary artery disease. Role of coronary clinical presentation and extent of coronary vessels involvement: the COBRA trial. Eur Heart J 27:2632–2639
13. Dong JY, Zhang YH, Qin LQ (2011) Erectile dysfunction and risk of cardiovascular disease: meta-analysis of prospective cohort studies. J Am Coll Cardiol 58:1378–1385
14. Gandaglia G, Briganti A, Jackson G et al (2014) A systematic review of the association between erectile dysfunction and cardiovascular disease. Eur Urol 65:968–978
15. Inman BA, Sauver JL, Jacobson DJ et al (2009) A population-based, longitudinal study of erectile dysfunction and future coronary artery disease. Mayo Clin Proc 84:108–113
16. Chew KK, Finn J, Stuckey B et al (2010) Erectile dysfunction as a predictor for subsequent atherosclerotic cardiovascular events: findings from a linked-data study. J Sex Med 7:192–202
17. Riedner CE, Rhoden EL, Fuchs SC et al (2011) Erectile dysfunction and coronary artery disease: an association of higher risk in younger men. J Sex Med 8:1445–1453
18. Jackson G (2007) The importance of risk factor reduction in erectile dysfunction. Curr Urol Rep 8:463–466
19. Vlachopoulos C, Ioakeimidis N, Terentes-Printzios D et al (2008) The triad: erectile dysfunction – endothelial dysfunction – cardiovascular disease. Curr Pharm Des 14:3700–3714
20. Vlachopoulos C, Rokkas K, Ioakeimidis N et al (2007) Inflammation, metabolic syndrome, erectile dysfunction, and coronary artery disease: common links. Eur Urol 52:1590–1600
21. Vlachopoulos C, Jackson G, Stefanadis C et al (2013) Erectile dysfunction in the cardiovascular patient. Eur Heart J 34:2034–2046
22. Nehra A, Jackson G, Miner M et al (2012) The Princeton III consensus recommendations for the management of erectile dysfunction and cardiovascular disease. Mayo Clin Proc 87:766–778
23. Jackson G, Nehra A, Miner M et al (2013) The assessment of vascular risk in men with erectile dysfunction: the role of the cardiologist and general physician. Int J Clin Pract 67:1163–1172
24. Jackson G (2013) Erectile dysfunction and asymptomatic coronary artery disease: frequently detected by computed tomography coronary angiography but not by exercise electrocardiography. Int J Clin Pract 67:1159–1162

The Prognostic Role of Erectile Dysfunction for Cardiovascular Events

9

Dimitrios Terentes-Printzios
and Charalambos Vlachopoulos

Abbreviations

ABI	Ankle-brachial index
CAC	Coronary artery calcium
CAD	Coronary artery disease
CCTA	Coronary computed tomography angiography
CfPWV	Carotid-femoral pulse wave velocity
CI	Confidence intervals
CV	Cardiovascular
CVD	Cardiovascular disease
ED	Erectile dysfunction
HF	Heart failure
IL-6	Interleukin-6
IMT	Intima-media thickness
MACE	Major adverse cardiac events
ONTARGET	ONgoing Telmisartan Alone and in combination with ramipril global endpoint trial
PSV	Peak systolic velocity
RR	Relative risk
SCORE	Systematic coronary risk evaluation
TOM	Testosterone in older men with mobility limitations
TRANSCEND	Telmisartan randomized assessment study in ACE intolerant subjects with cardiovascular disease
VITAL	Vitamins and lifestyle

D. Terentes-Printzios (✉) • C. Vlachopoulos
1st Department of Cardiology, Cardiovascular Diseases and Sexual Health Unit,
Athens Medical School, Athens, Greece
e-mail: dimitristerentes@yahoo.gr; cvlachop@otenet.gr

9.1 Introduction

Erectile dysfunction (ED) is a universal clinical problem with thousands of new cases per year [1]. Cardiovascular disease (CVD) and ED share common risk factors [2], while evidence-based studies have identified pathophysiological links, such as endothelial dysfunction, inflammation, and low testosterone [3], thus identifying ED as an appealing candidate marker for future events. Screening and diagnosing ED is essential for primary prevention since ED assessment offers a low-cost, easy alternative to several investigational cardiovascular biomarkers [4] and could describe the risk over and beyond traditional risk factors, particularly for those patients belonging into the intermediate cardiovascular risk category [5]. ED may precede clinically overt CVD by 2–5 years providing a valuable time window to earlier modification of risk factors and potentially improve outcomes [4].

A number of studies and meta-analyses examined the ability of ED to predict the risk of future fatal and nonfatal cardiovascular events and all-cause mortality [5, 6]. Integration of current knowledge makes evident that presence of ED increases the risk for future cardiovascular events, myocardial infarction, stroke, and all-cause mortality [5, 6]. Evidence points towards a grading effect of the severity of ED in the predictive ability of this condition for clinical outcome [7].

Several vascular and circulatory biomarkers such as aortic stiffness [8] and testosterone [9], along with baseline cardiovascular risk and reliable diagnosis of ED with a validated questionnaire, have demonstrated an essential role in the determination of the predictive ability of ED [4, 5]. Of special interest is the effect of pharmacological treatment of ED on prognosis. Several studies have implicated that improvement of ED and ED-associated comorbidities either by pharmacological or lifestyle interventions might also have a per se beneficial impact on cardiovascular risk [5, 10].

9.2 Pathophysiological Links of Erectile Dysfunction and Cardiovascular Events

Vasculogenic ED may result from impairment of endothelial dependent and/or independent smooth muscle relaxation (i.e., functional vascular ED, early stages), occlusion of the penile arteries by atherosclerosis (i.e., structural vascular ED, late stages), or a combination of these processes [3]. Vasculogenic ED or primarily vasculogenic ED (i.e., in cases that the cause of ED is multifactorial along with hormonal disturbances or diabetic neuropathy) should be regarded as harbinger of incident or future cardiovascular disease. Risk factors associated with ED are classical CV risk factors related to atherosclerosis including age, hypercholesterolemia, hypertension, insulin resistance and diabetes, smoking, obesity, metabolic syndrome, sedentary lifestyle, and depression [2]. Moreover, both atherosclerosis and ED have been linked to endothelial dysfunction and inflammation and low testosterone levels [3, 11–13]. Men with ED, which is largely due to impaired nitric oxide bioavailability rather than atherosclerosis in the penile vasculature, are found to have endothelial dysfunction and subclinical atherosclerosis in other vascular beds as well [13].

ED seems to precede manifestation (or documentation) of coronary artery disease (CAD) in about two-thirds of cases by a mean time interval of 2–3 years and a cardiovascular event (myocardial infarction and stroke) by 3–5 years, although longer time frames have been reported [14–16]. A plausible explanation is proposed by the "artery size" hypothesis [17]. According to this hypothesis, for a given atherosclerotic burden, the smaller penile arteries suffer obstruction earlier than the larger coronary arteries; hence, ED may be symptomatic before a coronary event. Furthermore, in theory, the longer the ED duration, the longer the time of exposure to risk factors and to disease processes and thus the greater the risk of subclinical or future CVD. Therefore, while the accumulating plaque burden does not induce flow-limiting obstruction, it may be the cause of acute CV events in susceptible patients. Endothelial dysfunction and increased oxidative stress are also essential factors in the genesis of myocardial ischemia and acute cardiovascular events through changes in plaque compositions that eventually may influence plaque stability and coronary thrombosis [3].

9.3 Erectile Dysfunction as a Marker of Prevalent CAD

Association of ED with prevalent CAD goes both ways [18]. According to several cross-sectional studies, one to two out of three CAD patients are diagnosed with ED [12]. On the other hand, ED patients have increased risk for asymptomatic CAD [12]. The percentage of ED patients with positive exercise stress tests or significant coronary stenosis by conventional or computed tomography coronary angiography can be as high as 50 % [12]. In fact, the most compelling evidence comes from a prospective angiographic study, showing that almost one out of five men without symptoms for CAD, presenting with vasculogenic ED as their only symptom, have significant coronary artery stenosis [19]. Finally, the severity of the ED correlates with the severity of the CAD and consequently with gravity of prognosis [16].

9.4 Erectile Dysfunction as a Prognostic Marker of Cardiovascular Events

The results of numerous experimental, cross-sectional and retrospective studies created the spark for the link between ED and CV events that warranted conduction of prospective studies. The Prostate Cancer Prevention Trial in 2005 [20] was the first large prospective study to confirm researchers' assumptions and offer them both answers as well as further questions on the subject. In particular, men included in the placebo arm of the trial with baseline or "incidental" ED developed during the follow-up had 1.45-fold higher risk to experience a CV event compared to individuals without ED. However, these results were limited by lack of validated questionnaires, by the heterogeneity of CV events used as endpoints, and by the high rate of patients who developed ED during follow-up (65 % after 7 years). Most of these limitations were dealt with in a population-based study by Banks et al. [7], evaluating the association between ED and future CV endpoints in a large Australian cohort of 95,038 men. Interestingly, ED severity showed a gradual association with CV endpoints that was even stronger in patients with prior CVD. Particularly, individuals with a known history of CVD complaining of severe ED had a roughly twofold higher probability of experiencing CV events compared to those without ED. This was confirmed also in patients without a known history of CVD [7].

ED has been investigated as a predictor of clinical outcome also in men at high CV risk, such as patients with CAD, heart failure (HF), and diabetes [10, 21–24]. Diabetics are the best studied group among them. Three prospective studies investigated the relationship between ED and CV events in diabetics and all three came to the same conclusion that ED is an important predictor of CV events in diabetes [10, 21, 24]. In fact, the pooled odds ratio in diabetics was estimated in a recent meta-analysis at 1.74 (95 % confidence interval [CI]: 1.34–2.27) for CV events and 1.72 (95 % CI: 1.5–1.98) for CAD [25]. In accordance, a sub-study of the ONgoing Telmisartan Alone and in combination with Ramipril Global Endpoint Trial (ONTARGET)-Telmisartan Randomized AssessmeNt Study in ACE iNtolerant subjects with cardiovascular Disease (TRANSCEND) trials [23] confirmed the predictive role of ED in a population at high risk for CVD. Finally, a small prospective study showed a trend for increased mortality in patients with HF and ED compared to HF patients without ED [22].

However, an independent association between ED and CVD is not a universal finding of prospective studies. Hotaling et al. [26] in the large prospective VITamins and Lifestyle (VITAL) study involving 31,296 men failed to show an association between ED and CV mortality. Possible explanations for this result are the enrollment of a low CV risk population and the fact that men were diagnosed with ED using a single question. In addition, Ponholzer et al. [27] also did not show a statistically significant association between ED and CV events in a population of 2,506 men with a mean age of 45 years. However, this study was also hampered by several limitations such as the investigation of mainly young individuals at low CV risk, the assessment of outcome merely based on the information regarding hospital admissions, as well as the short follow-up period. Furthermore, Araujo et al. [28] investigated the predictive role of ED over Framingham risk score. The authors, despite showing that ED is independently associated with increased CVD incidence, did not find a significant improvement in the prediction of who will and will not develop CVD beyond that offered by traditional risk factors. These neutral studies casted doubt on the association between ED and CV endpoints.

In order to clear this doubt, an overall robust quantitative estimate of the predictive value of ED for different outcomes as well estimation of the possible publication bias was warranted. Recently, three meta-analyses [5, 6, 29] showed that ED significantly increases the risk of CVD and that this increase is independent of conventional CV risk factors. In the most recent and most

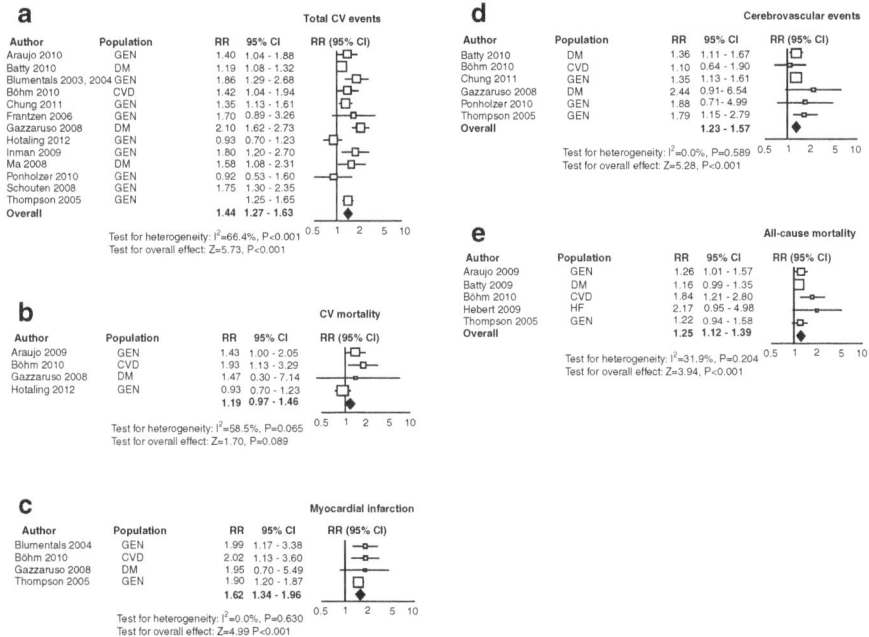

Fig. 9.1 Relative risk and 95 % confidence interval for erectile dysfunction and total cardiovascular events (**a**), cardiovascular mortality (**b**), myocardial infarction (**c**), cerebrovascular events (**d**), and all-cause mortality (**e**) (With permission from Vlachopoulos et al. [5]). *CV* cardiovascular, *CVD* cardiovascular disease, *DM* diabetes mellitus, *HF* heart failure, *GEN* general population

comprehensive meta-analysis [5], we analyzed results from almost 100,000 participants included in 14 studies with a mean follow-up of over 6 years. We showed that patients with ED had a significantly increased risk by 44 % for CV events, 62 % for myocardial infarction, and 25 % for overall mortality compared to those without ED (Fig. 9.1). Interestingly, the relative risk (RR) for future adverse events was higher at younger ages and intermediate-CVD-risk populations [5]. Furthermore, the assessment of ED by a structured validated questionnaire was associated with higher RR of CVD as compared to when the diagnosis of ED was made with a single question [5]. Importantly, publication bias could not have affected our results in a meaningful manner.

9.5 The Role of Biomarkers in Prognosis of Cardiovascular Events in Erectile Dysfunction

As already stated, ED carries by itself an independent risk for both prevalent CAD and future CV events. Several tests that measure the general atherosclerotic burden (not necessarily obstructive) either in the coronary circulation (i.e., coronary calcium score by electron-beam computed tomography) or in extra-coronary vessels (i.e., ankle-brachial index, carotid intima-media thickness) along with functional arterial indices (flow-mediated dilatation) or mixed (functional and structural) arterial indices (aortic stiffness and wave reflection indices) are also considered surrogate markers of CVD [4, 13, 30]. ED has been associated with all the above mentioned markers of overall atherosclerotic burden (Table 9.1). It would be extremely clinically useful to identify potential biomarkers that would predict future CV event in the ED population. These biomarkers of generalized vascular disease discussed above are potential such candidates. However, to the best of our knowledge, carotid-femoral pulse wave velocity (cfPWV) is the only biomarker of generalized vascular disease that independently predicts future major adverse cardiac events (MACE) in ED and has the ability to reclassify patients in the proper CV risk group over and beyond traditional CV risk factors [8]. cfPWV is a validated noninvasive assessment of aortic stiffness, which has been shown to have an independent predictive value for cardiovascular events and all-cause mortality [31–33]. In addition, pulse pressure, a crude index of arterial stiffness, has also been shown to predict outcome in ED patients [34]. It should be noted that the rest abovementioned indices have not shown a predictive ability specifically in ED patients since relevant studies are lacking. However, based on their ability in various populations, they are expected to show such performance in ED patients.

Hormonal testing (testosterone or prolactin) has been shown to be an independent predictor of CV events in ED patients. In specific, while total testosterone levels <8 nmol/L are associated with increased chance of MACE, for each 10 ng/mL increment of prolactin levels (in ED patients without pathological hyperprolactinemia, prolactin <735 mU/L or 35 ng/ mL), the risk for MACE is decreased by 5 % [8, 35]. We also demonstrated in a group of hypertensive patients consisting primarily of patients with ED that the predictive ability of total testosterone is incremental to Framingham risk score and has the potential to reclassify these patients to their appropriate CV risk group [36]. Furthermore, albuminuria (micro- or macro-), as assessed by albumin/creatinine ratio >3.5 mg/mmol and albumin excretion ratio >30 mg/day, predicts outcome in diabetic patients with and without ED [10, 21]. Interestingly, assessment of both flaccid and dynamic peak systolic velocity (PSV) (flaccid PSV < 13 cm/s and dynamic PSV < 25 cm/s) in penile Doppler is a prognostic marker for incident major CV events [37].

Finally, office-based assessment of cardiovascular risk using conventional risk factor algorithms, such as Framingham risk score and Systematic COronary Risk Evaluation (SCORE), is important for initial risk stratification [4]. In 2012 the Third Princeton Consensus Conference addressed the role of screening and lifestyle modifications in ED patients according to CVD risk [38]. On the foundations of Princeton III recommendations, a practical clinical algorithm has been recently proposed [4] (Fig. 9.2). Therefore, inclusion of such biomarkers and CV risk scores in the assessment of ED patients may aid in identifying which asymptomatic ED patient should be further investigated and how aggressively should be treated [4].

Table 9.1 Prognostic markers of cardiovascular disease in the patient with erectile dysfunction

Biomarkers	Association with vasculogenic ED	Overall CV predictive value	Association with CV prevalence in ED	CV predictive value in ED	Response to treatment	Applicability	Cost-effectiveness
Testosterone	+++	++	+	+	+	++++	++++
hsCRP	++	+++	+	−	+	++++	++++
Fibrinogen, IL-6	+++	++	+	−	+	++	+++
Carotid IMT	+++	+++	+	−	+	++	+++
Aortic stiffness (PWV)	+++	+++	+	++	++	++	+++
ABI	++	+++	+	−	−	+++	++++
CCTA	++	+++	+	−	−	+	+
CAC	++	++++	+	−	−	+	+
Endothelial dysfunction	+++	++	+	−	++	++	+++
Albuminuria (micro- or macro-)	+	+++	+	+	−	++++	++++
Penile color Doppler	++++	−	+	+	++	+	++

Association with ED, applicability, response to treatment, prognostic value, and cost-effectiveness of biomarkers (scored from 0 to 4+)
ABI ankle-brachial index, *CAC* coronary artery calcium, *CCTA* coronary computed tomography angiography, *CVD* cardiovascular disease, *ED* erectile dysfunction, *IL-6* interleukin-6, *IMT* intima-media thickness, *PWV* pulse wave velocity

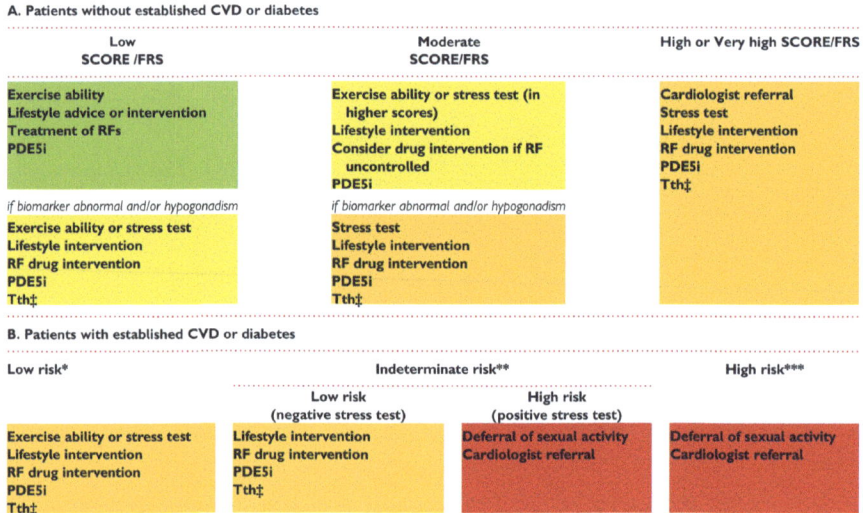

Fig. 9.2 Management of ED patient with (**a**) and without (**b**) cardiovascular disease (With permission from Vlachopoulos et al. [4]). *Low-risk patients include those with complete revascularization (e.g., via coronary artery bypass grafting, stenting, or angioplasty), patients with asymptomatic controlled hypertension, those with mild valvular disease, and patients with left ventricular dysfunction/heart failure (NYHA classes I and II) who achieved five metabolic equivalents of the task (*METS*) without ischemia on recent exercise testing. **Indeterminate risk patients include diabetics, those with mild or moderate stable angina pectoris, past myocardial infarction (2–8 weeks) without intervention awaiting exercise electrocardiography, congestive heart failure (NYHA class III), and noncardiac sequelae of atherosclerotic disease (e.g., peripheral artery disease and a history of stroke or transient ischemic attack); this patient with ED may require assessment for additional vascular disease using carotid intima-media thickness or ankle-brachial index and subsequent reclassification to low or high risk. ***High-risk patients include those with unstable or refractory angina pectoris, uncontrolled hypertension, congestive heart failure (NYHA class IV), recent myocardial infarction without intervention (2 weeks), high-risk arrhythmia (exercise-induced ventricular tachycardia, implanted internal cardioverter defibrillator with frequent shocks, and poorly controlled atrial fibrillation), obstructive hypertrophic cardiomyopathy with severe symptoms, and moderate to severe valve disease, particularly aortic stenosis. ‡Where appropriate *CVD* cardiovascular disease, *FRS* Framingham risk score, *PDE5i* phosphodiesterase type 5 inhibitors, *RF* risk factor, *Tth* testosterone therapy; *NYHA* New York Heart Association

9.6 The Effect of Treatment of Erectile Dysfunction on Prognosis of Cardiovascular Events

Improvement of ED by lifestyle interventions, common to those recommended for reduction of CVD risk, might per se be beneficial in terms of erectile function and prognosis. After the initial ED evaluation and prior to administration of specific ED treatment, exercise ability should be considered to estimate CV risk associated with sexual activity [39]. A recent meta-analysis of 14 studies established a significant association between acute cardiac events and episodic physical or/and sexual activity that was attenuated among individuals with high levels of habitual physical activity.

Of special interest is the effect of pharmacological treatment of ED, as it appears that this may also have a beneficial impact on risk [40]. Indeed, Frantzen et al. [41] showed that 2 years after the introduction of sildenafil, the RR of the incidence of CVD among men with ED compared with healthy men significantly decreased from 1.7 to 1.1. Furthermore, Gazzaruso et al. [10] showed that type 5 phosphodiesterase inhibitors offer a marginal protection against the development of major adverse cardiac events in CAD diabetic patients with ED.

Testosterone treatment for hypogonadal ED patients as well as its effect on cardiovascular outcomes is a highly debated subject. Systematic reviews and meta-analyses of testosterone therapy show a neutral or small unfavorable effect on cardiovascular outcomes [42, 43]. However, the Testosterone in Older Men With Mobility Limitations (TOM) trial [44], which randomized community-dwelling men 65 years and older with limitations in mobility and total serum testosterone levels lower than 350 ng/dL to placebo or testosterone gel for 6 months showed more cardiovascular events in the testosterone arm. However, the clinical applicability of these findings is limited by the usage of an off-label, high, and rapid escalation dosing regimen and by the inclusion of frail elderly men with impaired mobility. Furthermore, in a recent retrospective study [45] testosterone users were found to have an increased risk of cardiovascular outcomes; however, the study is hampered by methodological shortcomings in analysis and credibility of data report. Based on these results testosterone treatment must be reserved for patients who (1) are symptomatic (ED or reduced libido) of testosterone deficiency and (2) they have biochemical evidence of low testosterone (total testosterone <8 nmol/L or 230 ng/dL) with respect to its contraindications and limitations as well as close follow-up [4, 38].

Drugs used in cardiovascular disease prevention and treatment, such as drugs of the renin-angiotensin-aldosterone system and statins, apart from reducing cardiovascular risk appear to have a beneficial effect on ED itself. It is rational to believe that these drugs will have a beneficial effect in cardiovascular outcomes of ED patients as well [46]. Limited data have demonstrated a significant role of statins in improving the prognosis of diabetics with CAD that included a significant proportion of ED patients [10]. Undoubtedly, more data are needed and future follow-up studies should ideally collect information on ED treatment and investigate their effect on prognosis [47].

Conclusion

In summary, CVD and ED share common risk factors, while evidence-based studies have identified pathophysiological links, such as endothelial dysfunction and inflammation. ED also confers an independent risk for future CV events. The usual 3-year time frame between the onset of ED symptoms and a CV event offers an opportunity for risk mitigation and potentially improvement of outcomes. Current literature and guidelines [48] support implementation of ED into clinical practice and stress the need to establish standardized methods to diagnose ED and to investigate the potential effect of use of biomarkers and ED treatment on CV events and all-cause mortality.

Glossary

Ankle-brachial index It is the ratio of the blood pressure in the lower legs (posterior tibial artery or dorsalis pedis artery) to the blood pressure in the arms (brachial artery).
Arterial stiffness It is the reduced capability of an artery to expand in response to pressure changes.
Pulse wave velocity It is the distance traveled (Δx) by the pressure wave divided by the time (Δt) for the wave to travel that distance.
Vascular biomarkers Biomarkers that originate from changes in function or structure of blood vessels such as aortic stiffness, carotid intima-media thickness, coronary artery calcium calcification, and endothelial function.
Vasculogenic ED It is diagnosed when the peak systolic velocity (PSV) is less than 35 cm/s and/or when the end-diastolic velocity (EDV) is greater than 5 cm/s in penile Doppler.

References

1. Feldman HA, Goldstein I, Hatzichristou DG, Krane RJ, McKinlay JB (1994) Impotence and its medical and psychosocial correlates: results of the Massachusetts Male Aging Study. J Urol 151(1):54–61
2. Weber MF, Smith DP, O'Connell DL, Patel MI, de Souza PL, Sitas F, Banks E (2013) Risk factors for erectile dysfunction in a cohort of 108 477 Australian men. Med J Aust 199(2):107–111
3. Vlachopoulos C, Ioakeimidis N, Terentes-Printzios D, Stefanadis C (2008) The triad: erectile dysfunction–endothelial dysfunction–cardiovascular disease. Curr Pharm Des 14(35): 3700–3714
4. Vlachopoulos C, Jackson G, Stefanadis C, Montorsi P (2013) Erectile dysfunction in the cardiovascular patient. Eur Heart J 34(27):2034–2046
5. Vlachopoulos CV, Terentes-Printzios DG, Ioakeimidis NK, Aznaouridis KA, Stefanadis CI (2013) Prediction of cardiovascular events and all-cause mortality with erectile dysfunction: a systematic review and meta-analysis of cohort studies. Circ Cardiovasc Qual Outcomes 6(1):99–109
6. Dong JY, Zhang YH, Qin LQ (2011) Erectile dysfunction and risk of cardiovascular disease: meta-analysis of prospective cohort studies. J Am Coll Cardiol 58(13):1378–1385
7. Banks E, Joshy G, Abhayaratna WP, Kritharides L, Macdonald PS, Korda RJ, Chalmers JP (2013) Erectile dysfunction severity as a risk marker for cardiovascular disease hospitalisation and all-cause mortality: a prospective cohort study. PLoS Med 10(1):e1001372
8. Vlachopoulos C, Ioakeimidis N, Aznaouridis K, Terentes-Printzios D, Rokkas K, Aggelis A, Panagiotakos D, Stefanadis C (2014) Prediction of cardiovascular events with aortic stiffness in patients with erectile dysfunction. Hypertension 64(3):672–678
9. Corona G, Monami M, Boddi V, Cameron-Smith M, Fisher AD, de Vita G, Melani C, Balzi D, Sforza A, Forti G, Mannucci E, Maggi M (2010) Low testosterone is associated with an increased risk of MACE lethality in subjects with erectile dysfunction. J Sex Med 7:1557–1564
10. Gazzaruso C, Solerte SB, Pujia A, Coppola A, Vezzoli M, Salvucci F, Valenti C, Giustina A, Garzaniti A (2008) Erectile dysfunction as a predictor of cardiovascular events and death in diabetic patients with angiographically proven asymptomatic coronary artery disease: a potential protective role for statins and 5-phosphodiesterase inhibitors. J Am Coll Cardiol 51:2040–2044

11. Vlachopoulos C, Aznaouridis K, Ioakeimidis N, Rokkas K, Vasiliadou C, Alexopoulos N, Stefanadi E, Askitis A, Stefanadis C (2006) Unfavourable endothelial and inflammatory state in erectile dysfunction patients with or without coronary artery disease. Eur Heart J 27(22):2640–2648
12. Vlachopoulos C, Rokkas K, Ioakeimidis N, Stefanadis C (2007) Inflammation, metabolic syndrome, erectile dysfunction, and coronary artery disease: common links. Eur Urol 52(6):1590–1600
13. Vlachopoulos C, Aznaouridis K, Ioakeimidis N, Rokkas K, Tsekoura D, Vasiliadou C, Stefanadi E, Askitis A, Stefanadis C (2008) Arterial function and intima-media thickness in hypertensive patients with erectile dysfunction. J Hypertens 26(9):1829–1836
14. Hodges LD, Kirby M, Solanki J, O'Donnell J, Brodie DA (2007) The temporal relationship between erectile dysfunction and cardiovascular disease. Int J Clin Pract 61(12):2019–2025
15. Inman BA, Sauver JL, Jacobson DJ, McGree ME, Nehra A, Lieber MM, Roger VL, Jacobsen SJ (2009) A population-based, longitudinal study of erectile dysfunction and future coronary artery disease. Mayo Clin Proc 84:108–113
16. Montorsi P, Ravagnani PM, Galli S, Rotatori F, Veglia F, Briganti A, Salonia A, Dehò F, Rigatti P, Montorsi F, Fiorentini C (2006) Association between erectile dysfunction and coronary artery disease. Role of coronary clinical presentation and extent of coronary vessels involvement: the COBRA trial. Eur Heart J 27(22):2632–2639
17. Montorsi P, Ravagnani PM, Galli S, Rotatori F, Briganti A, Salonia A, Rigatti P, Montorsi F (2005) The artery size hypothesis: a macrovascular link between erectile dysfunction and coronary artery disease. Am J Cardiol 96(12B):19M–23M
18. Gandaglia G, Briganti A, Jackson G, Kloner RA, Montorsi F, Montorsi P, Vlachopoulos C (2014) A systematic review of the association between erectile dysfunction and cardiovascular disease. Eur Urol 65(5):968–978
19. Vlachopoulos C, Rokkas K, Ioakeimidis N, Aggeli C, Michaelides A, Roussakis G, Fassoulakis C, Askitis A, Stefanadis C (2005) Prevalence of asymptomatic coronary artery disease in men with vasculogenic erectile dysfunction: a prospective angiographic study. Eur Urol 48:996–1002; discussion 1002–1003
20. Thompson IM, Tangen CM, Goodman PJ, Probstfield JL, Moinpour CM, Coltman CA (2005) Erectile dysfunction and subsequent cardiovascular disease. JAMA 294:2996–3002
21. Ma RC, So WY, Yang X, Yu LW, Kong AP, Ko GT, Chow CC, Cockram CS, Chan JC, Tong PC (2008) Erectile dysfunction predicts coronary heart disease in type 2 diabetes. J Am Coll Cardiol 51:2045–2050
22. Hebert K, Lopez B, Macedo FY, Gomes CR, Urena J, Arcement LM (2009) Peripheral vascular disease and erectile dysfunction as predictors of mortality in heart failure patients. J Sex Med 6:1999–2007
23. Böhm M, Baumhäkel M, Teo K, Sleight P, Probstfield J, Gao P, Mann JF, Diaz R, Dagenais GR, Jennings GL, Liu L, Jansky P, Yusuf S, ONTARGET/TRANSCEND Erectile Dysfunction Substudy Investigators (2010) Erectile dysfunction predicts cardiovascular events in high-risk patients receiving telmisartan, ramipril, or both: the ONgoing Telmisartan Alone and in combination with Ramipril Global Endpoint Trial/Telmisartan Randomized AssessmeNt Study in ACE iNtolerant subjects with cardiovascular Disease (ONTARGET/TRANSCEND) Trials. Circulation 121:1439–1446
24. Batty GD, Li Q, Czernichow S, Neal B, Zoungas S, Huxley R, Patel A, de Galan BE, Woodward M, Hamet P, Harrap SB, Poulter N, Chalmers J, ADVANCE Collaborative Group (2010) Erectile dysfunction and later cardiovascular disease in men with type 2 diabetes: prospective cohort study based on the ADVANCE (Action in Diabetes and Vascular Disease: Preterax and Diamicron Modified-Release Controlled Evaluation) trial. J Am Coll Cardiol 56:1908–1913
25. Yamada T, Hara K, Umematsu H, Suzuki R, Kadowaki T (2012) Erectile dysfunction and cardiovascular events in diabetic men: a meta-analysis of observational studies. PLoS ONE 7(9):e43673
26. Hotaling JM, Walsh TJ, Macleod LC, Heckbert S, Pocobelli G, Wessells H, White E (2012) Erectile dysfunction is not independently associated with cardiovascular death: data from the vitamins and lifestyle (VITAL) study. J Sex Med 9(8):2104–2110

27. Ponholzer A, Gutjahr G, Temml C, Madersbacher S (2010) Is erectile dysfunction a predictor of cardiovascular events or stroke? A prospective study using a validated questionnaire. Int J Impot Res 22:25–29
28. Araujo AB, Hall SA, Ganz P, Chiu GR, Rosen RC, Kupelian V, Travison TG, McKinlay JB (2010) Does erectile dysfunction contribute to cardiovascular disease risk prediction beyond the Framingham risk score? J Am Coll Cardiol 55:350–356
29. Guo W, Liao C, Zou Y, Li F, Li T, Zhou Q, Cao Y, Mao X (2010) Erectile dysfunction and risk of clinical cardiovascular events: a meta analysis of seven cohort studies. J Sex Med 7: 2805–2816
30. Vlachopoulos C (2012) Progress towards identifying biomarkers of vascular aging for total cardiovascular risk prediction. J Hypertens 30(Suppl):S19–S26
31. Vlachopoulos C, Aznaouridis K, Stefanadis C (2010) Prediction of cardiovascular events and all-cause mortality with arterial stiffness: a systematic review and meta-analysis. J Am Coll Cardiol 55:1318–1327
32. Vlachopoulos C, Aznaouridis K, Stefanadis C (2013) Aortic stiffness for cardiovascular risk prediction: just measure It, just Do It! J Am Coll Cardiol 63(7):647–649
33. Ben-Shlomo Y, Spears M, Boustred C, May M, Anderson SG, Benjamin EJ, Boutouyrie P, Cameron J, Chen CH, Cruickshank JK, Hwang SJ, Lakatta EG, Laurent S, Maldonado J, Mitchell GF, Najjar SS, Newman AB, Ohishi M, Pannier B, Pereira T, Vasan RS, Shokawa T, Sutton-Tyrell K, Verbeke F, Wang KL, Webb DJ, Hansen TW, Zoungas S, McEniery CM, Cockcroft JR, Wilkinson IB (2013) Aortic pulse wave velocity improves cardiovascular event prediction: an individual participant meta-analysis of prospective observational data from 17,635 subjects. J Am Coll Cardiol 63(7):636–646
34. Corona G, Monami M, Boddi V, Rastrelli G, Melani C, Balzi D, Sforza A, Forti G, Mannucci E, Maggi M (2011) Pulse pressure independently predicts major cardiovascular events in younger but not in older subjects with erectile dysfunction. J Sex Med 8(1):247–254
35. Corona G, Rastrelli G, Boddi V, Monami M, Melani C, Balzi D, Sforza A, Forti G, Mannucci E, Maggi M (2011) Prolactin levels independently predict major cardiovascular events in patients with erectile dysfunction. Int J Androl 34(3):217–224
36. Vlachopoulos C, Ioakeimidis N, Terentes-Printzios D, Aznaouridis K, Rokkas K, Aggelis A, Synodinos A, Lazaros G, Stefanadis C (2013) Plasma total testosterone and incident cardiovascular events in hypertensive patients. Am J Hypertens 26(3):373–381
37. Corona G, Monami M, Boddi V, Cameron-Smith M, Lotti F, de Vita G, Melani C, Balzi D, Sforza A, Forti G, Mannucci E, Maggi M (2010) Male sexuality and cardiovascular risk. A cohort study in patients with erectile dysfunction. J Sex Med 7:1918–1927
38. Nehra A, Jackson G, Miner M, Billups KL, Burnett AL, Buvat J, Carson CC, Cunningham GR, Ganz P, Goldstein I, Guay AT, Hackett G, Kloner RA, Kostis J, Montorsi P, Ramsey M, Rosen R, Sadovsky R, Seftel AD, Shabsigh R, Vlachopoulos C, Wu FC (2012) The Princeton III consensus recommendations for the management of erectile dysfunction and cardiovascular disease. Mayo Clin Proc 87(8):766–778
39. Dahabreh IJ, Paulus JK (2011) Association of episodic physical and sexual activity with triggering of acute cardiac events: systematic review and meta-analysis. JAMA 305(12): 1225–1233
40. Vlachopoulos C, Terentes-Printzios D, Ioakeimidis N, Rokkas K, Stefanadis C (2009) PDE5 inhibitors in non-urological conditions. Curr Pharm Des 15(30):3521–3539
41. Frantzen J, Speel TG, Kiemeney LA, Meuleman EJ (2006) Cardiovascular risk among men seeking help for erectile dysfunction. Ann Epidemiol 16:85–90
42. Carson CC 3rd, Rosano G (2012) Exogenous testosterone, cardiovascular events, and cardiovascular risk factors in elderly men: a review of trial data. J Sex Med 9(1):54–67
43. Xu L, Freeman G, Cowling BJ, Schooling CM (2013) Testosterone therapy and cardiovascular events among men: a systematic review and meta-analysis of placebo-controlled randomized trials. BMC Med 11:108
44. Basaria S, Coviello AD, Travison TG, Storer TW, Farwell WR, Jette AM, Eder R, Tennstedt S, Ulloor J, Zhang A, Choong K, Lakshman KM, Mazer NA, Miciek R, Krasnoff J, Elmi A,

Knapp PE, Brooks B, Appleman E, Aggarwal S, Bhasin G, Hede-Brierley L, Bhatia A, Collins L, LeBrasseur N, Fiore LD, Bhasin S (2010) Adverse events associated with testosterone administration. N Engl J Med 363(2):109–122
45. Vigen R, O'Donnell CI, Barón AE, Grunwald GK, Maddox TM, Bradley SM, Barqawi A, Woning G, Wierman ME, Plomondon ME, Rumsfeld JS, Ho PM (2013) Association of testosterone therapy with mortality, myocardial infarction, and stroke in men with low testosterone levels. JAMA 310(17):1829–1836
46. Nehra A, Jackson G, Miner M, Billups KL, Burnett AL, Buvat J, Carson CC, Cunningham GR, Goldstein I, Guay AT, Hackett G, Kloner RA, Kostis J, Montorsi P, Ramsey M, Rosen RC, Sadovsky R, Seftel AD, Vlachopoulos C, Wu FC (2013) Diagnosis and treatment of erectile dysfunction for reduction of cardiovascular risk. J Urol 189(6):2031–2038
47. Miner M, Seftel AD, Nehra A, Ganz P, Kloner RA, Montorsi P, Vlachopoulos C, Ramsey M, Sigman M, Tilkemeier P, Jackson G (2012) Prognostic utility of erectile dysfunction for cardiovascular disease in younger men and those with diabetes. Am Heart J 164(1):21–28
48. Perk J, De Backer G, Gohlke H, Graham I, Reiner Z, Verschuren WM, Albus C, Benlian P, Boysen G, Cifkova R, Deaton C, Ebrahim S, Fisher M, Germano G, Hobbs R, Hoes A, Karadeniz S, Mezzani A, Prescott E, Ryden L, Scherer M, Syvänne M, Scholte Op Reimer WJ, Vrints C, Wood D, Zamorano JL, Zannad F, Bax J, Baumgartner H, Ceconi C, Dean V, Deaton C, Fagard R, Funck-Brentano C, Hasdai D, Hoes A, Kirchhof P, Knuuti J, Kolh P, McDonagh T, Moulin C, Popescu BA, Reiner Z, Sechtem U, Sirnes PA, Tendera M, Torbicki A, Vahanian A, Windecker S (2012) European guidelines on cardiovascular disease prevention in clinical practice (version 2012): the fifth joint task force of the European Society of Cardiology and other societies on cardiovascular disease prevention in clinical practice (constituted by representatives of nine societies and by invited experts). Eur J Prev Cardiol 19(4):585–667

Erectile Dysfunction in Chronic Kidney Disease

Bojan Jelaković, Margareta Fištrek Prlić, and Mario Laganović

10.1 Introduction

Chronic kidney disease (CKD) is a growing health problem worldwide affecting approximately 15 % of the adult population [1]. The risk of dying is severalfolds higher than the risk of starting with renal replacement therapy (RRT), CVDs being the main cause of death [2]. Among various risk factors and mechanisms, nitric oxide (NO) deficiency is particularly interesting [3]. Currently with advances in medical care, the survival of CKD patients has been prolonged, and physical functioning and quality of life (QoL) became more important [4]. CKD patients are likely to reveal various sexual dysfunctions prior to dialysis. Symptoms of this disturbing disability are reported with increasing frequency as renal function declines [5]. Approximately 75 % of men undergoing dialysis have erectile dysfunction (ED) which is much higher than in other chronic diseases. ED is the main sexual problem associated with mental QoL in CKD men [5–8]. The causes of such high prevalence are multifactorial and include physiological, psychological and iatrogenic factors. The pathogenesis of sexual and ED in CKD has been attributed to several risk factors, but to none of them conclusively. Importantly, ED as a serious handicap for normal life should be considered as a marker of endothelial dysfunction and atherosclerosis as well as an indicator of possible silent coronary heart disease.

B. Jelaković, MD, PhD (✉) • M.F. Prlić, MD • M. Laganović, MD, PhD
Department for Nephrology, Hypertension, Dialysis and Transplantation,
School of Medicine University of Zagreb,
University Hospital Centre Zagreb, Kišpatićeva 12, Zagreb 10000, Croatia
e-mail: jelakovicbojan@gmail.com; margareta.fistrek@gmail.com; mlaganovic@gmail.com

© Springer International Publishing Switzerland 2015
M. Viigimaa et al. (eds.), *Erectile Dysfunction in Hypertension and Cardiovascular Disease: A Guide for Clinicians*,
DOI 10.1007/978-3-319-08272-1_10

10.2 Endocrine Alterations in Men with Chronic Kidney Disease Related to Erectile Dysfunction

The reasons for gonadal dysfunction in CKD patients are not entirely clarified. A combination of primary testicular failure and secondary pituitary hypothalamic dysfunction has been implicated. Disturbances in the pituitary-gonadal axis can be detected already in mild to moderate CKD progressively worsening as the kidney function declines, being present even after initiation of dialysis [8]. Successful kidney transplantation restores the hypothalamic-pituitary axis and pulsatile gonadotropin-releasing hormone (GnRH) and luteinising hormone (LH) release [9]. Gonadal abnormalities which are apparent in end-stage-renal disease (ESRD) further deteriorate after starting with RRT. Impaired spermatogenesis and testicular damage with decreased volume of ejaculate, oligo- or azoospermia and low percentage of motility were reported [10]. Histologic analyses revealed decreased later stages of spermatogenesis which are hormonally dependent [9]. In addition to morphological changes, normal estradiol concentration and absence of Leydig cell hypertrophy indicate that functional hypogonadism should be also considered.

Reduced levels of total and free testosterone presented already in patients with moderate CKD are attributed to the Leydig cell dysfunction [11]. While metabolic clearance rate is similar to the values observed in non-CKD men, decreased production is probably the most important reason. Emotional state, muscle mass and sleep deprivation could additionally affect and decrease testosterone values in CKD patients. In more than 70 % of patients undergoing dialysis, serum testosterone is in the hypogonadal range [12]. Testosterone is not substantially cleared during haemodialysis, and the method of dialysis does not alter total or free testosterone [11, 13]. Low levels of testosterone can contribute to decreased libido, ED, oligospermia, infertility, delayed ejaculation and affect the musculoskeletal system. Men with low testosterone levels are, regardless of kidney function, at increased risk of coronary artery disease which might suggest a possible preventive role for testosterone therapy [14, 15]. On the contrary, total plasma oestrogen concentrations are often elevated. Approximately 30 % of men undergoing chronic haemodialysis reported gynecomastia [8].

Early stages of CKD are associated with increased levels of LH very probably as a consequence of diminished release of testosterone from the Leydig cells and loss of the negative feedback. In addition, renal clearance of LH is reduced, and dialysis does not correct LH values [10]. In uremic patients, the pulsatile release of GnRH is altered [5, 8, 11, 12]. Dialysis has no effect, while restoration was observed after kidney transplantation. The follicle-stimulating hormone (FSH) level is also elevated in men with CKD, as well as the LF/FSH ratio. Seminiferous tubule and Sertoli cells are damaged in CKD; consecutively less inhibin is secreted which diminishes negative feedback resulting in increased FSH secretion.

Increased plasma prolactin levels are common finding in men with CKD (prevalence rate of 25–55 %) [16]. While the kidney plays a little role in prolactin metabolism, increased secretion is more important than reduced degradation. Increased secretion may be related to the development of secondary hyperparathyroidism

(hyperparathyroidism stimulates prolactin secretion) and is associated with loss of libido, low testosterone levels and infertility. Bromocriptine reduces prolactin secretion; however, effects on libido and sexual function are inconsistent.

Endocrine abnormalities, particularly low testosterone and hyperprolactinaemia, diminish libido contributing thereby to ED.

10.3 Vascular Disease and Neuropathy as Causes of Erectile Dysfunction in Chronic Kidney Disease

CKD is a chronic CVD. Atherosclerosis and arteriosclerosis are accelerated in CKD patients being present in the whole arterial vascular tree including the internal iliac, pelvic and pudendal arteries. Occlusive atherosclerotic disease of cavernous artery was found in up to 78 % of dialysed patients, while corporeal veno-occlusive dysfunction was reported in 90 % [17]. The role of penile haemodynamics in CKD is not completely elucidated. Importantly, progressive occlusive disease is manifested early in the penile bed before involving larger coronary vessels. Thus, ED was proposed to serve as marker for coronary heart disease preceding symptomatic CVD for several years [18, 19]. In addition to reduction in arterial inflow, veno-occlusive dysfunction is present in many patients worsening ED by venous leakage and decreased ability to achieve and maintain erection [17]. As in non-CKD men, ED is associated with many CV risk factors starting with endothelial dysfunction and ending with hypertension, atherosclerosis and diabetes. In the non-CKD population silent coronary disease in patients with ED ranged between 8 and 56 %, and it was proposed that ED may be a harbinger or silent coexistent or subsequent coronary artery disease [18, 20, 21]. Thus, in CKD men with ED the search for CV risk factors should be undertaken, and coronary artery disease should be ruled out. Older age, associated comorbidity, diabetes, prostate disease, peripheral arteriopathy and some antihypertensive drugs have been found to be associated with ED in patients on RRT. It is well accepted that endothelial dysfunction has an important role already in early CKD stages which remained after RRT was introduced [4–6, 18, 20]. As mentioned previously, in CKD patients NO deficiency deserves particular attention. The expression of NO synthase has been shown to be alternated with associated changes in IGF-1 resulting in decreased NO availability and consequently decreased regional blood flow. Reduced L-arginine synthesis, enhanced activity of arginases and impaired proximal tubule reabsorption of filtered L-arginine are causes of less availability of systemic NO in CKD patients [22]. Additionally, patients undergoing dialysis lose L-arginine [23]. In patients with more advanced stages of CKD, accumulated asymmetrical dimethyl arginine (ADMA) inhibits nitric oxide synthase (NOS) contributing to the NO deficit state as well [24, 25]. While CKD is a state of oxidative stress, a great part of NO synthesised by the kidneys and endothelial cells is converted to peroxynitrite.

Sensory and motor neuropathy which are frequently present in CKD patients, particularly those with diabetic nephropathy, are important contributors of ED. Haemodialysis patients are reported to have an abnormal response to Valsalva manoeuvre; they have impaired nocturnal penile tumescence (NPT) and bulbocavernosus reflex as neurophysiological evidence for autonomic and peripheral neuropathy. Abnormal Valsalva manoeuvre correlates with abnormal NPT and a lower number of sexual intercourses [26]. Dysfunction of the pelvic autonomic system decreases sensation and arousal stimuli [27].

10.4 Psychosocial Factors and Quality of Life in Chronic Kidney Disease

CKD and RRT per se have negative impact on QoL causing distress and interpersonal difficulties. Drop in self-esteem, anxiety and depression can cause or increase problems in sexual function. Changes in body shape and image (catheter, fistula, oedema, fetor, etc.) also importantly contribute to the desire and sexual function [28]. Symptoms of depression which are highly prevalent in patients undergoing dialysis are independently associated with sexual dysfunction [29]. Those who are most depressed have the most severe degree of sexual dysfunction. Depressive symptoms were found to be an independent factor for sexual function in men undergoing haemodialysis [29, 30]. However, this might be the chicken-egg situation. Very probably, common factors are responsible for both. Higher sexual desire and intercourse satisfaction predicted higher level in physical, social and general health scores. Long survival on dialysis itself is associated with the decrease of QoL, and this could influence the sexual life of those patients. Lew-Starowicz et al. revealed in multiple regression analysis that anxiety in men independently predicted the lower quality of sexual life [32]. They concluded that sexual disability which correlated with anxiety seriously impacts QoL in dialysed patients. Marital conflicts, more frequently presented in dialysed patients, are related to worsening of the socioeconomic situation. Nearly 60 % of couples affected by dialysis listed sexual issue as an important problem, while 40 % reported never having intercourse.

10.5 Erectile Dysfunction in Chronic Kidney Disease

The exact prevalence of ED in CKD is not established. However, according to some small studies, it is significantly higher than in the age-adjusted general population. It was reported that even 80 % of men undergoing dialysis have some degree of ED [5–7, 33–37]. Varying degrees of reported prevalence of ED (41–93 %) depend on the CKD stage. The high prevalence of ED in CKD patients is related to frequently present comorbidities (atherosclerosis, diabetes and hypertension) which per se are associated with ED. Additionally, CKD itself contributes to the progression of this disability, and RRT can only partly restore derangements. ED in CKD patients recognises a multifactorial aetiology; organic and psychological factors are closely related. Psychological and metabolic factors, ageing, diabetes, hypertension, atherosclerosis, CVD, physical status and pharmacological therapy are predisposing factors for ED in CKD patients.

It is well established that the prevalence of ED increases by ageing. In CKD patients, symptoms of ED appear earlier in the life span. Messina et al. and Rosas et al. reported on the higher prevalence of ED in CKD patients younger than 50 years [34, 36]. Higher prevalence of ED in younger patients with CKD might be considered as a marker of earlier systemic vascular ageing. Hypertension, the second most important cause of end-stage renal disease (ESRD), is present in up to 85 % of patients on RRT. In the general population, hypertension is associated with higher prevalence of ED. However, the relationship between hypertension and ED in a population of patients with CKD is not completely elucidated [36]. In the general population diabetics had twice the odds of having ED than age-matched nondiabetics. Higher prevalence of diabetes among the ESRD population importantly contributes to higher prevalence of ED. There are no data supporting a direct role of dyslipidaemia on ED.

The relationship between CVD and ED is well documented. It is now accepted that many of the risk factors for CVD as well as for CKD are the same risk factors for ED which can be considered a symptom or sign of global endothelial dysfunction and atherosclerosis. It was questioned whether the onset of ED can be used as an effective predictor of CVD. Some authors reported that ED may be present 3–5 years before coronary events [37]. Coronary artery calcium score was significantly higher among dialysed patients with severe ED than in those without this problem [38].

Bellinghieri et al. reported that sexual dysfunction is inversely associated with glomerular filtration rate (GFR) [39]. It was shown that both sexual and ED are improved after successful kidney transplantation [5, 40]. Those facts point on that CKD per se may contribute to ED. As already mentioned, NO availability is lower in CKD patients which could affect both endothelial dysfunction and ED. Haemodialysis is one of many factors causing sexual dysfunction in ESRD patients. The prevalence of ED among patients undergoing haemodialysis was almost three times higher than in controls [34, 35]. Duration and adequacy of dialysis had no relationship to severity and prevalence of ED [31]. The relationship between anaemia and ED in CKD patients was reported, and diminished oxygen delivery to the penile tissue, due to low haemoglobin levels, has been associated with decreased NO synthesis. It was observed that erythropoietin therapy improves erectile and sexual function [41, 42]. Data on the beneficial effect that dialysis might have on ED are still inconsistent [5–7, 32–34, 44, 66, 67].

CKD patients need multifactorial drug therapy. Some drugs are known to be related to ED – diuretics, some antihypertensives, antidepressants, H2 antagonists, digoxin, alpha-methyldopa, reserpine, fibrates and metoclopramide. On the contrary, ACE inhibitors were found to be inversely associated with ED [31].

10.6 Diagnostic Approach/Evaluation of Erectile Dysfunction in a Patient with Chronic Kidney Disease

ED is a major health issue of modern life that is often underdiagnosed because of patients' shame and physicians' unawareness [43]. In many societies cultural, religious and even legal factors are still boundaries trying to keep this important part of life a private issue. Physicians and nurses should face this problem as experts and scientists aiming to help a patient to have a better QoL. Sexuality may not be easily discussed, and being aware of this inherent limitation, health-care providers have to find the proper way to approach this problem in each patient. Elucidation of sexual function and general questions about QoL should be an obligate and regular element of taking history and clinical exam. Basically, diagnostic approach for sexual and ED in CKD patients is alike to all other patients. The International Index of Erectile Function (IIEF) is a validated questionnaire which could be used in CKD patients. Sexual difficulties should be interpreted in the context of the patient's life, demands and expectations. However, some specific issues should be taken into account helping to elucidate the cause of ED in CKD patients. It is important to distinguish between problems with libido and ED. The lack of secondary sexual characteristics and small soft testicles suggest hypogonadism as a cause of ED. Vascular and neurogenic causes are more likely to be associated with normal-sized testicles. The concomitant presence of CV or cerebrovascular disease indicates that vascular causes might be the crucial factor for ED. Medical therapy should be carefully analysed as various drugs could contribute to ED. Adequacy of dialysis, correction of anaemia and electrolyte status should be reviewed. In patients with normal nocturnal erections during the REM sleeping phase, psychological factors should be evaluated and then proper therapy proposed. NPT testing could help in discriminating between organic and psychological causes of ED based on assumption that men with psychological cause will have erection during the sleep. Patients with psychogenic ED should be further evaluated with psychological testing. The presence or absence of sexual dysfunction in spouses and marital relationship as well as some socioeconomic problems must be considered. Doppler study will provide information on penile blood flow. Some authors proposed penile Doppler velocimetry with PGE1 test [44]. Prolonged latency time of bulbocavernosus reflex suggests that neurogenic mechanisms are involved. Hormonal analyses (prolactin, testosterone, LH/FSH) have to be included in diagnostic algorithm. It must not be forgotten that the majority of CKD patients have more than one causative factor for ED and each patient should be approach as an individual.

The algorithm proposed for evaluation and treatment of ED in CKD patients is shown in Fig. 10.1.

10.7 Treatment of Erectile Dysfunction in a Patient with Chronic Kidney Disease

Undoubtedly, restoration of sexual function is of utmost significance aiming to increase patients' QoL. However, treatment of ED is frequently frustrating and requires multifaceted approach. Achieving success is even harder in CKD patients. Treatment options include psychosexual therapy, management of endocrine disorders, correction of anaemia, avoidance of certain medications, drug therapy, transurethral or intracavernosal therapy, vacuum devices and surgical treatment. For those undergoing dialysis optimal delivery and optimisation of dialysis dose as well

10 Erectile Dysfunction in Chronic Kidney Disease

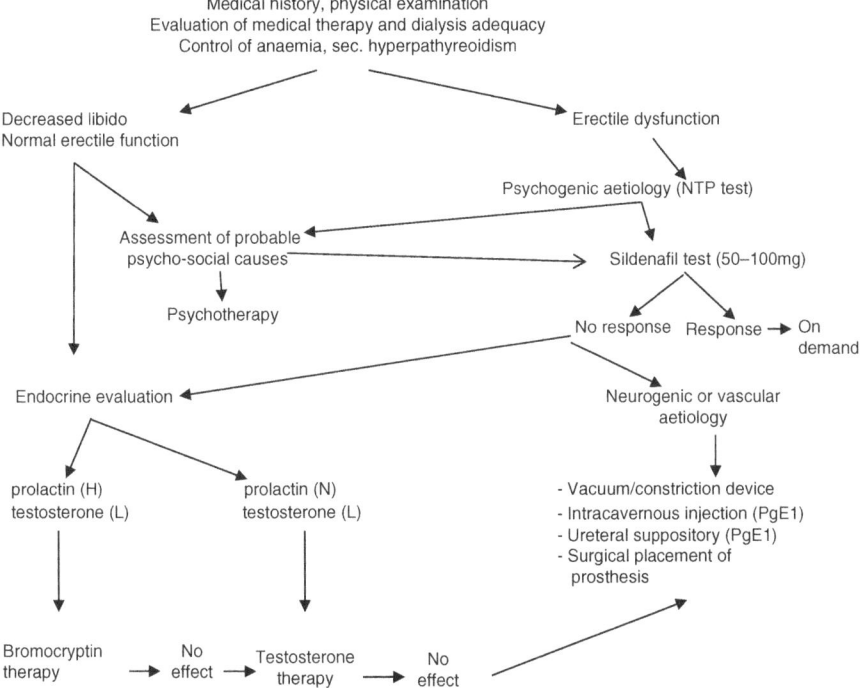

Fig. 10.1 Evaluation and therapy of erectile dysfunction in patients with chronic kidney disease (Data from Palmer [8] and Bellinghieri [44])

as correction of all metabolic alterations and anaemia are of utmost importance. The concept of lifestyle measures should be promoted (smoking cessation, regular physical activity, achieving optimal body mass index). With starting dialysis some of symptoms are improved but without achieving normalisation. Kidney transplantation can have additional beneficial effect, but not in all patients. The patient's nutritional status should be monitored. In patients whom psychogenic cause is suspected, psychotherapy could be advised (rational emotional and/or group therapy).

Poor effectiveness of testosterone replacement therapy was reported in dialysis patients [45, 46]. The effect on libido is more pronounced than the effect on erectile function [46]. The response may be modulated by the patient's nutritional status, activity level and growth hormone values. It has been recommended that this treatment should be initiated only in patients with clear clinical manifestations of biochemically confirmed hypogonadism [47]. Although data related to CV risk are inconclusive (risk for dyslipidaemia and sleep apnea), testosterone should be used with caution, and transdermal application (testosterone enanthate and cypionate) should be preferred. Side effect profile is similar in CKD patients as in other non-CKD hypogonadal patients.

Erythropoietin therapy is associated with lower probability of ED and improved sexual life in haemodialysis patients [41, 42, 48, 49]. Erythropoietin therapy increased global QoL decreasing sensation of fatigue and increasing exercise tolerance. It can lead to normalisation of the pituitary-gonadal feedback mechanism reducing LH, FSH and prolactin and increasing testosterone levels [49]. It is not resolved whether these endocrine changes are solely the result of correction of the anaemia or a direct effect of erythropoietin.

It might be questioned whether deficit in systemic and kidney NO synthesis could decrease the efficacy of PDE-5 inhibitors in CKD patients. However, improvement (60–85 %) in sexual performance and satisfaction was reported in patients undergoing haemodialysis using 50 mg of sildenafil [50, 51]. Nevertheless, in addition to some morphological changes, alterations in NO metabolism in advanced stages of CKD could be the reason of observing somewhat less responses in CKD patients. Sildenafil is the most known and widely used PDE-5 inhibitor which is mostly excreted in the faeces and only 13 % in the urine. Sildenafil pharmacokinetics do not appear to be affected by mild to moderate renal impairment, and clearance of sildenafil is neither reduced in patients with severe CKD nor cleared by haemodialysis [52]. It has similar efficacy in patients on haemodialysis and peritoneal dialysis [53]. The occurrence of side effects is similar to other patients and men groups. Hypotension is the most important problem, but intradialytic hypotension was not reported. However, some authors propose its use on non-dialysis days. Other PDE-5 inhibitors have been approved as well. As in the general population PDE-5 inhibitors are not indicated in patients receiving nitrates. They could be advised to patients with recent coronary events, uncontrolled hypertension and uncompensated heart failure only after the patient achieves normal result on maximal exercise stress testing. The dopamine agonist apomorphine is not contraindicated in patients either on nitrates or on antidepressants. Regarding relative deficiency of NO in CKD patients and its contribution to increased CV risk, some authors raised the question whether treatment with PDE-5 inhibitors could be promising therapy for the CV outcome and not only for improving erectile function.

Vacuum constrictor devices, intraureteral prostaglandins (alprostadil), intracavernous injections of vasoactive agents and penile prosthesis could be used in CKD patients as in all other men having ED. However, intracavernous injections should be cautiously used in uremic patients because of frequently presented platelet dysfunction.

Although some studies did not prove kidney transplantation to have beneficial effect on sexual and ED [43, 54–56], majority of authors [57–61] indicated that this therapy has a positive impact on sexual life. Renal transplantation reverts to normal hormonal alterations [58, 60]. It was reported that libido and penile tumescence are increased by 73 % [61]. However, Tsujimura et al. found that regardless of hormone profiles that had largely returned to normal after transplantation, only 30 % reported an improvement in sexual function [62]. Frequency of intercourse increased only by 37 %, indicating that some of the risk factors for sexual and ED remained after renal transplantation [63, 64]. The possible reasons for the absence of beneficial effect of kidney transplantation on sexual function in some patients are graft dysfunction, compromised penile vascularity, side effects of immunosuppressive and antihypertensive drugs, pre-existing hypertension or diabetes, smoking or some psychological problems (anxiety of the function of the graft). Pourmand et al. reported lower probability of erectile function improvement among patients whose graft was anastomosed to the common iliac artery (this is the source of major blood supply of the penis) [43]. No differences in sexual function were reported between patients treated with cyclosporine or tacrolimus [65]. Kaufman et al. reported that early renal transplantation may have a beneficial effect on the penile vasculopathy [17]. The Cochrane review and meta-analysis of Vecchio et al. based on analyses of data obtained in more than 320 patients concluded that PDE-5 inhibitors and zinc replacement are promising interventions for treating sexual dysfunction in CKD patients [66, 67]. However, they underlined that evidence is limited which points to an unmet need for studying interventions.

Conclusion

ED in CKD patients is a challenging issue. Nephrologists as well as all affiliated physicians and nurses should be aware of the high prevalence of various forms of sexual dysfunction in CKD patients and the impact this has on the QoL. There is a need for screening for sexual and ED as some, or maybe most, abnormalities could be cured or at last improved. Assessment of sexual function should be incorporated into the routine evaluation of all CKD patients. As ED could be considered as a symptom of endothelial dysfunction, all patients with this complaint must be carefully assessed for all other CV risk factors and silent coronary artery disease. As Holley and Schmidt concluded patients at all levels of CKD, socioeconomic status and gender deserve better QoL [68].

References

1. Coresh J M.D., Selvin E, Stevens LA, Manzi J, Kusek JW, Eggers P, Van Lente F, Levey AS (2007) Prevalence of chronic kidney disease in the United States. J Am Med Assoc 298(17):2038–2047
2. Go AS, Chertow GM, Fan D, McCulloch CE, Hsu CY (2004) Chronic kidney disease and the risks of death, cardiovascular events, and hospitalization. N Engl J Med 351(13):1296–1305
3. Modlinger PS, Wilcox CS, Aslam S (2004) Nitric oxide, oxidative stress, and progression of chronic renal failure. Semin Nephrol 24(4):354–365
4. Leão R, Sousa L, Azinhais P, Conceição P, Jorge Pereira B, Borges R, Grenha V, Retroz E, Temido P, Cristo L, Sobral F (2010) Sexual dysfunction in uraemic patients undergoing haemodialysis: predisposing and related conditions. Andrologia 42:166–175
5. Navaneethan SD, Vecchio M, Johnson DW, Saglimbene D, Graziano G, Pellegrini F, Lucisano G, Craig JC, Ruospo M, Gentile G, Manfreda VM, Querques M, Stroumza P, Torok M, Celia E, Gelfman R, Ferrari JN, Bednarek-Skublewska A, Dulawa J, Bonifati C, Hegbrant J et al (2010) Prevalence and correlates of self-reported sexual dysfunction in CKD: a meta-analysis of observational studies. Am J Kidney Dis 56(4):670–685
6. Lai CF, Wang YT, Hung KY, Peng YS, Lien YR, Wu MS, Chang CH, Chiang SS, Yang CS, Shiah CJ, Lu CS, Yang CC, Chuang HF, Wu KD, Tsai TJ, Chen WY (2007) Sexual dysfunction in peritoneal dialysis patients. Am J Nephrol 27(6):615–621
7. Makarem AR, Karami MY, Zekavat OR (2011) Erectile dysfunction among hemodialysis patients. Int Urol Nephrol 43(1):117–123
8. Palmer BF (1999) Sexual dysfunction in uremia. J Am Soc Nephrol 10:1381–1388

9. Palmer BF (2004) Outcomes associated with hypogonadism in men with chronic kidney disease. Adv Chronic Kidney Dis 4:342–347
10. Prem AR, Punekar SV, Kalpana M, Kelkar AR, Acharya VN (1996) Male reproductive function in uraemia: efficacy of haemodialysis and renal transplantation. Br J Urol 78(4):635–638
11. De Vries CP, Gooren LJG, Oe PL (1984) Haemodialysis and testicular function. Int J Androl 7:97–103
12. Handelsman DJ (1985) Hypothalamic-pituitary gonadal dysfunction in renal failure, dialysis, and renal transplantation. Endocr Rev 6:151–182
13. Altman JJ (1988) Sex hormones in chronic renal failure of the diabetic. Ann Endocrinol (Paris) 49(4–5):412–417
14. Malkin CJ, Pugh PJ, Jones RD, Jones TH, Channer KS (2003) Testosterone as a protective factor against atherosclerosis-immunomodulation and influence upon plaque development and stability. J Endocrinol 178(3):373–380
15. Liu PY, Death AK, Handelsman DJ (2003) Androgens and cardiovascular disease. Endocr Rev 24:313–340
16. Gómez F (1980) Endocrine abnormalities in patients undergoing long-term hemodialysis: the role of prolactin. Am J Med 68:522–530
17. Kaufman JM, Hatzichristou DG, Mulhall JP, Fitch WP, Goldstein I (1994) Impotence and chronic renal failure: a study of the hemodynamic pathophysiology. J Urol 151(3):612–618
18. Montorsi P, Ravagnani PM, Galli S, Rotatori F, Briganti A, Salonia A, Rigatti P, Montorsi F (2005) The artery size hypothesis: a macrovascular link between erectile dysfunction and coronary artery disease. Am J Cardiol 96(12B):19–23
19. Ponholzer A, Temml C, Obermayr R et al (2005) Is erectile dysfunction an indicator for increased risk of coronary heart disease and stroke? Eur Urol 48:512–518
20. Gazzaruso C, Giordanetti S, De Amici E, Bertone G, Falcone C, Geroldi D, Fratino P, Solerte SB, Garzaniti A (2004) Relationship between erectile dysfunction and silent myocardial ischemia in apparently uncomplicated type 2 diabetic patients. Circulation 110:22–26
21. Lewis RW, Fugl-Meyer KS, Corona G, Hayes RD, Laumann EO, Moreira ED Jr, Rellini AH, Segraves T (2010) Definitions/epidemiology/risk factors for sexual dysfunction. J Sex Med 7:1598–1607
22. Tizianello A, De Ferrari G, Garibotto G, Gurreri G, Robaudo C (1980) Renal metabolism of amino acids and ammonia in subjects with normal renal function and in patients with chronic renal insufficiency. J Clin Invest 65:1162–1173
23. Baylis C (2006) Arginine, arginine analogs and nitric oxide production in chronic kidney disease. Nat Rev Nephrol 2:209–220
24. Vallance P, Leone A, Calver A, Collier J, Moncada S (1992) Endogenous dimethylarginine as an inhibitor of nitric oxide synthesis. J CVPharmacol 20:60–62
25. Ravani P, Tripepi G, Malberti F, Testa S, Mallamaci F, Zoccali C (2005) Asymmetrical dimethylarginine predicts progression to dialysis and death in patients with chronic kidney disease: a competing risks modeling approach. J Am Soc Nephrol 16:2449–2455
26. Kersh ES, Kronfield SJ, Unger A, Popper RW, Cantor S, Cohn K (1974) Autonomic insufficiency in uremia as a cause of hemodialysis-induced hypotension. N Engl J Med 290:650–653
27. Campese VM, Procci WR, Levitan D et al (1982) Autonomic nervous system dysfunction and impotence in uremia. Am J Nephrol 2:140–143
28. Finkelstein FO, Shirani S, Wuerth D, Finkelstein SH (2007) Therapy insight: sexual dysfunction in patients with chronic kidney disease. Nat Clin Pract Nephrol 3(4):200–207
29. Peng YS, Chiang CK, Hung KY, Chiang SS, Lu CS, Yang CS, Wu KD, Yang CC, Lin RP, Chang CJ, Tsai TJ, Chen WY (2007) The association of higher depressive symptoms and sexual dysfunction in male haemodialysis patients. Nephrol Dial Transplant 22(3):857–861
30. Theofilou PA (2012) Sexual functioning in chronic kidney disease: the association with depression and anxiety. Hemodial Int 16(1):76–81
31. Rosas SE, Joffe M, Franklin E, Strom BL, Kotzker W, Brensinger C, Grossman E, Glasser DB, Feldman HI (2003) Association of decreased quality of life and erectile dysfunction in hemodialysis patients. Kidney Int 64:232–238

32. Lew-Starowicz M, Gellert R (2009) The sexuality and quality of life of hemodialyzed patients—ASED multicenter study. J Sex Med 6(4):1062–1071
33. Steele TE, Wuerth D, Finkelstein S, Juergensen D, Juergensen P, Kliger AS, Finkelstein FO (1996) Sexual experience of the chronic peritoneal dialysis patient. J Am Soc Nephrol 7:1165–1168
34. Rosas SE, Joffe M, Franklin E, Strom BL, Kotzker W, Brensinger C, Grossman E, Glasser D, Feldman HI (2001) Prevalence and determinants of erectile dysfunction in hemodialysis patients. Kidney Int 59(6):2259–2266
35. Tomada N, Natividade P, Vendeira P, Loureiroi A, Rei M (2003) Prevalencia da Disfunctia Erectilnuma Unidade de Hemodialise. Acta Urologica 20(3):45–49
36. Messina LE, Claro JA, Archimedes N, Andrade E, Ortiz V, Srougi M (2007) Erectile dysfunction in patients with chronic renal failure. Int Braz J Urol 33(5):673–678
37. Jackson G, Padley S (2008) Erectile dysfunction and silent coronary artery disease: abnormal computed tomography coronary angiogram in the presence of normal exercise ECGs. Int J Clin Pract 62(6):973–976
38. Inci K, Hazirolan T, Aki FT, Oruc O, Tombul T, Tasar C, Erkan I, Bakkaloglu M, Turgan C, Ergen A (2008) Coronary artery calcifications in hemodialysis patients and their correlation with the prevalence of erectile dysfunction. Transplant Proc 40(1):77–80
39. Bellinghieri G, Santoro D, Mallamace A, Savica V (2008) Sexual dysfunction in chronic renal failure. J Nephrol 21(13):113–117
40. Al Khallaf H (2010) Analysis of sexual functions in male nondiabetic hemodialysis patients and renal transplant recipients. Transpl Int 23(2):176–181
41. Lawrence IG, Price DE, Howlett TA, Harris KP, Feehally J, Walls J (1997) Erythropoietin and sexual dysfunction. Nephrol Dial Transplant 12(4):741–747
42. Beusterien KM, Nissenson AR, Port FK, Kelly M, Steinwald B, Ware JE Jr (1996) The effects of recombinant human erythropoietin on functional health and well-being in chronic dialysis patients. J Am Soc Nephrol 7(5):763–773
43. Pourmand G, Emamzadeh A, Moosavi S, Mehrsai A, Taherimahmoudi M, Nikoobakht M, Saraji A, Salem S (2007) Does renal transplantation improve erectile dysfunction in hemodialysed patients? What is the role of associated factors? Transplant Proc 39(4):1029–1032
44. Bellinghieri G, Santoro D, Lo Forti B, Mallamace A, De Santo RM, Savica V (2001) Erectile dysfunction in uremic dialysis patients: diagnostic evaluation in the sildenafil era. Am J Kidney Dis 38(Suppl 1):115–117
45. Lawrence IG, Price DE, Howlett TA, Harris KP, Feehally J, Walls J (1998) Correcting impotence in the male dialysis patient: experience with testosterone replacement and vacuum tumescence therapy. Am J Kidney Dis 31(2):313–319
46. Johansen KL (2004) Treatment of hypogonadism in men with chronic kidney disease. Adv Chronic Kidney Dis 11(4):348–356
47. Morales A, Lunenfeld B, International Society for the Study of the Aging Male Investigation, treatment and monitoring of late-onset hypogonadism in males (2002) Official recommendations of ISSAM. International Society for the Study of the Aging Male. Aging Male 5(2):74–86
48. Sobh MA, AbdelHamid IA, Atta MG, Refaie AF (1992) Effect of erythropoietin on sexual potency in chronic haemodialysis patients. A preliminary study. Scand J Urol Nephrol 26(2):181–185
49. Kokot F, Wiecek A, Schmidt-Gayk H, Marcinkowski W, Gilge U, Heidland A, Rudka R, Trembecki J (1995) Function of endocrine organs in hemodialyzed patients of long-term erythropoietin therapy. Artif Organs 19(5):428–435
50. Paul HR, McLeish D, Rao TKS, Friedman EA (1999) Initial experience with sildenafil for erectile dysfunction in maintenance hemodialysis (MD) patients. J Am Soc Nephrol 11:222A
51. Rosas SE, Wasserstein A, Kobrin S, Harold I, Feldman HI (2001) Preliminary observations of sildenafil treatment for erectile dysfunction in dialysis patients. Am J Kidney Dis 37(1):134–137
52. Grossman EB, Swan SK, Muirhead GJ et al (2004) The pharmacokinetics and hemodynamics of sildenafil citrate in male hemodialysis patients. Kidney Int 66:367–374

53. Sam R, Patel P (2006) Sildenafil in dialysis patients. Int J Artif Organs 29(3):264–268
54. Espinoza R, Gracida C, Cancino J, Ibarra A (2006) Prevalence of erectile dysfunction in kidney transplant recipients. Transplant Proc 38(3):916–917
55. Mirone V, Longo N, Fusco F, Verze P, Creta M, Parazzini F, Imbimbo C (2009) Renal transplantation does not improve erectile function in hemodialysed patients. Eur Urol 56(6):1047–1053
56. Rebollo P, Ortega F, Valdés C, Fernández-Vega F, Ortega T, García-Mendoza M, Gómez E (2003) Factors associated with erectile dysfunction in male kidney transplant recipients. Int J Impot Res 15:433–438
57. Saha M, Saha H, Niskanen L, Salmela K, Pasternack A (2002) Time course of serum prolactin and sex hormones following successful renal transplantation. Nephron 92:735–737
58. Akbari F, Alavi M, Esteghamati A, Mehrsai A, Djaladat H, Zohrevand R, Pourmand G (2003) Effect of renal transplantation on sperm quality and sex hormone levels. BJU Int 92(3):281–283
59. Barroso LVS, Miranda EP, Cruz NI, Medeiros MAS, Araújo ACO, Mota Filho FHA (2008) Analysis of sexual function in kidney transplanted men. Medeiros Transplant Proc 40(10):3489–3491
60. Burgos FJ et al (1997) Effect of kidney transplantation and cyclosporine treatment on male sexual performance and hormonal profile: a prospective study. Transplant Proc 29:227–228
61. Chu SH, Tay SK, Chiang YJ, Chuang CK, Chen HW, Chen CS, Chou CC, Huang CC (1998) Male sexual performance and hormonal studies in uremic patients and renal transplant recipients. Transplant Proc 30(7):3062–3063
62. Tsujimura A, Matsumiya K, Tsuboniwa N, Yamanaka M, Miura H, Kitamura M, Kishikawa H, Nishimura K, Ichikawa Y, Nagano S, Kokado Y, Takahara S, Okuyama A (2002) Effect of renal transplantation on sexual function. Arch Androl 48(6):467–474
63. Raiz L, Davies EA, Ferguson RM (2003) Sexual functioning following renal transplantation. Health Soc Work 28(4):264–272
64. Diemont WL, Vruggink PA, Meuleman EJ, Doesburg WH, Lemmens WA, Berden JH (2000) Sexual dysfunction after renal replacement therapy. Am J Kidney Dis 35(5):845–851
65. Kantarci G, Sahin S, Uras AR, Ergin H (2004) Effects of different calcineurin inhibitors on sex hormone levels in transplanted male patients. Transplant Proc 36:178
66. Vecchio M, Navaneethan SD, Johnson DW, Lucisano G, Graziano G, Saglimbene V, Ruospo M, Querques M, Jannini EA, Strippoli GF (2010) Interventions for treating sexual dysfunction in patients with chronic kidney disease. Cochrane Database Syst Rev (12):CD007747
67. Vecchio M, Navaneethan SD, Johnson DW, Lucisano G, Graziano G, Querquel M, Saglimbene V, Ruospo M, Bonifati C, Jannini EA, Strippoli GFM (2010) Treatment options for sexual dysfunction in patients with chronic kidney disease: a systematic review of randomized controlled trials. Clin J Am Soc Nephrol 5:985–995
68. Holley JL, Schmidt RJ (2010) Sexual dysfunction in CKD. Am J Kidney Dis 56(4):612–614

Erectile Dysfunction and Sleep Apnea

Jacek Wolf and Krzysztof Narkiewicz

11.1 Introduction

Undisturbed sleep and normal sexual activity comprise essential life needs guaranteeing continuity of the humankind. Recent analyses showed that both sleep and sexual activity started to precisely reflect detrimental influences of the environment, with special emphasis on the role of noncommunicable diseases. Inversely, line of evidence suggests that abnormal sleep and sexual dysfunction markedly determine our somatic and mental health. One of the most prevalent dyssomnias diagnosed in patients seeking medical advice due to poor sleep quality is obstructive sleep apnea (OSA), a condition with potent deleterious impact on cardiovascular control. Interestingly, symptomatology of the OSA syndrome described as early as 1970s [1] include signs of sexual dysfunction, yet the underlying mechanism linking these two conditions has been questioned until today.

In this chapter, we discuss the relationship between erectile dysfunction and one of the most prevalent sleep disorder, namely, obstructive sleep apnea.

11.2 Clinical Overview of Sleep-Disordered Breathing

Sleep-disordered breathing comprises different patterns of abnormal respiratory control during sleep among which obstructive sleep apnea (OSA) appears to be the most prevalent [2]. Other types of unstable breathing during sleep include different forms of central sleep apnea, hypoventilation syndromes, or overlapping syndromes seen in patients with established pulmonary diseases. Diagnosis of sleep-disordered

J. Wolf (✉) • K. Narkiewicz
Department of Hypertension and Diabetology,
Medical University of Gdańsk, Dębinki 7C, Gdańsk 80-952, Poland
e-mail: lupus@gumed.edu.pl; knark@gumed.edu.pl

breathing is based upon overnight study – polysomnography (PSG) or corresponding simplified method polygraphy (PG). Indices derived from PSG or PG recordings are widely accepted as disease markers that allow for detailed sleep apnea severity evaluation. Apnea-Hypopnea Index (AHI) equal or greater than five episodes per hour of sleep arbitrarily establishes the diagnosis. Pertaining to AHI, sleep apnea is further defined as mild (AHI 5–14.9), moderate (15–29.9), and severe (AHI ≥30).

Substantial symptoms of OSA consist of loud irregular snoring, witnessed periods of cessation of breathing, unrefreshing sleep, excessive daytime sleepiness, increased risk for car accidents, hypertension, and decreased libido. The epidemiological data suggest that every fourth adult man and every tenth woman in general, middle-aged population have the basis for sleep apnea diagnosis, where 4 and 2 % of males and females, respectively, may develop clinically overt OSA syndrome [3]. Importantly, OSA is much more prevalent in cardiovascular subpopulations where it remains highly under-recognized, especially in patients with resistant hypertension [4].

Management of different forms of sleep-disordered breathing comprises various modalities where noninvasive continuous positive airway pressure (CPAP) administered at night appears to have the highest applicability and long-term efficacy in OSA reversal. CPAP treatment not only efficiently reduces day- and nighttime symptoms improving quality of life but also decreases OSA-related morbidity and mortality. Unfortunately, adherence to CPAP therapy varies considerably across the OSA population [5].

11.3 Association of Obstructive Sleep Apnea with Selected Erectile Dysfunction Risk Factors

Obstructive sleep apnea and erectile dysfunction are tightly related to the degree of body fat content [6–8]. It is estimated that 70 % of OSA-affected patients have body mass index (BMI) greater than 25 kg/m^2, and the relationship between the content of the adipose tissue reflected in BMI and the severity of sleep apnea appears to be linear [6, 9]. In fact, obesity constitutes a major risk factor for incident sleep-disordered breathing, which is further emphasized by extremely high efficacy of bariatric surgery in sleep apnea amelioration [10]. It is important to mention that the relationship between obesity and sleep apnea appears to be reciprocal. One of the metabolic consequences of the sleep disruption is unfavorable shift in caloric intake and activity energy expenditure [11, 12]. Calvin et al. provided clear-cut evidence that subjects who are sleep deprived are predisposed to excessive food intake with subsequent inevitable weight gain. Specifically in sleep apnea, an abnormal satiety hormonal control which could explain this phenomenon was tested in many studies, yet the evidence is not consistent [13–15]. Interestingly, it has been postulated that BMI reflecting overall body fat is not the most accurate way to depict the interrelationship between sleep apnea and excess in adipose tissue. Analysis of body fat distribution evidenced that visceral adipose tissue to which substantial hormonal activity is attributed is much closer related to sleep apnea than peripheral fat content [16]. Both visceral adipose tissue and its negative correlate – lack of structured physical activity commonly clustering in OSA-patients – are well-recognized factors aggravating erectile function [17, 18].

Another detrimental consequence of central fat excess and sedentary lifestyle is increased type 2 diabetes mellitus (T2DM) morbidity – a very well-established and extremely potent risk factor of erectile dysfunction [19] (*see* Chap. 13). Remarkably, it is estimated that 58–86 % T2DM patients have sleep-disordered breathing [20, 21]. Although obesity has the great potential in moderating the coexistence between OSA and T2DM, other factors directly associated with untreated sleep apnea should not be disregarded in this relationship (intermittent hypoxia, systemic inflammation, neurohormonal changes, i.e., insulin metabolism or sympathetic nervous system overdrive) [9]. Overall, patients with untreated OSA are characterized by modest increases in insulin resistance and poorer glycemia control as reflected by higher HbA1C levels compared to T2DM patients free of sleep-disordered breathing. Anecdotal studies suggested that strength of this association is related to the degree of apnea severity, which persists even after controlling for confounding obesity [22]. Moreover, few short-term interventional studies supplement the concept of the causation role of OSA in worsening of diabetes control. The benefit from regular CPAP use in sleep apnea may additionally result in glucose decrease especially at night [23] and modest decline in HbA1C concentrations [24].

Among other known classical metabolic risk factors implicated in the deterioration of erectile function, evidence linking hypertension to sleep apnea is the most compelling [25–27]. Cross-sectional studies based on both office and ambulatory blood pressure measurements consistently show that patients with essential hypertension have a higher rate of undiagnosed sleep apnea [28] which is especially evident in resistant hypertension [29, 30]. Up to 84–90 % of individuals receiving multiple blood-lowering drug therapy may have concurrent undiagnosed OSA. The analysis of multiple reversible causes of secondary hypertension have shown that previously undiagnosed OSA markedly outnumbers a total of all other known conditions which are implicated in hypertension, including renovascular and kidney- or endocrine-related hypertension [31]. Animal models have evidenced mimicked obstructive sleep apnea as a potentially reversible cause of hypertension [32]. Importantly, this phenomenon has been replicated in human studies, where the effective reversal of OSA with nasal continuous positive airway pressure results in modest, yet sustained blood pressure fall [33]. Effective long-term CPAP treatment has been shown to improve blood pressure control in hypertensive patients, particularly when blood pressure is measured over 24 h [34, 35] and the benefit is greater in patients with more severe sleep apnea [36]. Importantly, CPAP-related blood pressure decrease is seen not only during sleep, but is also extended over the waking state.

11.4 OSA-Related Target Organ Damage

Taking into account vascular origin of the majority of ED cases, it is not surprising that these patients not only share the same pathophysiology but also develop similar complications (see Chap. 7). As compared to noncomplicated individuals, erectile dysfunction is strikingly prevalent in cardiovascular patients with already established target organ damage. What should be particularly stressed is the fact that clustering consequences of accelerated atherosclerosis further deteriorate erectile dysfunction, and this phenomenon apparently goes beyond additive effect of accumulated metabolic risk factors.

Several studies demonstrated that the number of complications primarily ascribed to hypertension alone may in part arise from untreated OSA. This is particularly evident for the main causes of premature cardiovascular mortality, including sudden cardiac deaths during sleep. Severe sleep apnea may also directly translate into nonfatal complications such as higher rate of incident coronary artery disease as well as poorer prognosis after myocardial infarction [37–39]. Another common problem in patients with OSA in comparison to their counterparts free of sleep-disordered breathing is the increased risk for the development of cardiac arrhythmias, as well as its higher reoccurrence rate seen after electrical cardioversion applied for, e.g., atrial fibrillation (AFib) [40–42] The practical clinical message for health professionals who manage patients with recurring AFib is that OSA diagnosis with subsequent CPAP commencement should improve rhythm control [43], as it may concurrently improve erectile function as these two pathologies are frequently coexistent [44]. Analogous associations were found with reference to cerebrovascular disease showing that OSA patients are characterized by an increased risk of a first-time stroke as well as a subsequent negative stroke outcome. The latter appears to be positively influenced by CPAP therapy [37, 45, 46]. Most probably, part of the aforementioned associations may be explained by concurrent drug treatment and disadvantageous metabolic profile; nevertheless, naturally associated with obstructive episodes mechanical stress, i.e., negative intrathoracic pressure swings, together with sympathetic overdrive, oxygen and CO_2 imbalances apparently aggravate these phenomena [47].

11.5 Association of Sexual Dysfunction with Obstructive Sleep Apnea

Although serum testosterone deficiency is not a sole determinant of erectile dysfunction, it is worth mentioning its possible link to sleep-disordered breathing. Few available studies provided an inconsistent evidence on gonadal function assessed by levels of testosterone in OSA male patients. With reference to circadian profile, peak in serum testosterone is seen at night only if accompanied by undisturbed sleep architecture for at least 3 h [48]. Sleep deprivation and abnormal sleep stages distribution is a common problem in OSA patients, which conceivably could translate to lower levels of testosterone. However, after adjustment for other risk factors (mainly obesity), there is no clear correlation between severity of OSA and the depression in gonadal function. Also studies with CPAP interventions produced conflicting results. Overall, short-to-moderate-term CPAP intervention may exert at worse neutral influence on objectively measured male hormones; however, advantageous associations were also reported [49–52]. Based on the available data, it is not likely that acute CPAP administration may directly affect gonadal function of clinical significance; however, an indirect impact mediated through other ED risk factors needs to be determined in long-term, sufficiently powered observations [53].

Severity of erectile dysfunction in the setting of sleep-disordered breathing was also addressed in several smaller cross-sectional, case-control, and interventional studies [54–58]. In general, there is a coherent evidence pointing at clustering of OSA with poor erection status in men, and this relationship appears to be tightly interrelated – the more severe the OSA, the greater erectile dysfunction these patients develop. Interestingly, first OSA syndrome definition proposed by Guilleminault et al. in late 1970s included impotence among typical manifestation of OSAs. For approximately four decades, relatively few studies addressed this problem and our understanding of this phenomenon is yet unsatisfactory.

Possible mechanisms linking OSA to impaired erectile function include repetitive nocturnal hypoxemias with its neuro-, and hormonal consequences. Low mean sleep time saturation may play a crucial role in the deterioration of ED in the setting of OSAS [59]. Patients with poorer saturation who experience more severe problems with penis erection present with neural dysfunction assessed with bulbocavernosus reflex, a widely accepted technique of documenting pudendal neuropathies [56]. Another aspect extensively explored in sleep apnea patients in terms of cardiovascular disease and erection problems is the functional status of endothelium. In fact, based on flow-mediated dilatation method, several cross-sectional studies and one-shot experiments employing CPAP suggested that untreated OSA results in endothelial dysfunction, and the nitric oxide bioavailability may be enhanced upon effective apnea elimination [60–63]. Other postulated mechanisms accompanying OSA which bear the potential to unfavorably modify erectile status include autonomic nervous system imbalances [64], shift in concentrations of vasoactive hormones and/or their precursors (adrenalin, noradrenalin, endothelin-1, aldosterone, angiotensin II) [65–69], low-grade systemic inflammation [70–72], or adverse influences on metabolism regulation promoting obesity and type 2 diabetes (see above).

Given the fact that OSA might play a causative role in worsening erection status in men, then reversal of apneic episodes at night should alleviate the problem, at least to some extent. Although overall CPAP has positive effect on erection status [55, 59, 73], minority of patients (up to 20 %) may experience further worsening of ED while on CPAP [74]. As it was stated above, one of the possible explanation of the discrepant results of the interventional studies with CPAP is unsatisfactory adherence of OSA patients to this treatment modality [75]. Also time of the observation may play the critical role. Interestingly, until today, there is no clear answer to the question of why only a fraction of affected OSA-patients suffer from cardiovascular disease, whereas others do not. Apparently, genetic propensities [76] as well as the elapsed time of the disease [26] should not be disregarded, but the problem seems to be more compound. Patients presenting a similar phenotype may in fact suffer from pathophysiologically different disorders [77, 78] where, e.g., the role of concomitant excessive daytime sleepiness reflecting the degree of sleep architecture disruption remains unclear in terms of cardiovascular morbidity [79]. Overall, these variables may significantly alter interventional studies outcomes including its impact on the erectile function. As of now health professionals should advocate sustained treatment with CPAP for patients with comorbid sleep apnea and ED, as it may not only reverse excessive daytime sleepiness but also enhance the erection status [74] and intimate and sexual relationships [57] in considerable proportion of patients.

Conclusions

Obstructive sleep apnea is highly prevalent in patients with erectile dysfunction, and the mechanisms implicated in this association appear to be very complex. The causation and the dose-response manner of the relationship between severity of obstructive sleep apnea and known risk factors predisposing to the development of erectile dysfunction has been suggested in multiple studies. Line of evidence linked OSA to obesity, hypertension, type 2 diabetes, and cerebrovascular and coronary diseases, all of which are tightly related to the aggravated erectile function. However, a direct negative influence of untreated sleep-disordered breathing on ED should not be disregarded. Since there is evidence showing advantageous effects of CPAP therapy on erectile performance in patients with OSA, the elimination of sleep apnea may constitute an important strategy in the management of these patients.

References

1. Guilleminault C, Eldridge FL, Tilkian A, Simmons FB, Dement WC (1977) Sleep apnea syndrome due to upper airway obstruction: a review of 25 cases. Arch Intern Med 137:296–300
2. American Academy of Sleep Medicine (2005) International classification of sleep disorders, 2nd edn. Diagnostic and coding manual. Westchester, IL: American Academy of Sleep Medicine
3. Young T, Palta M, Dempsey J et al (1993) The occurrence of sleep-disordered breathing among middle-aged adults. N Engl J Med 328:1230–1235
4. Logan AG, Perlikowski SM, Mente A et al (2001) High prevalence of unrecognized sleep apnoea in drug-resistant hypertension. J Hypertens 2001(19):2271–2277
5. Grote L, Hedner J, Grunstein R et al (2000) Therapy with nCPAP: incomplete elimination of Sleep Related Breathing Disorder. Eur Respir J 16:921–927
6. Newman AB, Nieto FJ, Guidry U, Lind BK, Redline S, Pickering TG, Quan SF, Sleep Heart Health Study Research Group (2001) Relation of sleep-disordered breathing to cardiovascular disease risk factors: the Sleep Heart Health Study. Am J Epidemiol 154:50–59
7. Feldman HA, Johannes CB, Derby CA, Kleinman KP, Mohr BA, Araujo AB, McKinlay JB (2000) Erectile dysfunction and coronary risk factors: prospective results from the Massachusetts male aging study. Prev Med 30:328–338
8. Hammoud AO, Gibson M, Peterson CM, Hamilton BD, Carrell DT (2006) Obesity and male reproductive potential. J Androl 27:619–626
9. Wolk R, Shamsuzzaman AS, Somers VK (2003) Obesity, sleep apnea, and hypertension. Hypertension 42:1067–1074
10. Buchwald H, Avidor Y, Braunwald E, Jensen MD, Pories W, Fahrbach K, Schoelles K (2004) Bariatric surgery: a systematic review and meta-analysis. JAMA 292:1724–1737
11. Baud MO, Magistretti PJ, Petit JM (2013) Sustained sleep fragmentation affects brain temperature, food intake and glucose tolerance in mice. J Sleep Res 22:3–12
12. Calvin AD, Carter RE, Adachi T, Macedo PG, Albuquerque FN, van der Walt C, Bukartyk J, Davison DE, Levine JA, Somers VK (2013) Effects of experimental sleep restriction on caloric intake and activity energy expenditure. Chest 144:79–86

13. Phillips BG, Kato M, Narkiewicz K et al (2000) Increases in leptin levels, sympathetic drive, and weight gain in obstructive sleep apnea. Am J Physiol 279:H234–H237
14. Patel SR, Palmer LJ, Larkin EK et al (2004) Relationship between obstructive sleep apnea and diurnal leptin rhythms. Sleep 27:206–210
15. Sánchez-de-la-Torre M, Mediano O, Barceló A, Piérola J, de la Peña M, Esquinas C, Miro A, Durán-Cantolla J, Agustí AG, Capote F, Marin JM, Montserrat JM, García-Río F, Barbé F (2012) The influence of obesity and obstructive sleep apnea on metabolic hormones. Sleep Breath 16:649–656
16. Dobrosielski DA, Patil SP (2013) Weight loss and obstructive sleep apnea: what lies AHEAD? SLEEP 36:627–629
17. Esposito KG, Giugliano F, Di Palo C, Giugliano G, Marfella R, D'Andrea F, D'Armiento M, Giugliano D (2004) Effect of lifestyle changes on erectile dysfunction in obese men: a randomized controlled trial. JAMA 291:2978–2984
18. Despres JP, Lemieux I (2006) Abdominal obesity and metabolic syndrome. Nature 444:881–887
19. Hermans MP, Ahn SA, Rousseau MF (2009) Erectile dysfunction, microangiopathy and UKPDS risk in type 2 diabetes. Diabetes Metab 35:484–489
20. Resnick HE, Redline S, Shahar E, Gilpin A, Newman A, Walter R, Ewy GA, Howard BV, Punjabi NM, Sleep Heart Health Study (2003) Diabetes and sleep disturbances: findings from the Sleep Heart Health Study. Diabetes Care 26:702–709
21. Foster GD, Sanders MH, Millman R, Zammit G, Borradaile KE, Newman AB, Wadden TA, Kelley D, Wing RR, Sunyer FX, Darcey V, Kuna ST, Sleep AHEAD Research Group (2009) Obstructive sleep apnea among obese patients with type 2 diabetes. Diabetes Care 32:1017–1019
22. Pillai A, Warren G, Gunathilake W, Idris I (2011) Effects of sleep apnea severity on glycemic control in patients with type 2 diabetes prior to continuous positive airway pressure treatment. Diabetes Technol Ther 13:945–949
23. Dawson A, Abel SL, Loving RT, Dailey G, Shadan FF, Cronin JW, Kripke DF, Kline LE (2008) CPAP therapy of obstructive sleep apnea in type 2 diabetics improves glycemic control during sleep. J Clin Sleep Med 4:538–542
24. Babu AR, Herdegen J, Fogelfeld L, Shott S, Mazzone T (2005) Type 2 diabetes, glycemic control, and continuous positive airway pressure in obstructive sleep apnea. Arch Intern Med 165:447–452
25. Lavie P, Herer P, Hoffstein V (2000) Obstructive sleep apnoea syndrome as a risk factor for hypertension: population study. BMJ 320:479–482
26. Peppard PE, Young T, Palta M et al (2000) Prospective study of the association between sleep-disordered breathing and hypertension. N Engl J Med 342:1378–1784
27. Nieto FJ, Young TB, Lind BK et al (2000) Association of sleep-disordered breathing, sleep apnea, and hypertension in a large community-based study. Sleep Heart Health Study. JAMA 283:1829–1836
28. Calhoun DA (2010) Obstructive sleep apnea and hypertension. Curr Hypertens Rep 12:189–195
29. Logan AG, Perlikowski SM, Mente A et al (2001) High prevalence of unrecognized sleep apnoea in drug-resistant hypertension. J Hypertens 19:2271–2277
30. Lloberes P, Lozano L, Sampol G et al (2010) Obstructive sleep apnoea and 24-h blood pressure in patients with resistant hypertension. J Sleep Res 19:597–602
31. Pedrosa RP, Drager LF, Gonzaga CC et al (2011) Obstructive sleep apnea: the most common secondary cause of hypertension associated with resistant hypertension. Hypertension 58:811–817
32. Brooks D, Horner RL, Kozar LF et al (1997) Obstructive sleep apnea as a cause of systemic hypertension. Evidence from a canine model. J Clin Invest 99:106–109
33. Fava C, Dorigoni S, Dalle Vedove F, Danese E, Montagnana M, Guidi GC, Narkiewicz K, Minuz P (2013) Effect of continuous positive airway pressure (CPAP) on blood pressure in patients with obstructive sleep apnea/hypopnea. A systematic review and meta-analysis (2014). Chest 145:762–771

34. Wilcox I, Grunstein RR, Hedner JA et al (1993) Effect of nasal continuous positive airway pressure during sleep on 24-hour blood pressure in obstructive sleep apnea. Sleep 16:539–544
35. Faccenda JF, Mackay TW, Boon NA et al (2001) Randomized placebo-controlled trial of continuous positive airway pressure on blood pressure in the sleep apnea–hypopnea syndrome. Am J Respir Crit Care Med 163:344–348
36. Pepperell JC, Ramdassingh-Dow S, Crosthwaite N et al (2002) Ambulatory blood pressure after therapeutic and subtherapeutic nasal continuous positive airway pressure for obstructive sleep apnoea: a randomised parallel trial. Lancet 359:204–210
37. Shahar E, Whitney CW, Redline S et al (2001) Sleep-disordered breathing and cardiovascular disease. Cross-sectional results of the Sleep Heart Health Study. Am J Respir Crit Care Med 163:19–25
38. Peker Y, Kraiczi H, Hedner J et al (1999) An independent association between obstructive sleep apnoea and coronary artery disease. Eur Respir J 13:179–184
39. Peker Y, Hedner J, Kraiczi H et al (2000) Respiratory disturbance index – an independent predictor of mortality in coronary artery disease. Am J Respir Crit Care Med 162:81–86
40. Guilleminault C, Connolly SJ, Winkle RA (1983) Cardiac arrhythmia and conduction disturbances during sleep in 400 patients with sleep apnea syndrome. Am J Cardiol 52: 490–494
41. Gami AS, Pressman G, Caples SM et al (2004) Association of atrial fibrillation and obstructive sleep apnea. Circulation 110:364–367
42. Mehra R, Benjamin EJ, Sahar E et al (2006) Association of nocturnal arrhythmias with sleep-disordered breathing. The Sleep Heart Health Study. Am J Respir Crit Care Med 173:910–916
43. Kanagala R, Murali NS, Friedman PA et al (2003) Obstructive sleep apnea and the recurrence of atrial fibrillation. Circulation 107:2589–2594
44. Szymański FM, Puchalski B, Filipiak KJ (2013) Obstructive sleep apnea, atrial fibrillation, and erectile dysfunction: are they only coexisting conditions or a new clinical syndrome? The concept of the OSAFED syndrome. Pol Arch Med Wewn 123:701–707
45. Yaggi HK, Concato J, Kernan WN, Lichtman JH, Brass LM, Mohsenin V (2005) Obstructive sleep apnea as a risk factor for stroke and death. N Engl J Med 353:2034–2041
46. Martinez-Garcia MA, Galiano-Blancart R, Roman-Sanchez P et al (2005) Continuous positive airway pressure treatment in sleep apnea prevents new vascular events after ischemic stroke. Chest 128:2123–2129
47. Johnson CB, Beanlands RS, Yoshinaga K et al (2008) Acute and chronic effects of continuous positive airway pressure therapy on left ventricular systolic and diastolic function in patients with obstructive sleep apnea and congestive heart failure. Can J Cardiol 24:697–704
48. Wittert G (2014) The relationship between sleep disorders and testosterone in men. Asian J Androl 16:262–265
49. Hoekema A, Stel AL, Stegenga B, van der Hoeven JH, Wijkstra PJ, van Driel MF, de Bont LG (2007) Sexual function and obstructive sleep apnea-hypopnea: a randomized clinical trial evaluating the effects of oral-appliance and continuous positive airway pressure therapy. J Sex Med 4:1153–1162
50. Bratel T, Wennlund A, Carlström K (1999) Pituitary reactivity, androgens and catecholamines in obstructive sleep apnoea. Effects of continuous positive airway pressure treatment (CPAP). Respir Med 93:1–7
51. Luboshitzky R, Lavie L, Shen-Orr Z, Lavie P (2003) Pituitary-gonadal function in men with obstructive sleep apnea. The effect of continuous positive airways pressure treatment. Neuro Endocrinol Lett 24:463–467
52. Grunstein RR, Handelsman DJ, Lawrence SJ, Blackwell C, Caterson ID, Sullivan CE (1989) Neuroendocrine dysfunction in sleep apnea: reversal by continuous positive airways pressure therapy. J Clin Endocrinol Metab 68:352–358
53. Knapp A, Myhill PC, Davis WA, Peters KE, Hillman D, Hamilton EJ, Lim EM, Davis TM (2014) Effect of continuous positive airway pressure therapy on sexual function and serum testosterone in males with type 2 diabetes and obstructive sleep apnoea. Clin Endocrinol (Oxf) 81:254–258

54. Budweiser S, Enderlein S, Jörres RA, Hitzl AP, Wieland WF, Pfeifer M, Arzt M (2009) Sleep apnea is an independent correlate of erectile and sexual dysfunction. J Sex Med 6:3147–3157
55. Taskin U, Yigit O, Acioglu E, Aricigil M, Toktas G, Guzelhan Y (2010) Erectile dysfunction in severe sleep apnea patients and response to CPAP. Int J Impot Res 22:134–139
56. Fanfulla F, Malaguti S, Montagna T, Salvini S, Bruschi C, Crotti P, Casale R, Rampulla C (2000) Erectile dysfunction in men with obstructive sleep apnea: an early sign of nerve involvement. Sleep 23:775–781
57. Reishtein JL, Maislin G, Weaver TE, Multisite Study group (2010) Outcome of CPAP treatment on intimate and sexual relationships in men with obstructive sleep apnea. J Clin Sleep Med 6:221–226
58. Margel D, Cohen M, Livne PM, Pillar G (2004) Severe, but not mild, obstructive sleep apnea syndrome is associated with erectile dysfunction. Urology 63:545–549
59. Gonçalves MA, Guilleminault C, Ramos E, Palha A, Paiva T (2005) Erectile dysfunction, obstructive sleep apnea syndrome and nasal CPAP treatment. Sleep Med 6:333–339
60. Carlson JT, Rangemark C, Hedner JA (1996) Attenuated endothelium-dependent vascular relaxation in patients with sleep apnoea. J Hypertens 14:577–584
61. Kraiczi H, Caidahl K, Samuelsson A et al (2001) Impairment of vascular endothelial function and left ventricular filling. Association with the severity of apnea-induced hypoxemia during sleep. Chest 119:1085–1091
62. Kato M, Roberts-Thomson P, Phillips BG et al (2000) Impairment of endothelium-dependent vasodilation of resistance vessels in patients with obstructive sleep apnea. Circulation 102:2607–2610
63. Bayram NA, Ciftci B, Keles T et al (2009) Endothelial function in normotensive men with obstructive sleep apnea before and 6 months after CPAP treatment. Sleep 32:1257–1263
64. Somers VK, Dyken ME, Clary MP, Abboud FM (1995) Sympathetic neural mechanisms in obstructive sleep apnea. J Clin Invest 96:1897–1904
65. Phillips BG, Narkiewicz K, Pesek CA et al (1999) Effects of obstructive sleep apnea on endothelin-1 and blood pressure. J Hypertens 17:61–66
66. Jordan W, Reinbacher A, Cohrs S et al (2005) Obstructive sleep apnea: Plasma endothelin-1 precursor but not endothelin-1 levels are elevated and decline with nasal continuous positive airway pressure. Peptides 26:1654–1660
67. Gjørup PH, Sadauskiene L, Wessels J et al (2007) Abnormally increased endothelin-1 in plasma during the night in obstructive sleep apnea: relation to blood pressure and severity of disease. Am J Hypertens 20:44–52
68. Moller DS, Lind P, Strunge B et al (2003) Abnormal vasoactive hormones and 24-hour blood pressure in obstructive sleep apnea. Am J Hypertens 16:274–280
69. Calhoun DA, Nishizaka MK, Zaman MA et al (2004) Aldosterone excretion among subjects with resistant hypertension and symptoms of sleep apnea. Chest 125:112–117
70. Shamsuzzaman AS, Winnicki M, Lanfranchi P et al (2002) Elevated C-reactive protein in patients with obstructive sleep apnea. Circulation 105:2462–2464
71. Kokturk O, Ciftci TU, Mollarecep E et al (2005) Elevated C-reactive protein levels and increased cardiovascular risk in patients with obstructive sleep apnea syndrome. Int Heart J 46:801–809
72. Yokoe T, Minoguchi K, Matsuo H et al (2003) Elevated levels of C-reactive protein and interleukin-6 in patients with obstructive sleep apnea syndrome are decreased by nasal continuous positive airway pressure. Circulation 107:1129–1134
73. Budweiser S, Luigart R, Jörres RA, Kollert F, Kleemann Y, Wieland WF, Pfeifer M, Arzt M (2013) Long-term changes of sexual function in men with obstructive sleep apnea after initiation of continuous positive airway pressure. J Sex Med 10:524–531
74. Margel D, Tal R, Livne PM, Pillar G (2005) Predictors of erectile function improvement in obstructive sleep apnea patients with long-term CPAP treatment. Int J Impot Res 17: 186–190
75. Treatment compliance with continuous positive airway pressure device among adults with obstructive sleep apnea (OSA): how many adhere to treatment? (2013) Harefuah 152:140–144. Abstract

76. Bostrom KB, Hedner J, Melander O et al (2007) Interaction between the angiotensin-converting enzyme gene insertion/deletion polymorphism and obstructive sleep apnoea as a mechanism for hypertension. J Hypertens 25:779–783
77. Younes M, Ostrowski M, Thompson W et al (2001) Chemical control stability in patients with obstructive sleep apnea. Am J Respir Crit Care Med 163:1181–1190
78. Xie A, Bedekar A, Skatrud JB et al (2011) The heterogeneity of obstructive sleep apnea (predominant obstructive vs pure obstructive apnea). Sleep 34:745–750
79. Kapur VK, Resnick HE, Gottlieb DJ (2008) Sleep disordered breathing and hypertension: does self-reported sleepiness modify the association? Sleep 31:1127–1132

Diabetes Mellitus and Erectile Dysfunction

12

Barbara Nikolaidou, Christos Nouris, Antonios Lazaridis, Christos Sampanis, and Michael Doumas

12.1 Introduction

Erectile dysfunction (ED), defined as the inability of the male to attain and maintain erection of the penis sufficient to permit satisfactory sexual intercourse [1], provokes diminishing effects on the patient's quality of life. This disorder was described in 5,000-year-old Egyptian scriptures [2], but only in the last few decades has it been consolidated as a distinct clinical entity. Evidence suggests that ED usually coexists and shares common pathophysiological pathways with several morbidities such as the metabolic syndrome, cardiovascular disease, and diabetes mellitus (DM). Specifically, in diabetic patients, ED is presented earlier, more frequently, and is more severe and resistant to treatment than in the general population, reflecting the challenge posed on the medical community implicated in the diagnosis and management of this disease.

B. Nikolaidou (✉) • A. Lazaridis • C. Sampanis
2nd Propedeutic Department of Internal Medicine, Aristotle University, Thessaloniki, Greece
e-mail: barbienn@yahoo.gr; spanbiol@hotmail.com; chsambanis@gmail.com

C. Nouris
Department of Anesthesiology and Intensive Care, Aristotle University, Thessaloniki, Greece
e-mail: xnouris@yahoo.gr

M. Doumas
2nd Propedeutic Department of Internal Medicine, Aristotle University, Thessaloniki, Greece

George Washington University, Washington, DC, USA
e-mail: michalisdoumas@yahoo.co.uk

12.2 Prevalence

Diabetes mellitus, a contemporary growing pandemic, plays a pivotal role in the appearance of cardiovascular and renal disease. It is responsible for the shortening of life expectancy with a huge financial cost of medical treatment. DM prevalence was estimated at 9.8 % in men and 9.2 % in women in 2008, showing an increase from 8.3 and 7.5 % in 1980, respectively [3]. In the USA alone, DM prevalence increased from 6.4 % (1999–2000) to 7.8 % (2003–2004) which might be attributed to vigilance and early diagnosis of the disease and is correlated to the ageing of the population [4], since prevalence regarding ages older than 65 approaches 21.2 % [5]. According to the World Health Organization, the number of people with type 2 DM is increasing worldwide. In 2013, 382 million people had DM and the number is estimated to rise to 592 million in 2035. Health expenditure concerning DM in 2013 was 548 billion US dollars [6]. Despite the medical progress in DM management, the complications of the disease provoke detrimental, sometimes even fatal, effects. Some of these include diabetic nephropathy, neuropathy, retinopathy, and finally, cardiovascular disease, the most important cause of death in patients suffering from DM [7]. Among different complications of DM, erectile dysfunction (ED) plays a key role not only because of its specific importance on quality of life but also because it shares a similar pathogenetic process with the cardiovascular complications of DM.

ED was underestimated for a long time, and only in the last few decades, physicians began looking into the problem through targeted studies. Nevertheless, the real prevalence of ED cannot be precisely estimated because physicians do not usually seek this disorder out. Available studies differ in quality due to the use of different definitions of ED, different study tools, different interpretations of results, and cultural disparities in the willingness to discuss sexual issues. Consequently, results cannot be applied to the general population. The precise prevalence concerning the general population is unclear and varies in different studies ranging from 7 to 53 %. However, it is estimated that 15–20 % of the general population suffers from ED [8]. In a recent study in which 22,839 men from eight different countries participated (Men's Attitudes to Life Events and Sexuality, MALES study), the prevalence of ED amounted to 16 % [9]. The numbers are much higher when it comes to specific population groups, like diabetics.

Diabetic men are two [10] to three times [11] more likely to develop ED than nondiabetic men. In addition, ED seems to appear 10 years earlier in DM patients than in the general population [12]. ED is associated with age both in the general population and in diabetic patients, thus in diabetics above the age of 60, prevalence reaches 95 % [13]. Men with DM experience more severe ED than nondiabetic men with ED, resulting in a worse disease-specific health-related quality of life [14]. Only few studies concern newly diagnosed diabetic patients [15–17] according to which 31–43 % suffer from ED. Most studies do not compare the prevalence of ED between type 1 and type 2 DM. Therefore, it is difficult to determine whether there are differences between the two major types of DM. It seems that no significant difference exists in prevalence of ED between the two types of DM after taking into account the effect of age [10, 18].

12.3 Risk Factors of Erectile Dysfunction

Age and duration of DM have been consistently shown to increase the risk of ED [19]. DM is the second greatest risk factor of ED, following age [11]. ED in DM is associated with the appearance of microvascular (retinopathy [20], neuropathy, and nephropathy) [21, 22] and macrovascular (cardiovascular disease) [19] complications in several studies. Poor glycemic control and high HbA1 levels are correlated to ED in some studies [21, 23, 24], but in other studies, such a correlation is not evident [25]. In the case that DM coexists with other diseases, such as hypertension [26] and cardiovascular disease, the possibility of appearance of ED is enhanced. Several cross-sectional and longitudinal studies have linked the development of ED, apart from DM, hypertension, and cardiovascular disease to hyperlipidemia [21, 27], obesity [28], insulin resistance, metabolic syndrome [23], lower urinary tract symptoms [29], and depression [30]. Lifestyle habits like smoking [21], sedentary life [31], and alcohol consumption have an additional negative effect on sexual function [32], but in some studies, moderate consumption of alcohol ameliorates ED [12, 18]. Several drugs contribute to the appearance of ED including antihypertensives (thiazide diuretics, b-blockers), antiarrhythmics (digoxin), psychotropics (tricyclic antidepressants, selective serotonin reuptake inhibitors, butyrophenones) and recreational substances (marijuana, opiates, cocaine) [33], and steroid agents [2]. The role of statins in the appearance of ED is still controversial [34]. Moreover, it has been proven that the number of medications administered is associated with the worsening of ED, even after comorbidities have been taken into account [35].

12.4 Pathophysiology

The pathophysiology of ED induced by DM is more complicated than in the general population. DM seems to affect different pathophysiological paths, in some cases more than one, simultaneously.

Diabetes mellitus as a chronic disease with multiple and serious complications is closely correlated to depression. According to a recent meta-analysis, patients suffering from DM present a twofold risk of depression [36]. Furthermore, ED worsens any preexisting depressive symptoms [37], which implies that it functions as a reinforcing mechanism. The development of ED can generate anxiety. Additionally, the lack of the partner's support can aggravate the condition. The sequence of these events leads to poor self-esteem and amplification of anxiety in both diabetic men and their partners, resulting in poor erectile function or worsening of the existing ED.

Vasculogenic ED is due to functional or structural impairment of the endothelium. Nitric oxide (NO) is synthesized from L-arginine by the endothelium of the penis arteries and nitrergic neurons, utilizing endothelial (eNOS) and neuronal (NOS) NO synthase, respectively. NO mediates relaxation of the corpus cavernosum and ultimately erection, through the formation of cyclic guanosine monophosphate (cGMP). One of the effector proteins for cGMP is cGMP-dependent protein kinase-1 (PKG-1) which is significantly reduced in diabetic rabbits [38]. DM is characterized by higher concentration of endothelin-1, a potent vasoconstrictor and pro-inflammatory peptide, which is associated with endothelial dysfunction. Furthermore, alterations in endothelin receptor sensitivity may enhance vasoconstrictor processes. Endothelin-1 has been involved in the RhoA/Rho kinase pathway whose consequent activation suppresses eNOS, decreasing the production of NO. Rho kinase is suggested to be upregulated in diabetics [39]. Moreover, data suggest that diabetic men present a different pattern of endothelial cell injury with differences in circulating endothelial microparticles and increased apoptotic activity compared to nondiabetic ED men [40].

Given that insulin has vasodilatory effects through NOS upregulation, insulin resistance is correlated to defective endothelial function and vasoconstriction [41]. Hyperglycemia in DM leads to the formation of advanced glycation end products (AGEs) which form covalent bonds with vascular collagen, leading to vascular thickening, decreased elasticity, endothelial dysfunction, and atherosclerosis [42]. Asymmetric dimethylarginine (ADMA), an endogenous analogue of L-arginine that competitively inhibits NOS, is elevated in DM and ED. High ADMA levels induce endothelial dysfunction and predict cardiovascular events [43]. Additionally, reduced production of NOS is induced by (a) overexpression of argininase II, an enzyme which is a NOS antagonist in the common substrate arginine, and (b) deficiency of NAPH, a necessary cofactor of NOS. The reduction of NADPH is also associated with the increased smooth muscle contractility by means of increased diacylglycerol and protein kinase C. Oxidative stress which is present in DM leads to the accumulation of free oxygen radicals and decreased levels of NO [44].

Autonomic neuropathy-induced ED is attributed to the reduction of the parasympathetic tone resulting in decreased NOS activity and consequent reduction in NO release from endothelial cells and non-adrenergic, non-cholinergic neurons. Further contributing mechanisms are increased oxidative stress, nerve hypoxia, and raised protein kinase C production [44]. Peripheral neuropathy involves impairment of sensory and motor neurons resulting in disrupted conduction of afferent and efferent impulses from and to the penis [45]. In some diabetic men, dysfunction of the penile nerves precedes neuropathy in the other peripheral nerves [46].

Hypogonadism is associated with DM, obesity, and ED. Prevalence of hypogonadism in the general population is quoted as 20 % of men aged 60–69 years, but in obesity and DM, it rises to 44 % [47]. According to a recent meta-analysis, DM can be considered independently associated with male hypogonadism [48]. Total testosterone is significantly lower in men with DM [49]. Patients with low testosterone concentrations present increased insulin resistance [50], poor glycemic control, and worsening of ED [51]. Testosterone is implicated in the process of NOS and phosphodiesterase type 5 (PDE5) production to the penis [52]. Possible mechanisms which interfere with hypogonadism in DM are: (a) low plasma concentration of sex hormone-binding globulin (SHBG), the major carrier of testosterone; (b) increased aromatase activity in visceral adipose tissue leading to decreased testosterone levels through conversion to estradiol; (c) reduced secretion of luteinizing hormone and testosterone due to DM-associated leptin resistance [31], and (d) high insulin resistance leading to a reduction in insulin action in hypothalamus resulting in hypogonadotropic hypogonadism [53]. ED and male hypogonadism are considered predictors of forthcoming metabolic disorders and cardiovascular events, although the specific pathologic pathways are not clear yet [48].

Other possible modalities which induce ED are hyperprolactinemia, hyperhomocysteinemia, disturbances of the thyroid gland, certain neurological disorders, and anatomical abnormalities of the penis [2, 54].

12.5 Management

In recent years, the introduction of numerous therapeutic strategies has revolutionized the management of patients with ED [2]. The substantial advances in the treatment of ED have led some authors to believe that a trial of oral therapy after taking a patient's history and performing a physical examination is all that is needed to treat ED [55]. However, this does not seem the case in men with DM who represent one of the most difficult to treat subgroups of ED patients [56]. Despite the considerable progress, the treatment of ED in diabetic patients remains difficult and complex [45].

Evidence suggests that ED presents substantial disparities in the diabetic population compared to nondiabetics which affect treatment options. The development of ED in diabetic men is complex and multifactorial [45] necessitating a holistic approach which incorporates several treatment modalities. Furthermore, diabetic ED is more resistant to treatment compared with nondiabetic ED. Diabetic men with ED may respond less to first-line treatments and are more likely to require more aggressive treatment [57].

Diagnostic evaluation plays a pivotal role in the management of DM patients with ED. The increased incidence and severity of ED in diabetic men [11] makes the diagnosis of ED a priority. Because men fail to volunteer their ED, health care professionals who treat patients with DM should raise the subject as part of their routine care [58]. Structured interviews [59] and self-reported questionnaires [60] are used by physicians as standardized sexual inventories to confront ED.

On the other hand, diabetic patients complaining of ED should be carefully investigated in terms of concomitant morbidities at an early stage. A strong and independent association between ED and cardiovascular disease has been established. ED is able to predict future cardiovascular events in diabetic patients [61] and appears to be strongly associated with the presence of silent CAD in apparently uncomplicated type 2 diabetes patients [62]. Thus, ED can mark the starting point for the evaluation and prevention of severe diseases. A minimal diagnostic evaluation must be performed in every DM patient suffering from ED [63]. The diagnostic approach includes an accurate medical and sexual history, a careful physical examination, and targeted laboratory tests of the patient's glycemic and lipid profile and testosterone levels [64]. The main goals of the assessment of ED are to identify the cause of the disorder and to ascertain risk factors and potentially life-threatening comorbid disorders.

The first step in the treatment of ED is the implementation of general measures to correct the modifiable risk factors. Lifestyle interventions such as smoking cessation, weight reduction, and increased physical activity can improve erectile function significantly [31]. Treatment of systematic diseases associated with ED is necessary. Obtaining good glycemic control is of paramount importance [65]. Prescription and over-the-counter medications that may have negative implications on sexual function should be avoided or switched to agents least likely to cause ED. Additionally, relationship counseling and psychotherapy may be useful for treating anxiety and depression.

Combined with general measures, oral therapies are regarded as the first-choice treatment strategy for ED. Phosphodiesterase type 5 inhibitors (PDE5i) are the mainstay of treatment of ED. They interfere with the NO-cGMP pathway resulting in prolonged relaxation of the cavernous smooth muscles and thus enhancing erectile function. Chronic use of PDE5i significantly improves endothelial function [66] and might reduce cardiovascular events [67]. Sildenafil, tadalafil, and vardenafil are worldwide available and have proven to be effective in diabetic men with ED [68]. However, the response to such treatment has been lower in diabetic than in nondiabetic subjects [69]. Diabetics require high doses of each agent and studies have shown an incremental clinical benefit with higher doses [70]. All three drugs indicate favorable safety profiles, but there is no sufficient information to single out the superior efficacy of any one of them [45, 58].

Testosterone plays an important part in maintaining adequate erectile function; however, testosterone replacement therapy is only recommended in DM men with ED who have proven low concentrations of bioavailable testosterone [71]. Despite the fact that antihypertensives are commonly associated with ED, recent data suggest that angiotensin receptor blockers [72] and nebivolol [73] could have a positive effect on erectile function. Statins seem to play a double-edged role in the treatment of ED, and there is controversial evidence about their effect on erectile function [74, 75]. Emerging evidence derived from a systematic review and meta-analysis revealed positive consequences of statins on erectile function [34].

Patients not responding to oral drugs may benefit from second- and third-line treatment. Intracavernosal injections and transurethral suppositories are used for the topical administration of vasoactive substances, such as alprostadil, papaverine, phentolamine, and vasoactive intestinal polypeptide, to the penile tissue. Vacuum constriction devices have been used as mechanical means of increasing and retaining blood in the penis for initiating erection but nearly half of the patients are not satisfied with this method [2]. Surgical implantation of penile artificial prosthesis is the last resort for treatment of ED and high satisfaction rates are reported.

Conclusions

Taking into consideration that sexual health is indissolubly associated with physical health, clinicians should persistently aim for the early diagnosis and proper management of ED in diabetic patients. A holistic approach composed of a careful medical history, a thorough clinical examination, basic laboratory tests, and composite and individualized treatment appears to be the gold standard for the management of ED in diabetics. In recent years, ED has drawn the attention of the scientific community, especially after having been recognized as a precursor of cardiovascular disease. Ongoing research on a molecular level has led to the better understanding of the physiology of the erectile mechanism and the pathophysiology of ED and has provided the basis for the introduction of novel and promising therapies.

References

1. NIH Consensus Conference. Impotence. NIH Consensus Development Panel on Impotence (1993) JAMA 270(1):83–90
2. Shamloul R, Ghanem H (2013) Erectile dysfunction. Lancet 381(9861):153–165
3. Danaei G et al (2011) National, regional, and global trends in fasting plasma glucose and diabetes prevalence since 1980: systematic analysis of health examination surveys and epidemiological studies with 370 country-years and 2.7 million participants. Lancet 378(9785):31–40
4. Ong KL et al (2008) Prevalence, treatment, and control of diagnosed diabetes in the U.S. National Health and nutrition examination survey 1999–2004. Ann Epidemiol 18(3):222–229
5. McDonald M et al (2009) Prevalence, awareness, and management of hypertension, dyslipidemia, and diabetes among United States adults aged 65 and older. J Gerontol A Biol Sci Med Sci 64(2):256–263
6. International Diabetes Federation (2013) IDF Diabetes Atlas, 6th edn. Brussels, Belgium: International Diabetes Federation. http://www.idf.org/diabetesatlas
7. Golden SH (2011) Emerging therapeutic approaches for the management of diabetes mellitus and macrovascular complications. Am J Cardiol 108(3 Suppl):59B–67B
8. Viigimaa M et al (2011) Hypertension and sexual dysfunction: time to act. J Hypertens 29(2):403–407
9. Rosen RC et al (2004) The multinational Men's Attitudes to Life Events and Sexuality (MALES) study: I. Prevalence of erectile dysfunction and related health concerns in the general population. Curr Med Res Opin 20(5):607–617
10. Bacon CG et al (2002) Association of type and duration of diabetes with erectile dysfunction in a large cohort of men. Diabetes Care 25(8):1458–1463
11. Feldman HA et al (1994) Impotence and its medical and psychosocial correlates: results of the Massachusetts male aging study. J Urol 151(1):54–61
12. Cho NH et al (2006) Prevalence of erectile dysfunction in Korean men with Type 2 diabetes mellitus. Diabet Med 23(2):198–203
13. El AY et al (2008) Diabetes and erectile dysfunction in Morocco: epidemiological study among outpatients. East Mediterr Health J 14(5):1090–1100
14. Penson DF et al (2003) Do impotent men with diabetes have more severe erectile dysfunction and worse quality of life than the general population of impotent patients? Results from the Exploratory Comprehensive Evaluation of Erectile Dysfunction (ExCEED) database. Diabetes Care 26(4):1093–1099
15. Corona G et al (2013) The SUBITO-DE study: sexual dysfunction in newly diagnosed type 2 diabetes male patients. J Endocrinol Invest 36(10):864–868
16. Junuzovic D, Hasanbegovic M, Masic I (2010) Risk factors for erectile dysfunction in patients with newly diagnosed diabetes mellitus. Med Arh 64(6):345–347
17. Al-Hunayan A et al (2007) The prevalence and predictors of erectile dysfunction in men with newly diagnosed with type 2 diabetes mellitus. BJU Int 99(1):130–134
18. Kalter-Leibovici O et al (2005) Clinical, socioeconomic, and lifestyle parameters associated with erectile dysfunction among diabetic men. Diabetes Care 28(7):1739–1744
19. Zheng H et al (2006) Predictors for erectile dysfunction among diabetics. Diabetes Res Clin Pract 71(3):313–319
20. Henis O et al (2011) Erectile dysfunction is associated with severe retinopathy in diabetic men. Urology 77(5):1133–1136

21. Fedele D et al (1998) Erectile dysfunction in diabetic subjects in Italy. Gruppo Italiano Studio Deficit Erettile nei Diabetici. Diabetes Care 21(11):1973–1977
22. Hermans MP, Ahn SA, Rousseau MF (2009) Erectile dysfunction, microangiopathy and UKPDS risk in type 2 diabetes. Diabetes Metab 35(6):484–489
23. Weinberg AE et al (2013) Diabetes severity, metabolic syndrome, and the risk of erectile dysfunction. J Sex Med 10(12):3102–3109
24. Awad H et al (2010) Erectile function in men with diabetes type 2: correlation with glycemic control. Int J Impot Res 22(1):36–39
25. Siu SC et al (2001) Prevalence of and risk factors for erectile dysfunction in Hong Kong diabetic patients. Diabet Med 18(9):732–738
26. Giuliano FA et al (2004) Prevalence of erectile dysfunction among 7689 patients with diabetes or hypertension, or both. Urology 64(6):1196–1201
27. Wei M et al (1994) Total cholesterol and high density lipoprotein cholesterol as important predictors of erectile dysfunction. Am J Epidemiol 140(10):930–937
28. Shaeer O, Shaeer K, The Global Online Sexuality Survey (GOSS): the United States of America in 2011 (2012) Chapter I: Erectile dysfunction among English-speakers. J Sex Med 9(12):3018–3027
29. Wiedemann A et al (2013) Men with type 2 diabetes and erectile dysfunction are a particular risk group for LUTS – results of the Witten diabetes survey. Aktuelle Urol 44(4):280–284
30. Giugliano F et al (2010) Determinants of erectile dysfunction in type 2 diabetes. Int J Impot Res 22(3):204–209
31. Malavige LS, Levy JC (2009) Erectile dysfunction in diabetes mellitus. J Sex Med 6(5):1232–1247
32. Derby CA et al (2000) Modifiable risk factors and erectile dysfunction: can lifestyle changes modify risk? Urology 56(2):302–306
33. Elbendary MA, El-Gamal OM, Salem KA (2009) Analysis of risk factors for organic erectile dysfunction in Egyptian patients under the age of 40 years. J Androl 30(5):520–524
34. Cai X et al (2014) The role of statins in erectile dysfunction: a systematic review and meta-analysis. Asian J Androl 16:461–466
35. Londono DC et al (2012) Population-based study of erectile dysfunction and polypharmacy. BJU Int 110(2):254–259
36. Anderson RJ et al (2001) The prevalence of comorbid depression in adults with diabetes: a meta-analysis. Diabetes Care 24(6):1069–1078
37. De Berardis G et al (2005) Longitudinal assessment of quality of life in patients with type 2 diabetes and self-reported erectile dysfunction. Diabetes Care 28(11):2637–2643
38. Chang S et al (2004) Downregulation of cGMP-dependent protein kinase-1 activity in the corpus cavernosum smooth muscle of diabetic rabbits. Am J Physiol Regul Integr Comp Physiol 287(4):R950–R960
39. Thorve VS et al (2011) Diabetes-induced erectile dysfunction: epidemiology, pathophysiology and management. J Diabetes Complicat 25(2):129–136
40. Esposito K et al (2008) Phenotypic assessment of endothelial microparticles in diabetic and nondiabetic men with erectile dysfunction. J Sex Med 5(6):1436–1442
41. Steinberg HO, Baron AD (2002) Vascular function, insulin resistance and fatty acids. Diabetologia 45(5):623–634
42. Petrie JR et al (1996) Endothelial nitric oxide production and insulin sensitivity. A physiological link with implications for pathogenesis of cardiovascular disease. Circulation 93(7):1331–1333
43. Tamler R (2009) Diabetes, obesity, and erectile dysfunction. Gend Med 6(Suppl 1):4–16
44. Bhasin S et al (2007) Sexual dysfunction in men and women with endocrine disorders. Lancet 369(9561):597–611
45. Phe V, Roupret M (2012) Erectile dysfunction and diabetes: a review of the current evidence-based medicine and a synthesis of the main available therapies. Diabetes Metab 38(1):1–13
46. Bleustein CB et al (2002) The neuropathy of erectile dysfunction. Int J Impot Res 14(6):433–439
47. Dhindsa S et al (2004) Frequent occurrence of hypogonadotropic hypogonadism in type 2 diabetes. J Clin Endocrinol Metab 89(11):5462–5468

48. Corona G et al (2011) Type 2 diabetes mellitus and testosterone: a meta-analysis study. Int J Androl 34(6 Pt 1):528–540
49. Ding EL et al (2006) Sex differences of endogenous sex hormones and risk of type 2 diabetes: a systematic review and meta-analysis. JAMA 295(11):1288–1299
50. Svartberg J et al (2004) The associations of endogenous testosterone and sex hormone-binding globulin with glycosylated hemoglobin levels, in community dwelling men. The Tromso Study. Diabetes Metab 30(1):29–34
51. El-Sakka AI, Sayed HM, Tayeb KA (2008) Type 2 diabetes-associated androgen alteration in patients with erectile dysfunction. Int J Androl 31(6):602–608
52. Traish AM et al (2003) Effects of medical or surgical castration on erectile function in an animal model. J Androl 24(3):381–387
53. Bruning JC et al (2000) Role of brain insulin receptor in control of body weight and reproduction. Science 289(5487):2122–2125
54. Al-Hunayan A et al (2008) Hyperhomocysteinemia is a risk factor for erectile dysfunction in men with adult-onset diabetes mellitus. Urology 71(5):897–900
55. Hackett G et al (2008) British society for sexual medicine guidelines on the management of erectile dysfunction. J Sex Med 5(8):1841–1865
56. Hatzimouratidis K, Hatzichristou D (2009) Erectile dysfunction and diabetes mellitus. Insulin 4:114–122
57. Walsh TJ et al (2014) Men with diabetes may require more aggressive treatment for erectile dysfunction. Int J Impot Res 26:112–115
58. Jackson G (2004) Sexual dysfunction and diabetes. Int J Clin Pract 58(4):358–362
59. Petrone L et al (2003) Structured interview on erectile dysfunction (SIEDY): a new, multidimensional instrument for quantification of pathogenetic issues on erectile dysfunction. Int J Impot Res 15(3):210–220
60. Rosen RC et al (1997) The international index of erectile function (IIEF): a multidimensional scale for assessment of erectile dysfunction. Urology 49(6):822–830
61. Batty GD et al (2010) Erectile dysfunction and later cardiovascular disease in men with type 2 diabetes: prospective cohort study based on the ADVANCE (Action in Diabetes and Vascular Disease: Preterax and Diamicron Modified-Release Controlled Evaluation) trial. J Am Coll Cardiol 56(23):1908–1913
62. Gazzaruso C, Coppola A, Giustina A (2011) Erectile dysfunction and coronary artery disease in patients with diabetes. Curr Diabetes Rev 7(2):143–147
63. Hatzimouratidis K et al (2010) Guidelines on male sexual dysfunction: erectile dysfunction and premature ejaculation. Eur Urol 57(5):804–814
64. Foresta C et al (2009) Clinical and metabolic evaluation of subjects with erectile dysfunction: a review with a proposal flowchart. Int J Androl 32(3):198–211
65. Klein R, Klein BE, Moss SE (2005) Ten-year incidence of self-reported erectile dysfunction in people with long-term type 1 diabetes. J Diabetes Complicat 19(1):35–41
66. Wrishko R et al (2009) Safety, efficacy, and pharmacokinetic overview of low-dose daily administration of tadalafil. J Sex Med 6(7):2039–2048
67. Reffelmann T, Kloner RA (2006) Cardiovascular effects of phosphodiesterase 5 inhibitors. Curr Pharm Des 12(27):3485–3494
68. Vardi M, Nini A (2007) Phosphodiesterase inhibitors for erectile dysfunction in patients with diabetes mellitus. Cochrane Database Syst Rev (1):CD002187
69. Bruzziches R et al (2008) Redefining the role of long-acting phosphodiesterase inhibitor tadalafil in the treatment of diabetic erectile dysfunction. Curr Diabetes Rev 4(1):24–30
70. Goldstein I et al (2003) Vardenafil, a new phosphodiesterase type 5 inhibitor, in the treatment of erectile dysfunction in men with diabetes: a multicenter double-blind placebo-controlled fixed-dose study. Diabetes Care 26(3):777–783
71. Isidori AM et al (2005) Effects of testosterone on sexual function in men: results of a meta-analysis. Clin Endocrinol (Oxf) 63(4):381–394
72. Ferrario CM, Levy P (2002) Sexual dysfunction in patients with hypertension: implications for therapy. J Clin Hypertens (Greenwich) 4(6):424–432

73. Cordero A et al (2010) Erectile dysfunction in high-risk hypertensive patients treated with beta-blockade agents. Cardiovasc Ther 28(1):15–22
74. El-Sisi AA et al (2013) Atorvastatin improves erectile dysfunction in patients initially irresponsive to Sildenafil by the activation of endothelial nitric oxide synthase. Int J Impot Res 25(4):143–148
75. Nurkalem Z et al (2014) The effect of rosuvastatin and atorvastatin on erectile dysfunction in hypercholesterolemic patients. Kardiol Pol 72:275–279

The Association Between Dyslipidemia and Its Treatment with Erectile Dysfunction

13

Andreas Pittaras, Konstantinos Avranas, Konstantinos Imprialos, Charles Faselis, and Peter Kokkinos

13.1 Introduction

Low-density lipoprotein cholesterol (LDL-C) plays a vital role in the atherosclerotic process, and currently dyslipidemia is considered to be one of the most important risk factors for CV events [1]. The introduction of statins in treatment protocols for patients with dyslipidemia was a major advance for the treatment of CV disease and effectively reduces LDL-C levels and CV events [2, 3]. Because of their effectiveness, 30 million individuals in the USA and up to 200 million individuals worldwide are currently on statin therapy. In addition, the role of statin therapy in primary and secondary prevention of CV events seems to be mediated by other mechanisms (beyond LDL-C reduction) as well. Statins exert beneficial effects even

A. Pittaras, MD (✉)
Cardiology Department, Asklepeion General Hospital,
22 El. Venizelou Street, Galatsi, 11147 Athens, Greece
e-mail: andreaspittaras@gmail.com

K. Avranas • K. Imprialos
2nd Propedeutic Department of Internal Medicine, Aristotle University,
49, Konstantinoupoleos Street, Thessaloniki 54643, Greece
e-mail: avranaskon@gmail.com; kostasimprialos@hotmail.com

C. Faselis
Cardiology Department, Veterans Affairs Medical Center,
VAMC and George Washington University,
50 Irving Str., NW-151-E, Washington, DC 20422, USA
e-mail: charles.faselis@va.gov

P. Kokkinos
Cardiology Department, Veterans Affairs Medical Center,
VAMC and Georgetown University and George Washington University,
50 Irving Str., NW-151-E, Washington, DC 20422, USA
e-mail: peter.kokkinos@va.gov

© Springer International Publishing Switzerland 2015
M. Viigimaa et al. (eds.), *Erectile Dysfunction in Hypertension and Cardiovascular Disease: A Guide for Clinicians*,
DOI 10.1007/978-3-319-08272-1_13

in patients with low, near-baseline LDL-C levels, even <80 mg/dl [4, 5]. Evidence also supports that statin-mediated health benefits are observed well before LDL-C levels decrease [6–9].

Erectile dysfunction (ED) is defined as the persistent inability to attain and/or maintain penile erection sufficient for sexual intercourse. ED is highly prevalent in the general male population and its prevalence increases with age. Traditionally, ED was considered to be either a psychological or an anatomic issue. Thus, the condition was managed by mental health professionals and urologists. However, advances in understanding the pathophysiology of ED in recent years lead the conclusion that origin of ED for the majority of patients is mainly vascular. Specifically, the reduced bioavailability of nitric oxide in the penile tissue in patients with atherosclerosis is the main pathological pathway of erectile dysfunction.

ED is highly prevalent in males with CV risk factors, especially in patients with arterial hypertension, diabetes mellitus, or obesity. The prevalence of ED in patients with dyslipidemia and the effects of statins on erectile function are not completely defined. This review aims to present available data on the relationship between dyslipidemia and ED and critically evaluate existing data about the effects of statins and other hypolipidemic agents on erectile function.

13.2 Epidemiology

In a Canadian Study of primary care physicians, ED was independently associated with cardiovascular disease. However, the study failed to highlight dyslipidemia as an independent risk factor [10]. On the contrary, Smith et al. [11] reported a high prevalence of newly diagnosed hypercholesterolemia and hypertriglyceridemia in men attending an ED clinic. In a large cohort of 272,325 patients with ED, the prevalence of hyperlipidemia was 20.2 %, and the age-specific prevalence ranged from 3.9 to 52.3 % [12]. In addition, ED was significantly more prevalent in individuals with dyslipidemia, coronary artery disease (CAD), and metabolic syndrome. In another study, ED was significantly more prevalent in patients who had both hypercholesterolemia and hypetriglyceridemia [13].

13.3 Pathophysiological Correlation Between ED and Dyslipidemia

Dyslipidemia-induced ED with high LDL-C concentrations as the major culprit has been proposed by Kim [14]. Similar erection response to intracavernous injection of papaverine, a smooth muscle relaxant, of patients with and without hyperlipidemia suggests that the endothelium-dependent relaxation is impaired in ED. This was further supported by in vitro experiments of cavernal tissue, where tissues taken from hyperlipidemic patients demonstrated impaired relaxation response to vasoactive agents, in comparison to tissues from normolipidemic individuals. Oxidized LDL inhibited this relaxation. The production of superoxide radical and the activity of total superoxide dismutase (SOD) (acts as a scavenger) in the hyperlipidemic group were both increased, suggesting a functional impairment of response to endothelial stimuli. Rao et al. [15] confirmed these findings, and others emphasized oxidized LDL as the major factor of impaired relaxation response, as well as the role of nitric oxide (NO), and its reduced generation or bioavailability in penile and vascular tissue [16]. Three experimental studies on rats and mice further support the aforementioned findings. Erectile responses to nerve electrical stimulation, in hypertriglyceridemic rats, was impaired following an increase in triglyceride levels by administration of 10 % fructose and restored when triglycerides were lowered [17]. High-cholesterol diet also had similar detrimental effects on erectile and endothelial function in rats [18, 19].

13.4 Statins and ED

13.4.1 Mechanism of Action

Statins are the cornerstone treatment against hypercholesterolemia. Statins lower blood cholesterol concentrations by inhibiting HMG-CoA reductase. This enzyme catalyzes the conversion of HMG-CoA into mevalonic acid, a cholesterol precursor, thus reducing the endogenous cholesterol synthesis. Apart from that, statins exhibit pleiotropic effects. They intervene intracellular molecular signaling pathways, antagonize accumulation of macrophages and inflammatory processes, and exert a protective action on endothelial cell function, increasing serum NO levels. Statins also reduce smooth muscle cell (SMC) proliferation, stabilize the atherosclerotic plaque, and inhibit platelet activation and coagulation process, hence reducing the cardiovascular risk. The well-established adverse effects are myopathy and elevation of liver enzymes [20]. Another, lately investigated possible adverse effect of statins is hypoandrogenemia, attributed to the inhibition of steroid hormones derived from cholesterol, including testosterone [21]. Statins might also decrease libido through central mechanisms [22].

13.4.2 Clinical Studies

The majority of interventional studies involve the use of atorvastatin in a relatively small number of patients. In general, these studies support that the use of statins improve penile rigidity and sexual function when compared to placebo [23–25]. There is also evidence to support that the effects of sildenafil on erectile function in hypercholesterolemic patients is enhanced when combined with statin therapy [26]. In addition, patients who do not respond to sildenafil exhibited a modest improvement in erectile function when treated with statins [27].

A prospective single-blind study compared the effect of atorvastatin and tadalafil on ED. Subjects ($n = 120$) were randomized to receive atorvastatin 10 mg/day, tadalafil 20 mg three times/week, a combination of the two for 3 months, or no medication. Mean improvement of IIEF score was significantly higher in both tadalafil group compared to control group ($p=0.0001$), and atorvastatin group compared to control group ($p=0.001$). The improvement in the tadalafil group was more profound than the atorvastatin group. There was no synergic effect of atorvastatin and tadalafil [28].

Not all studies reported favorable outcomes with statin therapy [29, 30]. In a randomized double-blind longitudinal study, 173 men with untreated ED were treated with 40 mg simvastatin daily ($n=90$) or placebo ($n=83$) for 6 months. Patients with high cardiovascular risk, hypertension, and angina and those already on ED or statin therapy were excluded. No significant difference in erectile function between the simvastatin and placebo groups ($p=0.27$) was noted [31].

A cross-sectional study of patients referred to a lipid clinic for dyslipidemia, and 339 age-matched men found that there were more impotent men in the group of patients treated with hypolipidemic drugs ($p=0.003$). Multivariate analysis showed that erectile dysfunction was dependent on treatment with fibrate derivatives (odds ratio, 1.46; 1.27–1.68) and statins (odds ratio, 1.51; 1.26–1.80) [32].

Cases of ED associated with statins were collected by the Spanish and French pharmacovigilance system. In the Spanish database, 38 cases were recognized, 93 % of which resolved after statin withdrawal. In the French database, 37 cases were reported, 85 % resolved after withdrawal and 5 cases exhibited a positive rechallenge [33].

In a prospective observational study including 80 men attending cardiovascular risk clinics, IIEF scores were measured prior to initiation and after 6 months of statin therapy. Prior to statin therapy, the mean IIEF score was 18.7, and 52 % had significant reduction of erectile function. After statin therapy, IIEF scores were reduced to 10.4 ($p<0.001$), and 22 % experienced new onset ED [34].

In a study of 1,899 men, there was no association between hyperlipidemia drug treatment and ED, except among younger men (<55) who had diabetes and/or CVD, where a strong association was observed (OR = 10.39, 95 % CI: 3.25, 33.20). In a statins-only analysis, the OR for treated hyperlipidemia was still substantial (OR = 8.86, 95 % CI: 2.69, 29.20), but no information was given regarding the type of statins and dosage [35].

Do et al. [36] assessed the same relation between statins and ED using a case/non-case method within the French Pharmacovigilance System Database. Among the total of spontaneous reports selected (110 685), exposure to statins was identified in 4,471 cases, of which 51 reports (1.1 %) concerned ED, whereas 431 (0.4 %) cases of ED were found in the 106 214 reports without exposure to statins ($p<0.0001$). No relationship was found between statin dosage, duration of statin therapy, and ED.

Corona et al. [37] reported that in a cohort of 3,484 men with ED, individuals who were treated with statins had significantly lower levels of total and free testosterone when compared to the rest of the sample ($p<0.0001$ for both). Statin treatment was also associated with reduced testis volume and a higher prevalence of hypogonadism-related symptoms and signs ($p<0.01$). Also, in the statins group, follicle-stimulating hormone levels were significantly higher compared to the untreated group, suggesting a possible mechanism for statin-related ED. These findings were confirmed by Cohen [38] who also noted an exacerbated free and total testosterone level reduction in individuals with preexisting hypoandrogenic anabolic deficiency state (decreased pregnenolone and DHEA concentrations).

In contrast to the aforementioned studies, a double-blind, randomized, placebo-controlled, clinical trial in patients with ED and endothelial dysfunction reported no significant difference in penile erection between those treated with simvastatin and the placebo group [39].

In another most recent prospective study, ED was assessed in a group treated with rosuvastatin 10–20 mg daily ($n=46$) and atorvastatin arm ($n=44$). The investigators reported no adverse effect on ED in those treated with atorvastatin, whereas the IIEF score was significantly lower after 6 months of rosuvastatin treatment ($p=0.019$). This is the first study to suggest that different types of statins may have a different effect on ED [40] (Table 13.1).

13.4.3 Experimental Data

In an experimental study (Wistar rats), it was found that pretreatment with atorvastatin increased the potency of sildenafil-induced relaxation ($p<0.01$), the plasma NOx concentrations, and sildenafil-induced hypotension and tachycardia [41]. These findings suggest a synergy through NO-mediated mechanisms, in the vascular relaxation. In another study, atorvastatin ameliorated sildenafil-induced penile erections in spontaneously hypertensive rats, by interfering with the Rho-kinase signaling pathway within the penis [42]. Atorvastatin benefits on erectile function were also observed in diabetic rats and diabetic rabbits [43]. Similar beneficial effects on erectile function were also observed with rosuvastatin in obese diabetic rats [44]. Simvastatin showed similar benefits in restoring erectile function when added to insulin, by inhibiting the RhoA-/Rho-kinase pathway [45].

13.5 Other Hypolipidemics and Erectile Dysfunction

Case reports or small series of patients who were treated with gemfibrozil suggest that ED might appear after 1–3 weeks of treatment and subside after withdrawal of the drug [46–49]. A review of clinical trial experience with fenofibrate reported ED as an adverse effect on 1.3 % of the patients [50].

In a single-center prospective randomized placebo-controlled parallel-group trial of 160 male patients with ED and dyslipidemia, niacin was associated with improvement of erectile function compared to placebo for 12 weeks [51]. In another single-blind, one-arm study of 54 men with untreated ED, niacin had beneficial effects on erectile function when given combined with propionyl-L-carnitine and L-arginine for 3 months [52].

Table 13.1 Comparative table of studies on statins and erectile function

Study, year	No. of patients	Study type	Study drugs	ED assessment	Outcome
Saltzman et al., 2004	9	Single-arm open-label	Atorvastatin	IIEF questionnaire, RigiScan	Improvement
Herrmann et al., 2006	12	Randomized, double-blind placebo-controlled	Atorvastatin	IIEF questionnaire	Improvement
Bank et al., 2006	35	Randomized, double-blind placebo-controlled	Atorvastatin, quinapril	IIEF questionnaire, endothelium-independent relaxation, Doppler blood flow	Improvement
Gokkaya et al., 2008	25	Single-arm open-label	Atorvastatin	IIEF questionnaire	Improvement
Dadkhah et al., 2010	131	Randomized, -blind placebo-controlled	Atorvastatin	IIEF questionnaire	Improvement
Gokce et al., 2012	120	Single-center, randomized, single-bind study	Atorvastatin Tadalafil	IIEF questionnaire Serum testosterone, nocturnal penile tumescence	Improvement
Pedersen et al., 1999 (comment on the Scandinavian Simvastatin Survival Study 1994)	4,444	Randomized, single-bind study	Simvastatin	IIEF questionnaire	No deterioration likely
Trivedi et al., 2013	173	Randomized, double-bind study	Simvastatin	IIEF questionnaire, male ED-specific quality of life, quality adjusted life years	Improvement
Bruckert et al., 1996	678	Crossover study	Simvastatin, pravastatin, fibrates, resins	Medical history	Hypolipidemic drugs as a possible cause of ED
Carvajal et al., 2006	38	Analysis of the cases of impotence of the Spanish and French pharmacovigilance system	Statins	Reports from patients	Possible cause of ED

Solomon et al., 2006	93	Prospective observational study	Statins	IIEF questionnaire	Possible cause
Hall et al., 2009	1,899	Observational crossover study	Hypolipidemics, meta-analysis on statins	IIEF questionnaire	Hypolipidemics, and statins may cause ED
Do et al., 2009	110,685	Case/non-case method on data within the French Pharmacovigilance System Database	Statins	Spontaneous reports	Statins
Corona et al., 2010	3,484	Crossover observational study	Statins	ANDROTEST, measurement of blood-testosterone	Statins may induce hypogonadism
Mastalir et al., 2005	41	Double-blind, randomized, placebo-controlled	Simvastatin	IIEF questionnaire, ED Index of Treatment Satisfaction	No relationship between simvastatin and ED
Nurkalem et al., 2014	90	Single-blind randomized	Atorvastatin, rosuvastatin	IIEF questionnaire	Atorvastatin increased ED Rosuvastatin showed no effect

Conclusions

This review sought to summarize available evidence regarding the relationship between ED and dyslipidemia. Most evidence support that dyslipidemia is associated with ED through induction of impaired relaxation response upon cavernal tissue. Hypercholesterolemia decreases the gene expression of endothelium-specific cell-to-cell junction proteins and decreased endothelial content in the corpus cavernosum. High levels of ox-LDL induce lower bioavailability of NO.

Available data regarding the effects of statins on erectile function is conflicting. Experimental data point towards a beneficial effect of statins on erectile function through several mechanisms. Clinical data, however, does not confirm these beneficial effects in all cases. Available clinical studies show positive, neutral, or even negative effects on erectile function. However, existing data is not of the highest quality. Many studies are observational with all inherent limitations of this study type, and available prospective randomized studies have usually small study samples and short follow-up. Moreover, the assessment of erectile function in other studies was not based on validated methods. Finally, information regarding a dose-dependent effect or within-class differences are inconclusive.

Information regarding other hypolipidemic agents, apart from statins, is scant and fragmented. Gemfibrozil appears to have detrimental effects on erectile function, while niacin might beneficially affect erectile function; however, available data needs to be confirmed by appropriately designed and adequately powered clinical trials.

References

1. Ference BA, Yoo W, Alesh I, Mahajan N, Mirowska KK, Mewada A et al (2012) Effect of long-term exposure to lower low-density lipoprotein cholesterol beginning early in life on the risk of coronary heart disease: a Mendelian randomization analysis. J Am Coll Cardiol 60(25):2631–2639
2. Ray KK, Seshasai SR, Erqou S, Sever P, Jukema JW, Ford I et al (2010) Statins and all-cause mortality in high-risk primary prevention: a meta-analysis of 11 randomized controlled trials involving 65,229 participants. Arch Intern Med 170(12):1024–1031
3. Taylor F, Huffman MD, Macedo AF, Moore TH, Burke M, Davey Smith G et al (2013) Statins for the primary prevention of cardiovascular disease. Cochrane Database Syst Rev 1:CD004816
4. Ridker PM, Danielson E, Fonseca FA, Genest J, Gotto AM Jr, Kastelein JJ et al (2008) Rosuvastatin to prevent vascular events in men and women with elevated C-reactive protein. N Engl J Med 359(21):2195–2207
5. Mihaylova B, Emberson J, Blackwell L, Keech A, Simes J, Barnes EH et al (2012) The effects of lowering LDL cholesterol with statin therapy in people at low risk of vascular disease: meta-analysis of individual data from 27 randomised trials. Lancet 380(9841):581–590
6. Di Sciascio G, Patti G, Pasceri V, Gaspardone A, Colonna G, Montinaro A (2009) Efficacy of atorvastatin reload in patients on chronic statin therapy undergoing percutaneous coronary intervention: results of the ARMYDA-RECAPTURE (Atorvastatin for Reduction of Myocardial Damage During Angioplasty) randomized trial. J Am Coll Cardiol 54(6):558–565
7. Vale N, Nordmann AJ, Schwartz GG, de Lemos J, Colivicchi F, den Hartog F et al (2011) Statins for acute coronary syndrome. Cochrane Database Syst Rev (6):CD006870
8. Athyros VG, Kakafika AI, Tziomalos K, Karagiannis A, Mikhailidis DP (2009) Pleiotropic effects of statins–clinical evidence. Curr Pharm Des 15(5):479–489

9. Athyros VG, Tziomalos K, Florentin M, Karagiannis A, Mikhailidis DP (2010) Statin loading in patients undergoing percutaneous coronary intervention for acute coronary syndromes: a new pleiotropic effect? Curr Med Res Opin 26(4):839–842
10. Grover SA, Lowensteyn I, Kaouache M, Marchand S, Coupal L, DeCarolis E et al (2006) The prevalence of erectile dysfunction in the primary care setting: importance of risk factors for diabetes and vascular disease. Arch Intern Med 166(2):213–219
11. Smith NJ, Sak SC, Baldo O, Eardley I (2007) The prevalence of newly diagnosed hyperlipidaemia in men with erectile dysfunction. BJU Int 100(2):357–361
12. Seftel AD, Sun P, Swindle R (2004) The prevalence of hypertension, hyperlipidemia, diabetes mellitus and depression in men with erectile dysfunction. J Urol 171(6 Pt 1):2341–2345
13. Gunduz MI, Gumus BH, Sekuri C (2004) Relationship between metabolic syndrome and erectile dysfunction. Asian J Androl 6(4):355–358
14. Kim SC (2000) Hyperlipidemia and erectile dysfunction. Asian J Androl 2(3):161–166
15. Rao K, Du GH, Yang WM (2006) Hyperlipidemia and erectile dysfunction. Zhonghua nan ke xue = Natl J Androl 12(7):643–646
16. Vrentzos GE, Paraskevas KI, Mikhailidis DP (2007) Dyslipidemia as a risk factor for erectile dysfunction. Curr Med Chem 14(16):1765–1770
17. Srilatha B, Adaikan PG (2006) Characterization of hypertriglyceridemia-induced erectile dysfunction. Urology 67(3):642–646
18. Ryu JK, Zhang LW, Jin HR, Piao S, Choi MJ, Tuvshintur B et al (2009) Derangements in endothelial cell-to-cell junctions involved in the pathogenesis of hypercholesterolemia-induced erectile dysfunction. J Sex Med 6(7):1893–1907
19. Demir O, Murat N, Soner BC, Demir T, Bal E, Can E et al (2010) Acute effects of hypercholesterolemic diet on erectile responses in rats. Urol Int 85(1):112–117
20. Stancu C, Sima A (2001) Statins: mechanism of action and effects. J Cell Mol Med 5(4):378–387
21. Rizvi K, Hampson JP, Harvey JN (2002) Do lipid-lowering drugs cause erectile dysfunction? A systematic review. Fam Pract 19(1):95–98
22. Tuccori M, Montagnani S, Mantarro S, Capogrosso-Sansone A, Ruggiero E, Saporiti A et al (2014) Neuropsychiatric adverse events associated with statins: epidemiology, pathophysiology, prevention and management. CNS Drugs. doi:10.1007/s40263-013-0135-1
23. Saltzman EA, Guay AT, Jacobson J (2004) Improvement in erectile function in men with organic erectile dysfunction by correction of elevated cholesterol levels: a clinical observation. J Urol 172(1):255–258
24. Herrmann HC, Levine LA, Macaluso J Jr, Walsh M, Bradbury D, Schwartz S et al (2006) Can atorvastatin improve the response to sildenafil in men with erectile dysfunction not initially responsive to sildenafil? Hypothesis and pilot trial results. J Sex Med 3(2):303–308
25. Bank AJ, Kelly AS, Kaiser DR, Crawford WW, Waxman B, Schow DA et al (2006) The effects of quinapril and atorvastatin on the responsiveness to sildenafil in men with erectile dysfunction. Vasc Med 11(4):251–257
26. Gokkaya SC, Ozden C, Levent Ozdal O, Hakan Koyuncu H, Guzel O, Memis A (2008) Effect of correcting serum cholesterol levels on erectile function in patients with vasculogenic erectile dysfunction. Scand J Urol Nephrol 42(5):437–440
27. Dadkhah F, Safarinejad MR, Asgari MA, Hosseini SY, Lashay A, Amini E (2010) Atorvastatin improves the response to sildenafil in hypercholesterolemic men with erectile dysfunction not initially responsive to sildenafil. Int J Impot Res 22(1):51–60
28. Gokce MI, Gulpinar O, Ozturk E, Gulec S, Yaman O (2012) Effect of atorvastatin on erectile functions in comparison with regular tadalafil use. A prospective single-blind study. Int Urol Nephrol 44(3):683–687
29. Pedersen TR, Faergeman O (1999) Simvastatin seems unlikely to cause impotence. BMJ 318(7177):192
30. Scandinavian Simvastatin Survival Study (1994) Randomised trial of cholesterol lowering in 4444 patients with coronary heart disease. Lancet 344(8934):1383–1389
31. Trivedi D, Kirby M, Wellsted DM, Ali S, Hackett G, O'Connor B et al (2013) Can simvastatin improve erectile function and health-related quality of life in men aged >/=40 years with

erectile dysfunction? Results of the erectile dysfunction and statins trial [ISRCTN66772971]. BJU Int 111(2):324–333
32. Bruckert E, Giral P, Heshmati HM, Turpin G (1996) Men treated with hypolipidaemic drugs complain more frequently of erectile dysfunction. J Clin Pharm Ther 21(2):89–94
33. Carvajal A, Macias D, Sainz M, Ortega S, Martin Arias LH, Velasco A et al (2006) HMG CoA reductase inhibitors and impotence: two case series from the Spanish and French drug monitoring systems. Drug Saf 29(2):143–149
34. Solomon H, Samarasinghe YP, Feher MD, Man J, Rivas-Toro H, Lumb PJ et al (2006) Erectile dysfunction and statin treatment in high cardiovascular risk patients. Int J Clin Pract 60(2):141–145
35. Hall SA, Kupelian V, Rosen RC, Travison TG, Link CL, Miner MM et al (2009) Is hyperlipidemia or its treatment associated with erectile dysfunction?: Results from the Boston Area Community Health (BACH) survey. J Sex Med 6(5):1402–1413
36. Do C, Huyghe E, Lapeyre-Mestre M, Montastruc JL, Bagheri H (2009) Statins and erectile dysfunction: results of a case/non-case study using the French pharmacovigilance system database. Drug Saf 32(7):591–597
37. Corona G, Boddi V, Balercia G, Rastrelli G, De Vita G, Sforza A et al (2010) The effect of statin therapy on testosterone levels in subjects consulting for erectile dysfunction. J Sex Med 7(4 Pt 1):1547–1556
38. Cohen PG (2011) Statins and male hypogonadism. J Sex Med 8(6):1826
39. Mastalir ET, Carvalhal GF, Portal VL (2011) The effect of simvastatin in penile erection: a randomized, double-blind, placebo-controlled clinical trial (Simvastatin treatment for erectile dysfunction-STED TRIAL). Int J Impot Res 23(6):242–248
40. Nurkalem Z, Yildirimturk O, Ozcan KS, Kul S, Canga Y, Satilmis S et al (2014) The effect of rosuvastatin and atorvastatin on erectile dysfunction in hypercholesterolemic patients. Kardiol Pol 72(3):275–279
41. Castro MM, Rizzi E, Rascado RR, Nagassaki S, Bendhack LM, Tanus-Santos JE (2004) Atorvastatin enhances sildenafil-induced vasodilation through nitric oxide-mediated mechanisms. Eur J Pharmacol 498(1–3):189–194
42. Fibbi B, Morelli A, Marini M, Zhang XH, Mancina R, Vignozzi L et al (2008) Atorvastatin but not elocalcitol increases sildenafil responsiveness in spontaneously hypertensive rats by regulating the RhoA/ROCK pathway. J Androl 29(1):70–84
43. Morelli A, Chavalmane AK, Filippi S, Fibbi B, Silvestrini E, Sarchielli E et al (2009) Atorvastatin ameliorates sildenafil-induced penile erections in experimental diabetes by inhibiting diabetes-induced RhoA/Rho-kinase signaling hyperactivation. J Sex Med 6(1):91–106
44. Wingard CJ, Moukdar F, Prasad RY, Cathey BL, Wilkinson L (2009) Reversal of voltage-dependent erectile responses in the Zucker obese-diabetic rat by rosuvastatin-altered RhoA/Rho-kinase signaling. J Sex Med 6(Suppl 3):269–278
45. Park K, Cho SY, Kim SW (2011) Erectile response to type 5 phosphodiesterase inhibitor could be preserved with the addition of simvastatin to conventional insulin treatment in rat model of diabetes. Int J Androl 34(5 Pt 2):e468–e474
46. Bain SC, Lemon M, Jones AF (1990) Gemfibrozil-induced impotence. Lancet 336(8727):1389
47. Bharani A (1992) Sexual dysfunction after gemfibrozil. BMJ Clin Res Ed 305(6855):693
48. Figueras A, Castel J, Capella D (1993) Gemfibrozil-induced impotence. Ann Pharmacother 27(7/8):982
49. James CW, Wu TS, McNelis KC (2002) Sexual dysfunction secondary to gemfibrozil. Pharmacotherapy 22(1):123–125
50. Blane GF (1989) Review of European clinical experience with fenofibrate. Cardiology 76(Suppl 1):1–10; discussion –3
51. Ng CF, Lee CP, Ho AL, Lee VW (2011) Effect of niacin on erectile function in men suffering erectile dysfunction and dyslipidemia. J Sex Med 8(10):2883–2893
52. Gianfrilli D, Lauretta R, Di Dato C, Graziadio C, Pozza C, De Larichaudy J et al (2012) Propionyl-L-carnitine, L-arginine and niacin in sexual medicine: a nutraceutical approach to erectile dysfunction. Andrologia 44(Suppl 1):600–604

Endocrine Disorders and Erectile Dysfunction

14

Konstantinos Tziomalos and Vasilios G. Athyros

14.1 Introduction

Endocrine disorders (except diabetes mellitus) represent an infrequent cause of erectile dysfunction. However, identification of an endocrine disorder in these patients is essential for three major reasons. First, it provides an opportunity for etiologic management of erectile dysfunction instead of symptomatic. Second, endocrine disorders associated with erectile dysfunction might also have important adverse sequelae on the general health and should therefore be timely identified and managed. Third, a limited panel of hormonal tests (i.e., serum total testosterone, thyrotropin, and prolactin levels) is frequently sufficient for reaching a diagnosis of these endocrine disorders.

In the present chapter, the endocrine disorders most frequently associated with erectile dysfunction are discussed, with emphasis on their prevalence in patients with erectile dysfunction, the diagnostic work-up, and the effects of their management on erectile function.

K. Tziomalos
First Propedeutic Department of Internal Medicine, Medical School, Aristotle University of Thessaloniki, AHEPA Hospital, 1 Stilponos Kyriakidi street, Thessaloniki 54636, Greece
e-mail: ktziomalos@yahoo.com

V.G. Athyros (✉)
Second Propedeutic Department of Internal Medicine, Medical School, Aristotle University of Thessaloniki, Hippokration Hospital, 15 Marmara street, Thessaloniki 55132, Greece
e-mail: vathyros@gmail.com

14.2 Hypogonadism

Even though there is no general agreement on the definition of low testosterone levels, in the general population, 24 % of men have morning serum total testosterone levels <300 ng/dl, i.e., levels currently considered diagnostic of hypogonadism [1]. Moreover, it is well established that serum total and free testosterone levels decline with aging in healthy men [2, 3]. Accordingly, the prevalence of low total testosterone levels increases in elderly men, affecting approximately 19, 28, and 49 % of men older than 60, 70, and 80 years, respectively [2]. However, only 27.7 % of men with low total testosterone levels have erectile dysfunction [1]. Moreover, serum total and free testosterone levels do not differ between patients with erectile dysfunction and age- and body mass index-matched healthy subjects [4, 5]. Indeed, even though androgens increase sexual desire, they do not play an important role in visually induced erections [6]. Accordingly, low testosterone levels do not appear to relate strongly to erectile dysfunction.

Despite the lack of a close relationship between hypogonadism and erectile dysfunction, measurement of serum total testosterone levels is currently recommended by most scientific societies in all patients with erectile dysfunction [7–9]. Among patients with erectile dysfunction, 4 % of those younger than 50 years and 9 % of those older than 50 years have low serum total testosterone levels [10]. In contrast, apparent signs of hypogonadism (i.e., small testes, gynecomastia, and reduced growth of body hair and beard) are rarely observed in patients with erectile dysfunction [11]. Indeed, if testosterone levels are measured only in patients with symptoms (e.g., low sexual desire) or signs suggestive of hypogonadism, 40 % of cases of low testosterone levels would be missed [10]. Total testosterone should be measured in the morning because serum testosterone levels exhibit a circadian variation and are higher in the morning [7]. Moreover, in patients with low testosterone levels, the diagnosis of hypogonadism should be confirmed by a second measurement, since as many as 30–40 % of patients will have normal levels on repeat testing [7, 8, 10, 12]. Testosterone measurements should not be performed in the presence of acute or subacute illnesses [7]. When total testosterone levels are near the lower limit of normal range and conditions that are associated with increased low sex-hormone-binding globulin (SHBG) levels are present, measurement of serum free testosterone levels might also be considered [7]. Common conditions that are characterized by higher SHBG levels and hence lower free testosterone levels include ageing, hyperthyroidism, and the use of estrogens, tamoxifen, and antiepileptic agents [7, 8]. It should emphasize that free testosterone levels should be measured only in reference laboratories because of the limited accuracy of many commercially available methods [7, 8]. In patients with documented low testosterone levels, serum luteinizing hormone, and follicle-stimulating hormone levels should also be measured to discriminate between primary and secondary hypogonadism [6–8]. In patients with secondary hypogonadism, measurement of serum prolactin levels and magnetic resonance imaging of the pituitary gland might be considered [7]. However, it should be mentioned that the prevalence of pituitary adenomas or hypothalamic lesions in these patients is low (3.1–6.7 %) [10, 13]. Accordingly, imaging might has to be reserved for patients with very low total testosterone levels (<100 ng/dl), panhypopituitarism, persistently elevated prolactin levels or symptoms suggestive of pituitary tumors (headache or visual field defects) [7].

Testosterone therapy can be considered in patients with erectile dysfunction who have low testosterone levels [7, 8]. However, it should be noted that administration of testosterone in placebo-controlled studies in patients with low testosterone levels exerted inconsistent effects on erectile function [14]. It is also unclear whether the combination of testosterone and phosphodiesterase-5 inhibitors improves erectile function in patients who do not respond to monotherapy with phosphodiesterase-5 inhibitors [7, 8, 15]. Several testosterone regimens are available (weekly or every 2 weeks im injections, patches, gel, pellets for sc implantation, and tablets for per os treatment), and the choice between them is individualized based on patient's preference and cost [7]. After initiation of testosterone therapy, efficacy of treatment, serum testosterone levels (aiming at levels in the mid-normal range), and hematocrit and serum prostate-specific antigen (PSA) levels should be evaluated at 3–6 months and then annually [7]. Testosterone treatment is contraindicated in patients with prostate cancer or uncontrolled heart failure, whereas patients with PSA levels >3 ng/ml should be evaluated by a urologist before initiation of testosterone therapy [7]. Moreover, older patients are at increased risk for prostate-related adverse events (cancer, PSA >4 ng/ml, biopsy, urinary retention, or worsening of symptoms associated with prostatic hyperplasia) [16] and potentially for cardiovascular events when treated with testosterone [17, 18]. Accordingly, these patients may opt to avoid testosterone therapy [7].

14.3 Prolactinoma

Sexual dysfunction due to decreased libido or erectile dysfunction is the commonest presenting symptom in men with prolactinomas [19]. More than half of men with prolactinomas report symptoms of erectile dysfunction [20]. However, given the rarity of prolactinomas, only 0.2–0.6 % of patients with erectile dysfunction has prolactinoma [10, 21]. The pathogenesis of erectile dysfunction in prolactinomas is unclear. Most patients with prolactinomas who report erectile dysfunction also have testosterone deficiency, which might contribute to erectile dysfunction [21]. Elevated prolactin levels suppress the release of gonadotropin-releasing hormone and consequently the secretion of luteinizing hormone [6]. Moreover, primary hypothyroidism might also be present in patients with prolactinomas and might also play a role in the pathogenesis of erectile dysfunction [19]. Administration of cabergoline, a D_2 selective dopamine receptor agonist, improved nocturnal penile tumescence in patients with prolactinoma [20]. Interestingly, this favorable effect of cabergoline was observed only in patients who achieved normalization of prolactin levels, even when testosterone levels were not normalized [20].

14.4 Hypothyroidism

Hypothyroidism is present in 5 % of patients with erectile dysfunction [22]. On the other hand, in a recent study, 84.1 % of patients with hypothyroidism had some degree of erectile dysfunction compared with 33.8 % of control subjects [23]. The severity of erectile dysfunction correlates inversely with serum thyrotropin levels, suggesting that thyroid dysfunction per se plays a direct role in the pathogenesis of erectile dysfunction [23]. Moreover, fatigue and mood disorders as well as low free testosterone levels are frequently present in patients with hypothyroidism and might also play a role [19, 24]. Treatment of hypothyroidism resulted in significant improvement in erectile function [23, 25].

14.5 Hyperthyroidism

Hyperthyroidism is present in 1 % of patients with erectile dysfunction [22]. On the other hand, 70.4 % of patients with hyperthyroidism had some degree of erectile dysfunction compared with 33.8 % of control subjects in a recent report [23]. The severity of erectile dysfunction correlates directly with serum thyroxine levels [23]. Similar to hyperthyroidism, fatigue and mood disorders are frequently present in patients with hyperthyroidism and might also play a role in the pathogenesis of erectile dysfunction [19]. Moreover, serum sex-hormone-binding globulin levels increase, resulting in reduced levels of free testosterone [24, 26]. Aromatization of testosterone to estrogens also increases [26]. Treatment of hyperthyroidism resulted in significant improvement in erectile function [23, 25].

References

1. Araujo AB, Esche GR, Kupelian V, O'Donnell AB, Travison TG, Williams RE, Clark RV, McKinlay JB (2007) Prevalence of symptomatic androgen deficiency in men. J Clin Endocrinol Metab 92:4241–4247
2. Harman SM, Metter EJ, Tobin JD, Pearson J, Blackman MR, Baltimore Longitudinal Study of Aging (2001) Longitudinal effects of aging on serum total and free testosterone levels in healthy men. Baltimore Longitudinal Study of Aging. J Clin Endocrinol Metab 86:724–731
3. Feldman HA, Longcope C, Derby CA, Johannes CB, Araujo AB, Coviello AD, Bremner WJ, McKinlay JB (2002) Age trends in the level of serum testosterone and other hormones in middle-aged men: longitudinal results from the Massachusetts male aging study. J Clin Endocrinol Metab 87:589–598
4. Korenman SG, Morley JE, Mooradian AD, Davis SS, Kaiser FE, Silver AJ, Viosca SP, Garza D (1990) Secondary hypogonadism in older men: its relation to impotence. J Clin Endocrinol Metab 71:963–969
5. Rhoden EL, Telöken C, Sogari PR, Souto CA (2002) The relationship of serum testosterone to erectile function in normal aging men. J Urol 167:1745–1748
6. Shamloul R, Ghanem H (2013) Erectile dysfunction. Lancet 381:153–165
7. Bhasin S, Cunningham GR, Hayes FJ, Matsumoto AM, Snyder PJ, Swerdloff RS, Montori VM, Task Force, Endocrine Society (2010) Testosterone therapy in men with androgen deficiency syndromes: an Endocrine Society clinical practice guideline. J Clin Endocrinol Metab 95:2536–2559

8. Buvat J, Maggi M, Gooren L, Guay AT, Kaufman J, Morgentaler A, Schulman C, Tan HM, Torres LO, Yassin A, Zitzmann M (2010) Endocrine aspects of male sexual dysfunctions. J Sex Med 7:1627–1656
9. Hatzimouratidis K, Amar E, Eardley I, Giuliano F, Hatzichristou D, Montorsi F, Vardi Y, Wespes E, European Association of Urology (2010) Guidelines on male sexual dysfunction: erectile dysfunction and premature ejaculation. Eur Urol 57:804–814
10. Buvat J, Lemaire A (1997) Endocrine screening in 1,022 men with erectile dysfunction: clinical significance and cost-effective strategy. J Urol 158:1764–1767
11. McVary KT (2007) Clinical practice. Erectile dysfunction. N Engl J Med 357:2472–2481
12. Brambilla DJ, O'Donnell AB, Matsumoto AM, McKinlay JB (2007) Intraindividual variation in levels of serum testosterone and other reproductive and adrenal hormones in men. Clin Endocrinol Oxf 67:853–862
13. Citron JT, Ettinger B, Rubinoff H, Ettinger VM, Minkoff J, Hom F, Kan P, Alloo R (1996) Prevalence of hypothalamic-pituitary imaging abnormalities in impotent men with secondary hypogonadism. J Urol 155:529–533
14. Boloña ER, Uraga MV, Haddad RM, Tracz MJ, Sideras K, Kennedy CC, Caples SM, Erwin PJ, Montori VM (2007) Testosterone use in men with sexual dysfunction: a systematic review and meta-analysis of randomized placebo-controlled trials. Mayo Clin Proc 82:20–28
15. Shabsigh R, Kaufman JM, Steidle C, Padma-Nathan H (2004) Randomized study of testosterone gel as adjunctive therapy to sildenafil in hypogonadal men with erectile dysfunction who do not respond to sildenafil alone. J Urol 172:658–663
16. Calof OM, Singh AB, Lee ML, Kenny AM, Urban RJ, Tenover JL, Bhasin S (2005) Adverse events associated with testosterone replacement in middle-aged and older men: a meta-analysis of randomized, placebo-controlled trials. J Gerontol A Biol Sci Med Sci 60:1451–1457
17. Basaria S, Coviello AD, Travison TG, Storer TW, Farwell WR, Jette AM, Eder R, Tennstedt S, Ulloor J, Zhang A, Choong K, Lakshman KM, Mazer NA, Miciek R, Krasnoff J, Elmi A, Knapp PE, Brooks B, Appleman E, Aggarwal S, Bhasin G, Hede-Brierley L, Bhatia A, Collins L, LeBrasseur N, Fiore LD, Bhasin S (2010) Adverse events associated with testosterone administration. N Engl J Med 363:109–122
18. Vigen R, O'Donnell CI, Barón AE, Grunwald GK, Maddox TM, Bradley SM, Barqawi A, Woning G, Wierman ME, Plomondon ME, Rumsfeld JS, Ho PM (2013) Association of testosterone therapy with mortality, myocardial infarction, and stroke in men with low testosterone levels. JAMA 310:1829–1836
19. Bhasin S, Enzlin P, Coviello A, Basson R (2007) Sexual dysfunction in men and women with endocrine disorders. Lancet 369:597–611
20. De Rosa M, Zarrilli S, Vitale G, Di Somma C, Orio F, Tauchmanova' L, Lombardi G, Colao A (2004) Six months of treatment with cabergoline restores sexual potency in hyperprolactinemic males: an open longitudinal study monitoring nocturnal penile tumescence. J Clin Endocrinol Metab 89:621–625
21. Delavierre D, Girard P, Peneau M, Ibrahim H (1999) Should plasma prolactin assay be routinely performed in the assessment of erectile dysfunction? Report of a series of 445 patients. Review of the literature. Prog Urol 9:1097–1101
22. Slag MF, Morley JE, Elson MK, Trence DL, Nelson CJ, Nelson AE, Kinlaw WB, Beyer HS, Nuttall FQ, Shafer RB (1983) Impotence in medical clinic outpatients. JAMA 249:1736–1740
23. Krassas GE, Tziomalos K, Papadopoulou F, Pontikides N, Perros P (2008) Erectile dysfunction in patients with hyper- and hypothyroidism: how common and should we treat? J Clin Endocrinol Metab 93:1815–1819
24. Krassas GE, Poppe K, Glinoer D (2010) Thyroid function and human reproductive health. Endocr Rev 31:702–755
25. Carani C, Isidori AM, Granata A, Carosa E, Maggi M, Lenzi A, Jannini EA (2005) Multicenter study on the prevalence of sexual symptoms in male hypo- and hyperthyroid patients. J Clin Endocrinol Metab 90:6472–6479
26. Soran H, Wu FC (2005) Endocrine causes of erectile dysfunction. Int J Androl 28(Suppl 2):28–34

The Metabolic Investigation of Erectile Dysfunction: Cardiometabolic Risk Stratification

15

Martin Miner

15.1 Introduction

Erectile dysfunction (ED), defined as the inability to maintain and achieve an erection sufficient for satisfactory intercourse, has a high prevalence and incidence worldwide [1]. A systematic review of epidemiologic evidence undertaken in 2002 showed a clear increase in prevalence in with advancing age, with rates for men younger than 40 years ranging from approximately from 2 to 9 %, compared with 18–86 % for those older than 80 years [2]. Although not life threatening, it may be a precursor or marker of more serious conditions, particularly coronary artery disease (CAD). Inman et al. [3] have shown when ED occurs in younger men, it is associated with a marked increase in the risk of future cardiac events and that overall ED may be associated with an approximately 80 % higher risk of subsequent CAD.

Sexual function is a complex, multifactorial process. The development of ED is attributable to both psychogenic factors and physiologic alterations in neural, vascular, hormonal, and metabolic perturbations, all mediated through endothelial and smooth muscle dysfunction. While this cascade of metabolic parameters can lead to early endothelial dysfunction and eventually, late cardiovascular events, this chapter will focus on the metabolic investigation of erectile dysfunction. Specifically, we will illustrate from our practice a clinical case and the value of the metabolic workup of the ED patient and the evolving concept of "cardiometabolic risk."

Cardiometabolic risk entails the risk of developing any of the following: type 2 diabetes (T2DM), cardiovascular disease (CVD), or metabolic syndrome (Met S). The assessment of cardiometabolic risk uses traditional risk factors such as smoking,

M. Miner, MD
Department of Family Medicine and Urology, Warren Alpert School of Medicine, Brown University, Providence, RI, USA

Men's Health Center, The Miriam Hospital, 164 Summit Ave, Providence, RI, USA
e-mail: martin_miner@brown.edu

high LDL-C cholesterol, hypertension, and elevated serum glucose as well as emerging risk factors closely related to abdominal obesity, especially intra-abdominal or visceral obesity. The relationship between traditional cardiovascular risk factors (hypercholesterolemia, hypertension, and smoking) and the occurrence of cardiovascular events is well understood. Our increasing understanding of the pathophysiology of cardiovascular disease is now defining value of a range of new cardiovascular risk factors. Risk stratification requires measurement tools of CVD risk that must be valid in the general male population, and measurement tests or biomarkers that help predict cardiac risk [4]. ED should become part of this CVD risk assessment.

Traditional models of cardiovascular risk such as Framingham Risk Score (FRS) are weighted toward age, and 80 % of men age 40–59 will have a low 10-year risk [5]. Incorporating some assessment of lifetime risk has been proposed as an added step to evaluate cardiovascular risk in this young middle-aged population noted by Inman with ED to be at particularly elevated CVS risk [3].

New data have emerged to justify a new version, though controversial, to better target lipid management therapies for the reduction of cardiovascular events in the adult population [6]. New guidelines have attempted to address the shortcomings of older risk models. ED guidelines such as Princeton III [7] have attempted to utilize evidence-based evaluation to further stratify men for cardiovascular (CVS) risk following the utilization of keen history taking and traditional risk models to establish the presence of predominantly vasculogenic ED and the volume of subclinical atherosclerotic burden which are markers for subsequent CVS events of MI and CVA in men [8]. These guidelines are an attempt to elaborate the following questions:

- Is a history of ED a harbinger for future cardiovascular risk? Is it best described as a risk marker or risk factor for future CVS events, and just what is the difference?
- Are there cost-effective, sensitive, and specific metabolic tests that might indicate increased cardiovascular risk?
- Will these tests delineate treatment based on identification of obstructive coronary artery disease (CAD) and atherosclerotic burden and thereby lower future CVS risk and improve erectile function?

15.2 The Metabolic Syndrome: A Cluster of Findings Increasing Risk of Type 2 DM and CVD (Its Relationship to ED)

Metabolic syndrome (Met S) is a complex disorder with high socioeconomic cost that is considered a worldwide epidemic. Met S is defined by a cluster of interconnected factors that directly increase the risk of coronary heart disease (CHD), other forms of cardiovascular atherosclerotic diseases (CVD), and type 2 DM. Its main components are dyslipidemia (elevated triglycerides and apolipoprotein B (apoB)-containing lipoproteins, and low high-density lipoproteins (HDL), hypertension, and deregulated glucose homeostasis, while abdominal obesity and insulin resistance (IR) have gained increasing attention as the core manifestations of the syndrome [9]. Recently, other abnormalities such as chronic proinflammatory and prothrombotic states, nonalcoholic fatty liver disease, and sleep apnea have been added to the entity of to the syndrome, making its definition even more complex. Besides the many components and clinical implications of Met S, there is still universally accepted pathogenic mechanism or clearly defined diagnostic criteria. Furthermore, there is still debate as to whether this entity represents a specific syndrome or is a surrogate of combined risk factors that put the individual at particular risk [10].

The most current definition incorporates the International Diabetes Federation (IDF) and American Heart Association/National Heart, Lung, and Blood Institute (AHA/NHLBI) definitions and requires a patient to have any three of the following five conditions [11]:

- Elevated waist circumference (ethnicity specific values, e.g., European males >94 cm [40 in.] and females >80 cm)
- Triglycerides 1.7 mmol/l or greater 150 mg/dL
- HDL-chol below 1.03 mmol/l [<40 mg/dL]
- BP >135/85 mmHg
- Fasting glucose >5.6 mmol/l [>100 mg/dL]

ED has been linked to multiple selected aspects of the metabolic syndrome, including type 2 diabetes mellitus [12, 13], increased fasting blood glucose [14, 15], arteriosclerotic disease manifestations [16–18], hypertension [13, 14, 19, 20], and obesity [13–15], and to the metabolic syndrome as defined by different health organizations [14, 15, 20, 21]. Moreover, Bal et al. [15] noted that the risk of ED increased in line with the number of factors of the Met S exhibited by a patient. Several interrelated mechanisms may explain the observed relationship between the Met S and ED. One obvious mechanism could be a low testosterone level, which has been shown to be associated with moderate and severe [22], possibly via a mechanism of diminished NO synthesis [23]. This hypothesis was supported by a report that testosterone treatment increases cavernosal expression of NO synthase mRNA in rats [24]. In this way, hypogonadism as a manifestation of the Met S could result in a diminished NO synthesis and subsequent ED. Another mechanism is peripheral arterial insufficiency due to an atherosclerotic disease. The presence of arterial vasculogenic ED is associated with ischemic heart disease in men >40 years old in several studies [25]. Furthermore, men with ED are twice as likely to have sustained a myocardial infarction compared with men without ED, and the risk becomes more pronounced with increasing age [26]. Increasing alpha adrenergic activity has been linked to several established aspects of the Met S and is an attractive potential mechanism that could explain the link between the Met S and ED. Evidence supporting this mechanism has come from a study demonstrating that patients with nonorganic ED have significantly higher sympathetic activity than those without ($p<0.05$) [27]. This mechanism has been supported by studies that have concluded that treatment with alpha-receptor antagonists, doxazosin [28], and alfuzosin [29, 30] may improve sexual function including ED. This mechanism is also attractive because it explains the link between ED and LUTS, which was confirmed by the Multinational Survey of the Aging Male (MSAM7) study [31]. This study included more than 14,000 men, aged 50–80 years, representative of the population of six European countries and the USA [32]. A fourth mechanism explaining the link between the Met S and ED involves increased activation of the Rho/Rhokinase pathway, acting downstream of norepinephrine and endothelin1 receptors. Diabetes and hypertension have been linked to increased activity in this pathway [28]. Increased activity in Rho/Rho-kinase pathway results in the inhibition of smooth muscle and subsequent smooth muscle contraction [33]. Although this mechanism has not been specifically demonstrated in erectile tissue, it adds to the body of evidence suggesting that ED is also an expression of the Met S and could arise via this mechanism [34].

There are several hypotheses concerning the mechanism linking the metabolic syndrome and male hypogonadism. Obesity, especially visceral obesity, is an established aspect of the metabolic syndrome. The activity of aromatase, an adipose enzyme that is involved in the irreversible conversion of testosterone into estradiol [35], is higher in men who are obese, and, consequently, they tend to have a decreased testosterone level and increased estradiol level [35, 36]. Thus, the metabolic syndrome provides an endocrine mechanism to explain the development of hypogonadotropic hypogonadism, as it is believed that the effect of estradiol on gonadotropin suppression is more potent than that of testosterone [37]. The findings of Zumoff and colleagues [38], who treated six obese men with oral testolactone (an aromatase inhibitor), support this conclusion. After 6 weeks, men treated with testolactone had higher levels of testosterone and LH and decreased levels of estrogen compared with their baseline levels [38].

The hypothalamic–pituitary–adrenal (HPA) axis provides yet another mechanism that could explain the link between the metabolic syndrome and hypogonadism. The HPA axis has been shown to be overactive in subjects suffering from the metabolic syndrome [39], and it is well established that cortisol inhibits the reproductive axis at several levels including secretion of GnRH and LH and also at the level of the testes themselves [40]. This emerging link between the metabolic syndrome and male hypogonadism via increased aromatase activity, hypogonadotropic hypogonadism, and increased activity of the HPA axis seems to suggest that male hypogonadism is also a urological aspect of the metabolic syndrome.

15.3 Novel Biomarkers (Metabolic and Imaging) to Clarify CVS Risk in the ED Patient

By definition, cardiac biomarkers are measurement tests that help predict cardiac risk [41]. They include traditional measurements of cardiovascular risk: the lipid panel, blood sugar, and blood pressure. They can include anthropomorphic measurements such as waist circumference (WC), body mass index (BMI), and other measures of visceral obesity. They can include imaging studies such as coronary artery calcification (CAC) as measured by electron-beam computed tomography or computed tomography or carotid intima–media thickness (CIMT) or carotid plaque. They can be surrogate measures of endothelial function such as peripheral arterial tonometry or serum asymmetric dimethylarginine (ADMA). They can be surrogate measures of arterial inflammation: highly sensitive C-reactive protein (hsCRP), TNF-alpha, adipokines, or Interleukin-6 (IL-6). They can measure insulin resistance and include fasting serum insulin, HOMA-IR, fasting glucose, or glycosylated A1C (HgBA1c). Lastly, they might include the measurement of the extremely artherogenic level of small, dense LDL particles (LDL-P), or Apolipoprotein B (apo-B) as measured by nuclear magnetic resonance.

Therefore, a range of important novel risk factors or biomarkers for cardiovascular disease are associated with the Met S, although not yet included within its definition. Most have yet to be validated for efficacy and cost-effective screening in both the asymptomatic and symptomatic ED patient. These include the above-noted chronic, low-grade inflammation, and disturbances in the secretion of bioactive substances from adipocytes ("adipokines") [42, 43], hsCRP, apo B, and vitamin D levels.

The cardiovascular risk factors associated with the metabolic syndrome, whether included within its diagnostic criteria or not, contribute to the progression of atherosclerotic cardiometabolic disease. Current diagnostic and therapeutic approaches do not adequately address these factors, and further clarification of the utility of these biomarkers in the ED patient is required.

We examine a few nontraditional markers and evaluate the quality of the evidence for their value as potential markers for cardiometabolic disease and thereby, in the ED patient. These have been graded according to the recommendations of the Centre for Evidence-Based Medicine: (http://www.cebm.net/levels_of_evidence.asp) [44]. Levels of evidence have been determined by consensus of the author following review of the present literature.

15.3.1 Waist Circumference (Intra-abdominal Adiposity) (IAA) in Men with ED: Level of Evidence = 1a

Intra-abdominal adiposity (IAA) drives the progression of multiple risk factors directly, through the secretion of excess free fatty acids and inflammatory adipokines and decreased secretion of adiponectin. The important contributions of IAA to dyslipidemia and insulin resistance provide an indirect, though clinically important, link to the genesis and progression of atherosclerosis and cardiovascular disease [45–47]. Presence of excess IAA is an important determinant of cardiometabolic risk. IAA is associated with insulin resistance, hyperglycemia, dyslipidemia, hypertension, and prothrombotic/proinflammatory states. Excess IAA typically is accompanied by elevated levels of C-reactive protein and free fatty acids (FFAs), as well as decreased levels of adiponectin. Abdominal obesity has been shown to be associated with the inflammation cascade, with adipose tissue expressing a number of inflammatory cytokines. Inflammation is now believed to play a role in the development of atherosclerosis and type 2 DM. Elevated levels of CRP are considered to be predictive of cardiovascular disease and insulin resistance [47, 48].

These components help to explain why excess abdominal adiposity is considered to be a great threat to cardiovascular and metabolic health. Abdominal obesity is associated with multiple cardiometabolic risk factors, including dyslipidemia [49], elevated blood glucose [50], and inflammation [41] – all factors leading to the development of CVD and DM in male ED patients. DM is, after age, the greatest risk factor for ED [2]. Patients with DM were three times more likely to develop ED than those who did not have DM [13, 51]. The prevalence for ED in these patients was as high as 75 % [52–54]. The Cologne Male Survey noted a fourfold increase in ED in men with DM as compared to the general population [55]. In the Health Professionals Follow-up Study, which involved greater than 30,000 subjects, Bacon et al. [56] found duration of DM strongly associated with incidence of ED. Rhoden et al. [57] found higher glycosylated hemoglobin levels in patients with DM to be significantly associated with more severe ED ($p<0.05$). The risk of ED in men with DM is also significantly associated with other diabetic complications such as diabetic neuropathy ($p<0.05$) [58].

Adipocytes generate inflammatory cytokines, and patients with obesity and T2DM tend to have a higher inflammatory profile. Inflammatory markers, such as IL-6 [59, 60], TNF-apha [59], or hsCRP [41], are elevated and have been associated with impaired endothelial function, cardiovascular events, and ED [60, 61].

15.3.2 Testosterone Levels and Cardiometabolic Risk: Level of Evidence = 2a

Hypogonadism is a common condition in men – especially older men – that can affect both health status and quality of life. Mulligan et al. [62] examined the prevalence rates and odds ratios for selected comorbidities associated with low testosterone levels in 2,162 primary care patients. They observed that the odds ratios of having low levels (hypogonadism is both the presence of low levels and clinical signs and symptoms) were increased in the presence of certain risk factors. The odds ratios for the presence of hypogonadism (the odds of having hyopogonadism if one has this risk factor versus not having the risk factor) being of 2.38 for obesity, 2.09 for diabetes, 1.84 for hypertension, and 1.47 for hyperlipidemia [62].

Research to date strongly and consistently shows testosterone replacement therapy (TT), at least over the short term (up to ~3 years), has positive effects on body composition – decreasing fat mass and increasing muscle mass – which in turn can reduce the risk for Met S and type 2 DM [63]. Evidence is moderately consistent for TT improving bone mineral density. Research to date also is strong showing TT has positive effects on various aspects of sexual function, though the specific effects differ from study to study. Most studies to date showed that TT increased sexual awareness and arousal, erectile function, and the frequency of spontaneous erections but was less consistent in enhancing actual sexual behavior and performance [64]. It is beyond the scope of this chapter to address the conflicting issues regarding testosterone and CVS events and mortality. One can simply say that studies thus far both positive and negative are cross-sectional and thereby, inconclusive. Yet, the authors feel it is vital to screen all men with ED for testosterone deficiency and thereby perhaps gain a sense of a man's overall health and stress. This is especially true in those men with a history of inadequate response to prior PDE5 inhibitors [65].

15.3.3 CAC Potential Role in ED Management: Level of Evidence = 1b

Coronary artery calcium (CAC) scores are better than carotid intima–media thickness (CIMT) as shown in a cohort of 44,052 asymptomatic patients referred for cardiovascular risk stratification. All-cause mortality rates (MRs) were calculated after stratifying by age groups and CAC score [66]. Another aim was to determine if coronary artery calcium (CAC) scoring is independently predictive of mortality in young adults and in the elderly population and if a young person with high CAC has a higher mortality risk than an older person with less CAC. Indeed, the value of CAC for predicting mortality extends to both elderly patients and those less than 45 years old. Elderly persons with no CAC have a lower MR than younger persons with high CAC [66].

In another MESA subanalysis, Detrano et al. [67] collected data on risk factors and performed coronary calcium scoring in an ethnically diverse population without cardiovascular disease at entry who were followed for a median of 3.8 years. They found that the adjusted risk of a CVD event was increased by a factor of 7.73 among participants with a CAC score of 101–300 compared to those individuals with no coronary calcium [67]. This risk increased to 9.67 among those with CAC scores exceeding 300 [67]. They noted that CAC scores are a strong predictor of incident CHD and provides predictive value beyond the standard Framingham risk data, regardless of race or ethnicity.

Thus, we propose the use of CAC scoring in men deemed at intermediate risk of CAD with ED according to the Framingham Risk Stratification or patients with low lifetime risk but one that might fall out of the present grading criteria [8]. The absence of CAC is conclusive of minimal to no risk of ASCVD in the following 10 years. The presence of CAC may help guide the clinician regarding appropriate primary prevention therapy and certainly is one of the strongest discriminatory tests for the intermediate-risk patient in CVD risk stratification.

15.3.4 The Role for Peripheral Arterial Tonometry (PAT) Assessment and Asymmetric Dimethylarginine (ADMA) as Markers of Endothelial Cell Function in Men with ED: Level of Evidence = 2a

Because endothelial dysfunction is considered the first step toward the generation of atherosclerotic plaque [68] and can be found in patients with cardiovascular risk factors [69, 70], the use of flow-mediated vasodilation (FMD) has long had a role in the evaluation of the pathology of erectile dysfunction. Indeed, Kaiser et al. [71] studied 30 men with ED and no other clinical cardiovascular disease and compared them with 27 age-matched controls without ED. The ED group had penile vascular disease present on Doppler ultrasound testing (mean peak systolic flow of 28 cm/s ± 3), an IIEF-5 score of 12.9 vs. 22.3 ($p=0.000001$) with a cutoff value for ED <21. While no significant differences were noted in fasting lipids, glucose, homocysteine, and CAC scores in the two groups, there was a significant difference in brachial artery flow-mediated vasodilation studies thereby illustrating the idea that ED appears to occur before the development of overt structural or functional systemic vascular disease and that abnormalities in the penile cavernosal nitric oxide/cyclic GMP vasodilator system may result in ED as an early clinical manifestation of vascular disease [72].

This led to the theory that endothelial dysfunction is believed to be the common initiator of ED and other atherosclerotic diseases. The importance of this study cannot be understated. Men with ED but no other clinical cardiovascular disease were found to have reduced flow-mediated vasodilation in the brachial artery in response to sublingual nitroglycerine, indicating endothelial dysfunction and abnormal smooth muscle relaxation. Evidence is accumulating that endothelial dysfunction is an early functional change thought to precede ASCVD changes in the cerebrovascular, coronary, and peripheral circulations [72].

Obesity is associated with increased activation of the rennin–angiotensin system, which in turn, leads to vasoconstriction and impaired endothelial function [73]. DM is associated with higher levels of asymmetric dimethylarginine (ADMA) [74]. ADMA is an endogenous analogue of L-arginine that competitively inhibits nitric oxide synthase (NOS) [75]. Elevated plasma ADMA levels signify impaired endothelial cell function [74, 75] and predict cardiovascular events [76–80]. A strong link of ADMA to CAD and ED has been reported [81].

Endothelial dysfunction is characterized by a reduction in endogenous nitric oxide activity that may be attributed to an elevation in ADMA levels [82]. Thus, it may be speculated that the elevation of endogenous ADMA may be associated with the systemic manifestations of endothelial dysfunction in patients with cardiovascular risk factors and ED [83].

15.3.5 Vitamin D and Cardiovascular Health: Level of Evidence = 2b

Vitamin D is known to have a well-defined role in bone and calcium metabolism, but it has also been implicated as a factor in cardiovascular health. Vitamin D deficiency as defined by the American Endocrine Society as less than 20 ng/ml affects nearly fifty percent of the world's population [84]. It has been observed that the incidence of cardiovascular disease increases with increasing distance from the equator, and correlation with vitamin D deficiency has been proposed as a mechanism [85]. Both the Framingham Offspring Study and the Health Professionals Follow-up Study showed an approximately doubled risk for cardiovascular events in vitamin

D-deficient subjects [84, 86]. Analysis of retrospectively collected data from 27,686 patients in the Intermountain Heart Collaborative Study Group (IHC) demonstrated that vitamin D levels were highly associated with coronary artery disease and myocardial infarction [87]. In the Multi-Ethnic Study of Atherosclerosis, lower 25(OH) D concentration was associated with an increased risk for incident coronary artery calcification, a measure of coronary atherosclerosis [88].

Study of the effects of the vitamin D receptor (VDR) has revealed potential mechanisms for the effects of vitamin D on vascular health. Vitamin D receptors are present in all of the key mediators of atherosclerosis including endothelial cells, vascular smooth muscle cells, and immune cells [89]. Vascular cell growth, migration, and differentiation along with immune response modulation and cytokine expression are tied to the activation of the VDR. Vitamin D is also directly involved in the systemic inflammatory response contributing to atherosclerosis [90]. Although interventional studies have not yet shown benefits of vitamin D supplementation in risk reduction, it is clearly evolving as an important marker of risk.

Most importantly, the use of these novel biomarkers and surrogates begs the question whether these markers or risk factors validate an organic cause for ED and whether modification of these markers/risk factors can improve both ED and lessen overall ASCVD risk? The honest answer is that we do not have clarification of this at present. There remains a disconnect between imaging surrogates and outcomes.

From the above evidence and our experience, we propose the following metabolic investigation of men with ED, including anthropomorphic and vital sign measurements:

- 2013 ASCVD AHA/ACC Risk Estimator to determine 10-year and lifetime ASCVD risk (MI and CVA) for men ages 40–59 years old [91].
- Waist circumference measured at the umbilicus.
- Blood pressure/heart rate.
- Fasting insulin and glucose levels.
- Baseline renal function (BUN/creatinine).
- Fasting lipid profile.
- Morning total testosterone level.
- Hs CRP.
- Vitamin D3 (OH).
- If there is any doubt with the use of the 2013 ASCVD Risk Estimator, then CT calcium scoring may clarify risk and treatment options.

When we examine the use of biomarkers, we must distinguish between screening to define a population at risk that we are not currently treating and reducing surrogate endpoints (e.g., MI, acute coronary syndrome, stroke). These questions, together with the issue posed by Thompson [92]. "Could erectile dysfunction serve as a surrogate measure of treatment efficacy in preventive interventions for cardiac disease?" can only be answered by further studies of cardiovascular disease prevention strategies in men with largely vasculogenic ED. Men with ED with or without CVS risk factors should be considered an "intermediate"-risk group for future cardiovascular

Table 15.1 Key points/potential pitfalls: what to avoid

1. Guidelines should never replace clinical judgment. They should aid and inform decision-making
2. Avoid layering tests. Testing should be ordered when specific information is required to aid in risk stratification and clinic decision-making
3. Lab testing should be interpreted in the appropriate context – checking morning samples of testosterone, repeating testosterone levels to confirm borderline results, checking two values of hsCRP, not screening during an acute illness. Results taken out of context can be misleading
4. Do not underestimate the value of lifestyle modification as an intervention. Estimation of risk can drive changes in behavior and promote health and wellness (over the usual paradigm of disease and treatment)

events. It is this group of men, particularly under the age of 60 years, who may benefit from utilization of some of these surrogate markers of cardiometabolic risk in a cost-effective manner to stratify them for subsequent aggressive treatment of preventative cardiovascular risk factors. These men, many of whom may be missed by the traditional Framingham risk criteria, may find the risk elaborated with prudent use of these biomarkers or imaging studies. Only further studies of men with vasculogenic ED and preventative measures will provide evidence as to which of the surrogate markers are impactful and efficacious in the delineation of such risk.

Conclusion

The metabolic investigation of erectile dysfunction involves primarily the investigation of metabolic sequela of visceral adiposity leading to type 2 DM or CVD. This is known as cardiometabolic risk. Older models of cardiovascular risk assessment (FRS) have generally underestimated risk in younger and middle-aged populations. The authors of the new risk models make adjustments for this and introduce the idea of balancing 10-year risk with lifetime risk to aid in decision-making in younger adults. Whether it is lifetime risk or ED that is used to enhance 10-year risk assessment, the concept is the same: to discern those who have started down the path of inflammation, endothelial dysfunction, and vulnerable plaque formation and thereby intervene somewhere upstream from the first ASCVD event. Lifetime risk may be something abstract to most patients, and current evidence does not support its use to guide pharmacotherapy. The value is to motivate therapeutic lifestyle changes. ED is something tangible. It affects mental health and quality of life. Young and middle-aged male patients with ED are likely to make changes that will have an immediate impact on both their CVS risk and overall sexual function (Table 15.1).

References

1. Hatzimouratidis K, Amar E, Eardley I et al (2010) Guidelines on male sexual dysfunction and premature ejaculation. Eur Urol 57:804–814

2. Prins J, Blanker MH, Bohnen AM et al (2002) Prevalence of erectile dysfunction: a systematic review of population –based studies. Int J Impot Res 14:422–432
3. Inman BA, St Sauver JL, Jacobson DJ et al (2009) A population-based, longitudinal study of erectile dysfunction and future coronary artery disease. Mayo Clin Proc 84:108–113.K
4. Marma AK, Berry JD, Ning H et al (2010) Distribution of 10-year and lifetime predicted risks for cardiovascular disease in US adults findings from the National Health and Nutrition Examination Survey 2003 to 2006. Circ Cardiovasc Qual Outcome 3:8–14
5. Dhaliwal SS, Welborn TA (2009) Central obesity and multivariable cardiovascular risk as assessed by the Framingham prediction scores. Am J Cardiol 103:1403–1407
6. Stone NJ, Robinson J, Lichtenstein AH et al (2014) 2013 ACC/AHA guideline on the treatment of blood cholesterol to reduce astherosclerotic cardiovascular risk in adults. J Am Coll Cardiol 63:2935–59
7. Nehra A, Jackson G, Miner M et al (2012) The Princeton III consensus recommendations for the management of erectile dysfunction and cardiovascular disease. Mayo Clin Proc 87(8):766–778
8. Miner M, Nehra A, Jackson G et al (2014) All men with vasculogenic ED require a cardiovascular workup. Am J Med 127(3):174–182
9. Castelli WP, Abbott RD, McNamara PM (1983) Summary estimates of cholesterol used to predict coronary heart disease. Circulation 67(4):730–734
10. Kassi E, Pervanidou P, Kaltsas G et al (2011) Metabolic syndrome: definitions and controversies. BMC Med 9:48–61
11. Alberti KG, Eckel RH, Grundy SM et al (2009) International Diabetes Task Force on Epidemiology and Prevention, National Heart, Lung and Blood Institute, American Heart Association, World Heart Federation, International Atherosclerosis Society, International Association for the Study of Obesity: harmonizing the metabolic syndrome: a joint interim statement of the International Diabetes Task Force on Epidemiology and Prevention; National Heart, Lung, and Blood Institute; American Heart Association; World Heart Federation; International Atherosclerosis Society; and International Association for the Study of Obesity. Circulation 120:1640–1645
12. Aslan Y, Sezgin T, Tuncel A et al (2009) Is type 2 diabetes mellitus a cause of severe erectile dysfunction in patients with metabolic syndrome. Urology 74:561–565
13. Saigal CS, Wessels H, Pace J et al; Urologic Diseases in America Project (2006) Predictors and prevalence of erectile dysfunction in a racially diverse population. Arch Intern Med 166:207–212
14. Demir T (2006) Prevalence of erectile dysfunction in patients with metabolic syndrome. Int J Urol 13:385–388
15. Bal K, Oder M, Sahin AS et al (2007) Prevalence of metabolic syndrome and its association with erectile dysfunction among urologic patients: metabolic backgrounds of erectile dysfunction. Urology 69:356–360
16. El Sakka AI, Morsy AM (2004) Screening for ischemic heart disease in patients with erectile dysfunction: role of penile Doppler ultrasonography. Urology 64:346–350
17. El-Sakka AI, Morsy AM, Fagih BI et al (2004) Coronary artery risk factors in patients with erectile dysfunction. J Urol 172:251–254
18. Jackson G (2009) Sexual response in cardiovascular disease. J Sex Res 46:233–236
19. Al Hunayan A, Al Mutar M, Kehind EO et al (2007) The prevalence and predictors of erectile dysfunction in men with newly diagnosed with type 2 diabetes mellitus. BJU Int 99:130–134
20. Tomada N, Tomada I, Botelho F et al (2011) Are all metabolic syndrome components responsible for penile hemodynamics impairment in patients with erectile dysfunction? The role of body fat mass assessment. J Sex Med 8:831–839
21. Kupelian V, Shabsig R, Araujo AB et al (2006) Erectile dysfunction as a predictor of the metabolic syndrome in aging men: results from the Massachusetts male aging study. J Urol 176:222–226
22. Corona G, Mannucci E, Ricca V et al (2009) The age related decline of testosterone is associated with different specific symptoms and signs in patients with sexual dysfunction. Int J Androl 32:720–728

23. Gorbachinsky I, Akpinar H, Assimos DG (2010) Metabolic syndrome and urologic diseases. Rev Urol 12:157–180
24. Reilly CM, Zamorano P, Stopper VS et al (1997) Androgenic regulation of NO availability in rat penile erection. J Androl 18:110
25. Shamloul R, Ghanem HM, Salem A et al (2004) Correlation between penile duplex findings and stress electrocardiography in men with erectile dysfunction. Int J Impot Res 16:235–237
26. Chen CJ, Kuo TB, Tseng YJ et al (2009) Combined cardiac sympathetic excitation and vagal impairment in patients with no organic erectile dysfunction. Clin Neurophysiol 120:348–352
27. Kirby RS, O'Leary MP, Carson C (2005) Efficacy of extended release doxazosin and doxazosin standard in patients with concomitant benign prostatic hyperplasia and sexual dysfunction. BJU Int 95:103–109
28. De Rose AF, Carmignani G, Corbu C et al (2002) Observational multicentric trial performed with doxazosin: evaluation of sexual effects on patients with diagnosed benign prostatic hyperplasia. Urol Int 68:95–98
29. Liguori G, Trombetta C, De Giorgi G et al (2009) Efficacy of combined oral therapy with tadalafil and alfuzosin: an integrated approach to management of patients with lower urinary tracts symptoms and erectile dysfunction. Preliminary report. J Sex Med 6:544–552
30. Kaplan SA, Gonzeles RR, Te AE (2007) Combination of alfuzosin and sildenafil is superior to monotherapy in treating lower urinary tract symptoms and erectile dysfunction. Eur Urol 51:1717–1723
31. McVary KT (2006) Lower urinary tract symptoms and sexual dysfunction: epidemiology and pathophysiology. BJU Int 97(Suppl 2):23–28
32. Rosen R, Altwein J, Boyle P et al (2003) Lower urinary tract symptoms and male sexual dysfunction: the multinational survey of the aging male (MSAM-7). Eur Urol 44(6):637–649
33. Faris JE, Smith MR (2010) Metabolic sequelae associated with androgen deprivation therapy for prostate cancer. Curr Opin Endocrinol Diabetes Obes 17:240–246
34. Hammarsten J, Peeker R (2011) Urologic aspects of the metabolic syndrome. Nat Rev Urol 8:483–494
35. Cohen PG (2008) Obesity in men: the hypogonadal estrogen receptor relationship and its effect on glucose homeostasis. Med Hypotheses 70:358–360
36. Vermeulen A, Kaufman JM, Deslypere JP et al (1993) Attenuated luteinizing hormone (LH) pulse amplitude but normal pulse frequency, and its relation to plasma androgens in hypogonadism of obese men. J Clin Endocrinol Metab 76:1140–1146
37. Cohen PG (1998) The role of estradiol in the maintenance of secondary hypogonadism in males in erectile dysfunction. Med Hypotheses 50:331–333
38. Zumoff B, Miller LK, Strain GW (1993) Reversal of the hypogonadotropic hypogonadism of obese men by administration of the aromatase inhibitor testolactone. Metabolism 52:1126–1128
39. Rosmond R, Dallman MF, Björntorp P (1998) Stress-related cortisol secretion in men: relationships with abdominal obesity and endocrine, metabolic and hemodynamic abnormalities. J Clin Endocrinol Metab 83:1853–1859
40. Chrousos G (1988) Stressors, stress, and neuroendocrine integration of the adaptive response. The 1997 Hans Selye Memorial Lecture. Ann N Y Acad Sci 851:311–335
41. Billups KL, Kaiser DR, Kelly AS et al (2003) Relation of C-reactive protein and other cardiovascular risk factors to penile vascular disease in men with erectile dysfunction. Int J Impot Res 15:231–236
42. Gelfand EV, Cannon CP, Rimonabant (2006) A cannabinoid receptor type 1 blocker for management of multiple cardiometabolic risk factors. JACC 47(10):1919–1926
43. Vasudevan AR, Ballantyne CM (2005) Cardiometabolic risk assessment: an approach to the prevention of cardiovascular disease and diabetes mellitus. Clin Conerstone 7(2–3):7–16
44. Centre for evidence-based medicine. http://www.cebm.net/levels_of_evidence.asp
45. Rathmann W, Haastert B, Herder C et al (2007) Differential association of adiponectin with cardiovascular risk markers in men and women? The KORA survey 2000. Int J Obes 31:770–776

46. Yamauchi T, Kamon J, Minokoshi Y et al (2002) Adiponectin stimulates glucose utilization and fatty-acid oxidation by activating AMP-activated protein kinase. Nat Med 8:1288–1295
47. Snijder MB, Heine RJ, Seidell JC et al (2006) Associations of adiponectin levels with incident impaired glucose metabolism and type 2 diabetes in older men and women. The Hoorn study. Diabetes Care 29:2498–2503
48. Silvestro A, Brevetti G, Schiano V et al (2005) Adhesion molecules and cardiovascular risk in peripheral arterial disease. Soluble vascular cell adhesion molecule-1 improves risk stratification. Thromb Haemost 93:559–563
49. Nikoobakht M, Nasseh H, Pourkasmaee M (2005) The relationship between lipid profile and erectile dysfunction. Int J Impot Res 17:523–526
50. Burke JP, Jacobson DJ, McGree ME et al (2007) Diabetes and sexual dysfunction: results from the Olmsted county study of urinary symptoms and health status among men. J Urol 177:1438–1442
51. Ponholzer A, Temml C, Mock K et al (2005) Prevalence and risk factors for erectile dysfunction in 2869 men using a validated questionnaire. Eur Urol 47:80–85
52. Fonseca V, Jawa A (2005) Endothelial and erectile dysfunction, diabetes mellitus, and the metabolic syndrome: common pathways and treatments? Am J Cardiol 96:13M–18M
53. Vinik A, Richardson D (1998) Erectile dysfunction in diabetes. Diabetes Rev 6:16–33
54. Fedele D, Coscelli C, Santeusanio F et al (1998) For the Gruppo Italiano Studio Deficit Erecttile nei Diabetici. Erectile dysfunction in diabetic subjects in Italy. Diabetes Care 21:1973–1977
55. Braun M, Wassmer G, Klotz T et al (2000) Epidemiology of erectile dysfunction: results of the 'Cologne male survey'. Int J Imp Res 12:305–311
56. Bacon CG, Hu FB, Giovannucci E et al (2002) Association and type and duration of diabetes with erectile dysfunction in a large cohort of men. Diabetes Care 25:1458–1463
57. Rhoden EL, Ribeiro EP, Riedner CE et al (2005) Glycosolated hemoglobin levels and the severity of erectile function in diabetic men. BJU Int 95:615–617
58. Gazzaruso C, Pujia A, Solerte SB et al (2006) Erectile dysfunction and angiographic extent of coronary artery disease in type II diabetic patients. Int J Impot Res 18:311–315
59. Naya M, Tsukamoto T, Morita K et al (2007) Plasma interleukin-6 and tumor necrosis factor-alpha can predict coronary endothelial dysfunction in hypertensive patients. Hypertens Res 30:541–548
60. Vlachopoulos C, Aznaouridis K, Ioakeimidis N et al (2006) Unfavourable endothelial and inflammatory state in erectile dysfunction patients with or without coronary artery disease. Eur Heart J 27:2640–2648
61. Giugliano F, Esposito K, Di Palo C et al (2004) Erectile dysfunction associates with endothelial dysfunction and raised proinflammatory cytokine levels in obese men. J Endocrinol Invest 27:665–669
62. Mulligan T, Frick MF, Zuraw QC et al (2006) Prevalence of hypogonadism in males at least 45 years: the HIM study. Int J Clin Pract 60:762–769
63. Buvat J, Maggi M, Guay A et al (2013) Testosterone deficiency in Men: systematic review and standard operating procedures for diagnosis and treatment. J Sex Med 10:245–284
64. Miner M, Canty D, Shabsigh R (2008) Testosterone replacement therapy in hypogonadal men: assessing benefits, risks, and best practices. Postgrad Med 120(3):130–152
65. Shabsigh R, Kaufman JM, Steidle C et al (2004) Randomized study of testosterone gel as adjunctive therapy to sildenafil in hypogonadal men with erectile dysfunction who do not respond to sildenafil alone. J Urol 172(2):658–663
66. Tota-Maharaj R, Blaha MJ (2012) Coronary artery calcium for the prediction of mortality in young adults <45 years old and elderly adults >75 years old. Eur Heart J 33:2955–2962
67. Detrano R, Guerci AD, Carr JJ et al (2008) Coronary calcium as a predictor of coronary events in four racial or ethnic groups. N Engl J Med 358:1336–1345
68. Cooke JP (2000) The endothelium: a new target for therapy. Vasc Med 5:49–53
69. Lekakis J, Papamichael C, Vemmos C et al (1998) Effects of acute cigarette smoking on endothelium-dependent arterial dilatation in normal subjects. Am J Cardiol 81:1225–1228

70. Higashi Y, Sasaki S, Nakagawa K et al (2001) Effect of obesity on endothelium-dependent, nitric oxide-mediated vasodilation in normotensive individuals and patients with essential hypertension. Am J Hypertens 14:1038–1045
71. Kaiser DR, Billups KL, Bank AL et al (2004) Impaired brachial artery endothelium-dependent and –independent vasodilation in men with erectile dysfunction and no other clinical cardiovascular disease. J Am Coll Cardiol 43:179–184
72. Shabsigh R (2005) Correlation between erectile dysfunction and metabolic syndrome. In: Sadovsky R (ed) Heart of the matter: erectile dysfunction as an early sign of vasculopathy. CogniMed Inc, Livingston, pp 14–21
73. Segura J, Ruilope LM (2007) Obesity, essential hypertension and rennin-angiotensin system. Public Health Nutr 10:1151–1155
74. Yamagishi S, Ueda S, Nakamura K et al (2008) Role of asymmetric dimethylarginine (ADMA) in diabetic vascular complications. Curr Pharm Des 25:2613–2618
75. Palmer RM, Ferrige AG, Moncada S (1987) Nitric oxide release accounts for the biological activity of endothelium-derived relaxing factor. Nature 327:524–526
76. Juonala M, Viikari J, Alfthan G et al (2007) Brachial artery flow-mediated dilation and asymmetrical dimethylarginine in the cardiovascular risk in young Finns study. Circulation 116:1367–1373
77. Ardigo D, Stuehlinger M, Franzini L et al (2007) ADMA is independently related to flow-mediated vasodilation in subjects at low cardiovascular risk. Eur J Clin Invest 37:263–269
78. Valkonen V, Paiva H, Salonen J et al (2001) Risk of acute coronary events and serum concentration of asymmetric dimethylarginine. Lancet 358:2127–2128
79. Mittermayer F, Krzyzanowska K, Exner M et al (2006) Asymmetric dimethylarginine predicts major adverse cardiovascular events in patients with advanced peripheral artery disease. Arterioscler Thromb Vasc Biol 26:2536–2540
80. Schnabel R, Blankenberg S, Lubos E et al (2005) Asymmetric dimethylarginine and the risk of cardiovascular events and death in patients with coronary artery disease: results from the AtheroGene study. Circ Res 97:e53–e59
81. Maas R, Wenske S, Zabel M et al (2005) Elevation of asymmetric dimethylarginine (ADMA) and coronary artery disease in men with erectile dysfunction. Eur Urol 48:1004–1011
82. Cooke JP (2000) Does ADMA cause endothelial dysfunction? Arterioscler Thromb Vasc Biol 20:2032–2037
83. Kielstein JT, Impraim B, Simmel S et al (2004) Cardiovascular effects of systemic nitric oxide synthase inhibition with ADMA in humans. Circulation 109:172–177
84. Judd S, Tangpricha V (1989) Vitamin D deficiency and risk for cardiovascular disease. Lancet 1:613
85. Hollick MF, Binkley NC, Heike BA et al (2011) Evaluation, treatment, and prevention of vitamin D deficiency: an endocrine society clinical practice guideline. J Clin Endocrinol Metab 96:1911–1930
86. Wallis D, Penckofer S, Sizemore G (2008) The "sunshine deficit" and cardiovascular disease. Circulation 118:1476–1485
87. Kuhn T, Kaaks R (2008) Plasma 25-hydroxyvitamin D and its genetic determinants in relation to incident myocardial infarction and stroke in the European Prospective Investigation into Cancer and nutrition (EPIC)-Germany study. Arch Int Med 168:1174–1180
88. Mullie P, Autier P (2010) Relation of vitamin D deficiency to cardiovascular disease. Am J Cardiol 106:963–968
89. de Boer I, Kestenbaum B, Shoben A et al (2009) 25-hyddroxyvitamin D levels inversely associate with risk for developing coronary artery calcification. J Am Soc Nephrol 20:1805–1812
90. Danik J, Manson J (2012) Vitamin D and cardiovascular disease. Curr Treat Options Cardiovasc Med 14:414–424
91. Goff DC Jr, Lloyd-Jones DM, Bennett G (2014) 2013 ACC/AHA guideline on the assessment of cardiovascular risk. J Am Coll Cardiol 63:2935–59
92. Thompson IM, Tamgen CM, Goodman PJ et al (2005) Erectile dysfunction and subsequent cardiovascular disease. JAMA 294:2296–3002

Erectile Dysfunction in the Elderly

Siegfried Meryn

16.1 Introduction

"It's far more important to know what person the disease has than what disease the person has." If this quote of Hippocrates, the father of modern medicine, was ever true, it is in the area of diagnosing and treating sexual dysfunction, particularly in the elderly. Human sexuality is how people experience and express themselves as sexual human beings. Sexuality is one of the most pervasive aspects of the human life cycle. For the majority of people, sexual enjoyment will imply sexual contacts and sexual intercourse with a partner.

Sexual expression usually starts when the hormones of puberty activate the somatic substrate of sexuality and does not really end until death. Human sexuality has aspects of an instinct and an insistent recurrent biological drive, but it is influenced by mental activity and by social, cultural, educational, legal, and normative characteristics of the environment in which subjects grow up and their personality develops. The palette of human sexual behavior has many more colors than the rainbow. The relevance of the above notion is that patients with sexual dysfunction face not only the problem itself but not rarely have strong feelings of embarrassment. The latter may be an impediment to seek proper medical treatment.

Although sexuality is very prevalent in our society today, at an individual level, patients and especially elder patients may still be apprehensive about discussing

S. Meryn (✉)
Department of Medical Education, Medical University of Vienna,
Spitalgasse 23, Vienna 1090, Austria
e-mail: siegfried.meryn@meduniwien.ac.at

details of their sexual practices and the anxieties they may harbor. Sexual problems are frequent among older adults, but these problems are infrequently discussed with physicians. An US Study found that a total of 38 % of men reported having discussed sex with a physician since the age of 50 [1].

The attending physician should choose his/her words carefully when taking an elder patient's history. It is of note that it is not only the language but also the healthcare provider's body language and facial expressions that can discourage information disclosure. Therefore, it is up to the physician to create an environment free from personal prejudice in order to best serve the patient. A useful strategy may be what has become known as "the parable method." With this method, the medical caregiver relates a "parable" or a story illustrating the point that the history of the patient is not very unique and that shame or guilt in the context of treating the problem might be counterproductive in achieving diagnostic and treatment goals. Examples are: "2 weeks ago, I had a similar patient and this person disclosed to me.... Is that also the case with you?"

The information the attending physician seeks thus becomes a less personal issue of the patient who finds relief in the fact that he or she is not the only person in the world facing this problem and that the attending physician obviously is at ease discussing the intimate aspects of the sexual practice that gave the patient reason to seek medical consultation.

An attitude free of prejudice and moral judgment is not the same as abstaining from information and education about sex.

The success of treating sexual dysfunction is as much determined by our expertise as our talent to discuss frankly with the patient the context of the disease.

16.2 The Epidemiology of Sexual Dysfunction in the Elderly

Until a century ago, people often did not live beyond the reproductive years, and sexuality of the elderly was a private issue but not a medical question that could frankly be discussed with healthcare providers. It was generally assumed that, with aging, loss of sexuality was natural and inevitable. And not life-threatening, little attention was given to sexual behavior and treatment of sexual dysfunctions in the older population. Over the last decades, life expectancy has considerably improved and also with the present-day spectacular treatment options for erectile dysfunction, men are seeking to maintain sexual activity into old age.

While the interest in sexuality in most aging men persists, a decline in sexual activity is typically seen with aging, which must be ascribed to declining general health and specific sexual dysfunctions. Several studies indicate that sexual health is a strong indicator of general health and, vice versa, that deterioration of general health has its impact on sexual function.

There are almost no medical guidelines for treating older adults with sexual dysfunction. Guidelines for treatment are often disease or symptom oriented (erectile dysfunction) and meant to serve essentially younger people, but a comprehensive treatment model for the aging is absent. Health policy organizations like the World

Health Organization in two recent reports pay no attention to sexual functioning and sexual health in the later years of life.

Elderly men continue to be sexually active throughout their lives. There is no true upper age limit for sexual activity. Several reports have, however, documented that the prevalence of sexual activities declines with age. A Swedish study [2] reported on sexual activity among a random selection of 319 men between 50 and 80 years. With aging there was a decline in frequency of desire, erections, orgasm, and intercourse, experienced as distress and negative impact on quality of life.

A French study found that though 66 % of men aged 70–79 reported being sexually active, but only 18 % of them reported one or more incidences of sexual intercourse per week. Studies of Australian and European men produced very similar results. In the Massachusetts Male Aging Study with a follow-up of 9 years also found an age-associated decline in most aspects of sexual functioning including sexual intercourse, erection, sexual desire, masturbation, satisfaction with sex, and difficulty with orgasm [3].

Having a partner, good health, good sexual self-esteem, enjoyable past experience, and an attitude that values the importance of sex in couple relationship were predictors. It was the ability to adapt to the limitations of aging less focused on performance and coitus that spelled the most successful sexuality in old age. People who are not fixated on penovaginal penetration and who are able to enjoy a wider range of sexual activities define their sex lives as better than others.

Recently, the concept of "sexually active life expectancy," defined as the "average number of years remaining spent as sexually active" was proposed. While life expectancy for men is shorter than for women, sexually active life expectancy is longer for men than for women, but men lose more years of a sexually active life as a result of poorer general health [4].

16.3 Conspiracy of Silence

The expression conspiracy of silence, or culture of silence, relates to a condition or matter which is known to exist but, by tacit communal unspoken consensus, is not talked about or acknowledged. Commonly such matters are considered personally embarrassing and/or culturally shameful to speak openly about.

In patients with cardiovascular disease, for instance, sexual dysfunction is frequently encountered. Several studies have established the link between erectile dysfunction (ED) and silent vascular disease, and as a consequence, ED may act as a marker for silent coronary artery disease (CAD) and therefore precede a coronary event in the elderly. In patients with established CAD, ED comes before CAD in the majority by an average of 2 up to 3 years. ED has the same risk factors in common as coronary artery disease. Patients with heart disease often fear triggering cardiovascular events when they want to engage in sexual activities which, by their nature, are more or less strenuous. This creates stress and anxiety negatively impacting the sexual lives of patients and their partners.

In a study in the Netherlands, a questionnaire addressing awareness, knowledge, and practice patterns about sexual dysfunction in cardiac patients was responded to by 54 % of the cardiologists. Only 16 % indicated to discuss sexual function regularly in the past year, and an estimated mean of 2 % of patients had been referred for help with a sexual problem. The majority (70 %) of cardiologists discussed/advised patients never or seldom about resuming sexual activity after myocardial infarction. The use of PDE5-inhibitors was checked by 19.4 % of the cardiologists. Important reasons not to discuss sexual function were lack of initiative of the patient (54 %), time constraints (43 %), and lack of training on dealing with sexual dysfunction (35 %). Sixty-three percent of the cardiologists stated they would be ready to refer patients to professionals providing sexual counseling when these professional services were better known to them and easily accessible. The conclusion is that sexuality is not routinely discussed in the cardiology practice. This lack of attention toward sexual matters is explained by ambiguities about responsibility for this part of healthcare, and further a lack of time, training and experience regarding the communication and treatment of sexual dysfunction [5].

Interestingly, more than 50 % of the cardiologists expect patients to take the initiative to discuss sexual matters. Several studies indicate that the majority of patients do not discuss their sexual problems with a healthcare provider. Men discussing sexual issues were more likely to have higher education. Sexuality is important for older adults, but interest in discussing aspects of sexual life is variable. Physicians should give their patient's opportunity to voice their concerns with sexual function and offer them alternatives for evaluation and treatment.

16.4 Polypharmacy

Polypharmacy refers to the effects of taking multiple medications concurrently to manage coexisting health problems, such as diabetes and hypertension. Too often, polypharmacy becomes problematic, such as when patients are prescribed too many medications by multiple healthcare providers working independently of each other. Also, drug interactions can occur if no single healthcare provider knows the patient's complete medication picture.

Among older adults, polypharmacy is a common problem. Currently, 44 % of men and 57 % of women older than age 65 take five or more medications per week; about 12 % of both men and women take ten or more medications per week. These agents include both prescription and over-the-counter preparations, such as vitamin and mineral supplements and herbal products. The latter, often labeled as natural, are rarely suspected of having undesired effects.

Older persons react differently to medications than younger persons. Although absorption rates for most drugs do not change with age, aging alters body fat and water composition: fat stores increase while total body water decreases. These changes can alter therapeutic drug levels, causing greater concentrations of water-soluble drugs and longer half-lives of fat-soluble drugs. Also, because the liver metabolizes many drugs, such age-related changes as reduced hepatic blood flow and liver size alter drug clearance. Subsequently, older patients may be more sensitive to some drugs and less sensitive to others. Classes of drugs that affect sexual functioning are antidepressants, antipsychotics, antiepileptics, antihypertensives, and cholesterol-lowering drugs. For review: http://www.netdoctor.co.uk/sexandrelationships/medicinessex.htm

A remarkable finding is that 5α-reductase inhibitors (finasteride, dutasteride), widely used in elderly for prostate problems and in younger for alopecia androgenica, may have sexual side effects. The prevalence rates of de novo erectile dysfunction of alpha reductase inhibitors have been estimated to amount to 5–9 %. One study found that the use of 5α- reductase inhibitors in men with sexual dysfunction does not significantly exacerbate preexisting ejaculatory or erectile difficulties but can further impair their sexual life by reducing sexual drive and spontaneous erection [6]. The explanation is not obvious. It is not certain whether the decreased circulating dihydrotestosterone (DHT) resulting from the use of 5α- reductase inhibitors leads to diminished sexual desire and/or orgasm. Patients receiving therapy with 5α-reductase inhibitors should be counseled as to potential sexual and psychological adverse effects.

16.5 Lower Urinary Tract Symptoms and Erectile Dysfunction

The most frequent urologic complaint in aging patients is lower urinary tract symptoms (LUTS). With increasing age, the prevalence of histological benign prostatic hyperplasia (BPH) increases from 8 % to 90 %. Parallel with LUTS, the prevalence of erectile function increases with aging. Until more than a decade ago, it was assumed that erectile dysfunction and LUTS are both inherent in the process of male aging but that they are nonrelated entities. The Multinational Survey of the Aging Male [7] provided evidence of a relationship between erectile dysfunction and LUTS. Other studies have confirmed this relationship. In men of all ages, the prevalence of ED is higher in men presenting LUTS, and the prevalence of ED is higher when the complaints of LUTS become more severe. In a recent review of 23 relevant studies correlating LUTS/BPH and ED [8], it was concluded that roughly one-third of men aged over 50 years present ED and LUTS/BPH simultaneously and that suffering from one of these two conditions has a high predictive value that the other condition is present as well. There is now increasing insight in the relationship between the pathological substrate of LUTS and erectile dysfunction. One of the underlying pathophysiological mechanisms of LUTS is the alteration of α-adrenergic receptor subtypes and an increase in α-adrenergic activity. The increased smooth muscle tone of the bladder neck and prostate capsule accounts for the symptoms of LUTS and can be relieved by α-adrenergic activity blockers. The relaxation of smooth muscle of the corpus cavernosum is pivotal for penile erection, and the higher than normal activation of α-adrenergic receptors through the sympathetic system causes early penile detumescence. Indeed it has been found that drugs that decrease smooth muscle tone through inhibition of α-adrenergic receptors may improve LUTS and ED at the same time. Alpha-adrenergic blockers, one of the main drugs to treat LUTS/BPH, facilitate relaxation of isolated fibers of smooth cavernous muscles.

Another mechanism for the relationship between LUTS and erectile dysfunction is the role that nitric oxide/cyclic GMP signaling plays in both erectile dysfunction and LUTS/BPH. Indeed, phosphodiesterase type 5 inhibitors ((PDE5) Is) are beneficial for the treatment of both conditions. Across the whole human lower urogenital tract, PDE5 gene and protein expression has been described, though with different patterns of appearance. The PDE5-Is on LUTS/BPH have probably several potential sites of actions such as the prostate and/or bladder and clinical improvement of patients with LUTS/BPH using these drugs, which traditionally enable erection [9] demonstrated that, at least from a therapeutical point of view, ED and LUTS/BPH can be treated in the same manner. It has been observed that sildenafil, tadalafil, and vardenafil reduced dose-dependent contraction of the muscle fibers of the three studied organs.

16.6 Penile Rehabilitation After Prostatectomy

Over the last decades, prostate cancer is diagnosed increasingly in younger men, and their concern is the preservation of erectile function after radical prostatectomy which is becoming an ever more important topic of discussion also among the elderly. A major step forward in the preservation of sexual function after radical prostatectomy was the development of the nerve-sparing procedure. Even during true nerve-sparing procedures, it is likely that nerves are affected by direct trauma, stretching, heating, ischemia, and local inflammation. This leads to neuropraxia, defined as a temporary block of nerve transmission despite an anatomical intact nerve fiber. There may be a slow recovery and erectile function may improve for up to 4 years after radical prostatectomy.

Penile rehabilitation after radical prostatectomy aims to reduce fibrotic changes in the corpus cavernosum after a prolonged period of penile flaccidity. It is plausible that tissue hypoxia is the inciting factor in these fibrotic changes, but the exact etiology of this process remains unknown. This disrupts the veno-occlusive mechanism, which is crucial in normal erectile function. While there is no proven mechanistic explanation, many practitioners believe that prolonged flaccidity of the corpus cavernosum accounts for the loss of erectile potency. They use some type of erectogenic treatment after radical prostatectomy aiming to enhance the return of sexual function [10].

Several studies have attempted to evaluate the efficacy of various pro-erectogenic modes of treatment used for early penile rehabilitation after radical prostatectomy. The results from studies with intracavernosal injections with prostaglandins and vacuum constriction devices indicate that an increased percentage of treated patients experience a return of natural erections compared in comparison with patients who received no treatment. However, the design of these studies has not been adequate since they have not included a proper placebo-controlled group, and the number of subjects evaluated has been limited. Longer, prospective, randomized, placebo-controlled studies are necessary to confirm the effectiveness of these treatments in improving long-term sexual function after radical prostatectomy.

More recent studies that have evaluated the chronic use of oral PDE-5 inhibitors suggest a beneficial effect on endothelial cell function among men suffering from erectile dysfunction due to a variety of causes. Studies point to increased oxygenation, activation of endothelial NO/cGMP, and nerve protection, as well as to more complicated cellular mechanisms, including activation of anti-apoptotic and antifibrotic factors. The data are still limited, but there might be a beneficial effect among post-prostatectomy patients, suggesting a possible role for these agents in enhancing the return of sexual function [10].

Conclusions

From puberty till the end of life sexuality remains a source of joy and concern in a man's life. Aging and its commonly associated illnesses have a profound effect on a man's sexual functioning. While symptom-oriented medical care for sexual problems has greatly improved over the past decades, comprehensive care for sexual functioning in old age is only starting to be addressed. In the medical discourse, both care providers and men themselves are hesitant to discuss sexual issues, putting the ball in one another's court. Specific aspects of sexual functioning in old age are the recognition that endothelial dysfunction is the common denominator linking vascular disease to ED and that ED may act as a marker of silent CAD and the polypharmacy, the use of multiple drugs with their potential side effects on sexual functions. Elderly men suffer from urological conditions such as LUTS which is causally related to erectile dysfunction. To restore/preserve sexual functions after prostatectomy penile rehabilitation may be necessary.

References

1. Lindau ST, Schumm L et al (2007) A study of sexuality and health among older adults in the United States. N Engl J Med 57:762–774
2. Helgason AR, Adolfsson J et al (1996) Sexual desire, erection, orgasm and ejaculatory functions and their importance to elderly Swedish men: a population-based study. Age Ageing 25(4):285–291
3. Araujo AB, Mohr BA et al (2004) Changes in sexual function in middle-aged and older men: longitudinal data from the Massachusetts Male Aging Study. J Am Geriatr Soc 52(9):1502–1509
4. Lindau ST, Gavrilova N (2010) Sex, health, and years of sexually active life gained due to good health: evidence from two US population based cross sectional surveys of ageing. Br Med J 340:c810
5. Nicolai MP, Both S et al (2013) Discussing sexual function in the cardiology practice. Clin Res Cardiol 102(5):329–336
6. Corona G, Rastrelli G et al (2012) Inhibitors of 5alpha-reductase-related side effects in patients seeking medical care for sexual dysfunction. J Endocrinol Invest 35(10):915–920
7. Rosen R, Altwein J et al (2003) Lower urinary tract symptoms and male sexual dysfunction: the multinational survey of the aging male (MSAM-7). Eur Urol 44(6):637–649

8. Seftel AD, de la Rosette J et al (2013) Coexisting lower urinary tract symptoms and erectile dysfunction: a systematic review of epidemiological data. Int J Clin Pract 67(1):32–45
9. Gacci M, Corona G et al (2012) A systematic review and meta-analysis on the use of phosphodiesterase 5 inhibitors alone or in combination with alpha-blockers for lower urinary tract symptoms due to benign prostatic hyperplasia. Eur Urol 61(5):994–1003
10. Fode M, Ohl DA et al (2013) Penile rehabilitation after radical prostatectomy: what the evidence really says. BJU Int 112(7):998–1008

Lifestyle Modification in Erectile Dysfunction and Hypertension

Margus Viigimaa

17.1 Introduction

Erectile dysfunction (ED) shares modifiable risk factors with hypertension. Moreover, hypertension is considered one of the most hazardous cardiovascular risk factors, and it is a frequent comorbidity of men with ED [1]. Lifestyle modifications should be the cornerstone of the therapy for ED and hypertension. Randomized clinical trials have shown lifestyle modification to be of clinical benefit in improving ED. Modifications in lifestyle can greatly reduce the risk of ED, and therefore, lifestyle changes and risk factor modification should accompany any specific pharmacotherapy or psychological therapy [2].

Clinical studies show that the blood-pressure lowering effects of lifestyle modifications can be equivalent to drug monotherapy [3]. Lifestyle measures should be instituted in all subjects with high-normal blood pressure and all patients who require drug treatment. It has been demonstrated that advice from health care professionals helps patients to make lifestyle changes.

Lifestyle measures to reduce the risk of SD, to reduce blood pressure, and to reduce the risk of blood pressure-related cardiovascular complications are: smoking cessation, weight reduction and maintenance, regular physical exercise, moderation of alcohol consumption, and dietary changes.

M. Viigimaa
North Estonia Medical Centre,
Tallinn University of Technology,
Ehitajate St. 5, Tallinn 19086, Estonia
e-mail: margus.viigimaa@regionaalhaigla.ee

17.2 Smoking Cessation

Smoking is linked with elevated rates of ED. It doubles the risk of SD [4]. Smoking is also a major risk factor for atherosclerotic cardiovascular disease. Although the rate of smoking is declining in Europe, it is still very common among individuals who have received little education. Widening education-related inequalities in smoking cessation rates have been observed in many European countries in recent years [5]. There is new evidence on the health effects of passive smoking, which strengthens the recommendation on passive smoking. It has been demonstrated that passive smoking also increases the risk of ED.

Smoking causes an acute increase in blood pressure and heart rate persisting for more than 15 min after smoking one cigarette. Studies using ambulatory blood pressure monitoring have shown that both untreated hypertensive and normotensive smokers present higher daily blood pressure values than nonsmokers. Tobacco use status should be established at each visit and hypertensive smokers and also patients with ED should be counselled regarding smoking cessation.

Several studies have investigated the effects of stopping smoking on sexual responding. A study by Pourmand et al. has found a significant correlation between smoking exposure and ED grade in men with ED [6]. There was an improvement in their ED severity in 25 % of ex-smokers and none of those who returned to smoking improved. Heavy smokers with ED showed a significant improvement in penile blood flow 24–36 h after smoking discontinuation [7]. Nocturnal penile tumescence and rigidity studies have shown significant improvement 24 h after smoking cessation.

Where necessary, smoking cessation medications, such as nicotine replacement therapy, bupropion, or varenicline should be considered. These drugs have been shown to be effective in clinical trials but are underused due to adverse effects, contraindications, low acceptability, and relatively high cost. A recent study by Harte and Meston enrolled smokers in an 8-week smoking cessation program involving a nicotine transdermal patch treatment and adjunctive counselling [8]. The study has shown that smoking cessation significantly enhances both physiological and self-reported indices of sexual health in long-term male smokers, irrespective of baseline erectile impairment. A meta-analysis of 36 trials comparing long-term cessation rates using bupropion versus control yielded a relative success rate of 1.69, whereas evidence of any additional effect of adding bupropion to nicotine replacement therapy was insufficient [9].

17.3 Weight Reduction and Maintenance

Obesity has shown to be a risk factor for ED, and cardiovascular disease risk factors are predictive of future erectile function and vice versa. The majority of men reporting ED symptoms (up to 80 %) are overweight or obese, and obese men have a consistently higher risk of sexual dysfunction than do men with a normal body weight [10]. However, it should also be noted that underweight (BMI 20 or less) may also be a risk factor for sexual dysfunction. Sexual dysfunction should be considered one of the numerous potentially reversible complications of obesity. The underlying mechanism of obesity-related sexual dysfunction is multifactorial. There are high rates of diabetes, metabolic syndrome, and hypertension in the obese, and these comorbidities have been clearly associated with sexual dysfunction. ED is threefold as common in diabetic men.

Hypertension is also closely correlated with excess body weight. In a meta-analysis the mean systolic and diastolic blood pressure reductions associated with an average weight loss of 5.1 kg were 4.4 and 3.6 mmHg, respectively [11]. Height, weight, and waist circumference should be measured and body mass index calculated for all hypertensives. Weight reduction should be recommended in all overweight hypertensive patients. Maintenance of a healthy body weight (body mass index 18.5–24.9 kg/m^2) and waist circumference (smaller than 102 cm for men and smaller than 88 cm for women) is recommended for nonhypertensive individuals to prevent hypertension and for hypertensive patients to reduce blood pressure [12]. Weight loss can also improve the efficacy of antihypertensive medications and the cardiovascular risk profile. Weight loss should employ a multidisciplinary approach that includes dietary education and regular exercise program.

Weight loss via diet or caloric reduction is the first-line prevention and treatment option of ED. A randomized, single-blind trial of 110 obese men has demonstrated that lifestyle changes, including a reduced calorie diet and increased exercise, are associated with improvement in sexual function in about one-third of obese men with erectile dysfunction at baseline [13]. This improvement was associated with amelioration of both endothelial function and markers of systemic vascular inflammation. Massachusetts Male Aging Study found that men who initiated physical activity in midlife had a 70 % reduced risk for erectile dysfunction relative to those who remained sedentary [14]. Gastric bypass surgery reliably induces substantial weight loss in the majority of the morbidly obese. It has been shown that substantial weight loss in patients underwent gastric bypass surgery normalizes sexual function in the morbidly obese males [15, 16].

17.4 Regular Physical Exercise

Exercise has been shown to affect ED prevalence and incidence. Higher levels of physical activity are associated with clinically significant lowering in the rate of ED. Erectile dysfunction in middle-aged men is often an early event in endothelial damage, and physical activity is able to improve both erectile and endothelial dysfunction [17]. Men who are sedentary are three times as likely to have ED, whereas moderate physical activity reduces the risk of ED by two-thirds, and in men with high physical activity, ED is reduced by over 80 % [18].

Epidemiological studies suggest that regular aerobic physical activity may be beneficial for both prevention and treatment of hypertension to lower cardiovascular risk and mortality. A meta-analysis of randomized controlled trials has shown that aerobic endurance training reduces resting systolic and diastolic blood pressures by

3.0/2.4 mmHg and in hypertensive group even by 6.9/4.9 mmHg [19]. For hypertensive patients, they should be advised to have 30–60 min of moderate intensity dynamic exercise (walking, jogging, cycling, or swimming) 4–7 days per week. Higher intensities of exercise are not being shown to be more effective. Intensive isometric exercise such as heavy weight lifting has marked pressure effect and should be avoided.

In a large meta-analysis of exercise and ED, which included seven cross-sectional analyses, there was an estimate of an approximate 40–60 % reduction in ED risk with moderate to higher levels of exercise [20]. In men less than 40 years of age, being sedentary was associated with a significantly increased risk of ED. Cardiovascular exercise may also provide reductions in risk or severity of ED of 40–50 % and even higher in men with diabetes and in men with other comorbidities such as hypertension [21]. Finally, there is some evidence that regular intercourse may be protective against developing ED. Sexual intercourse may preserve vascular function by maintaining cavernosal reactivity.

17.5 Moderation of Alcohol Consumption

The risk of ED also exists with excessive alcohol consumption, especially when combined with tobacco use or other heart-unhealthy behaviors [22]. In the Massachusetts Male Aging Study, excessive alcohol consumption (>600 mL/week) increased the probability of developing minimal impotence from 17 to 29 % [23]. Thus, clinicians should emphasize moderate or no intake for adequate sexual health. However, alcohol in moderation or infrequent consumption may provide some protection against ED, probably in part because of the long-term benefits of alcohol on high-density lipoprotein cholesterol.

The relationship between alcohol consumption, blood pressure levels, and the prevalence of hypertension is linear. Regular alcohol use raises blood pressure in treated hypertensive subjects. While moderate consumption may do no harm, the move from moderate to excessive drinking is associated both with raised blood pressure and with risk of stroke. The Prevention and Treatment of Hypertension Study (PATHS) has investigated effects of an alcohol treatment program on blood pressure. The intervention group had a 1.2/0.7 mm Hg greater reduction in blood pressure than the control group for the 6-month primary endpoint [24]. Hypertensive men who drink alcohol should be advised to limit their consumption to no more than 20–30 g ethanol per day and hypertensive women to no more than 10–20 g ethanol per day. Total alcohol consumption should not exceed 14 standard drinks per week for men and 9 standard drinks per week for women.

17.6 Dietary Changes

Patients with ED and hypertension should be advised to eat fresh fruits, vegetables, low-fat dairy products, dietary and soluble fiber, whole grains, and protein from plant sources that are reduced in saturated fat and cholesterol. Mediterranean type of diet especially has gained interest in recent years. The Mediterranean diet, rich in fruits, legumes, and vegetables, is a healthy dietary pattern, gaining widely recognition as a nonpharmaceutical mean of cardiovascular disease prevention, due to antioxidant anti-inflammatory properties. A number of studies and meta-analyses have reported on the cardiovascular protective effect of the Mediterranean diet [25]. Patients should be advised to eat fish twice a week and fruit and vegetables 300–400 g/day. Soymilk appeared to lower blood pressure when compared to skimmed cows' milk. Diet should accompany with other lifestyle changes. In patients with elevated blood pressure, compared to the DASH diet alone, the combination of the DASH diet with exercise and weight loss resulted in greater declines in blood pressure and left ventricular mass. Hypertensive patients should moderate coffee consumption. Caffeine consumption has long been associated with raised blood pressure and can demonstrate a dose-related increase of 5–15 mmHg systolic and 5–10 mmHg diastolic for several hours following consumption. Counselling by trained dieticians may be useful.

Folic acid, calcium, vitamin C, and vitamin E support the biochemical pathways leading to nitric oxide (NO) release and therefore improve sexual function. Folic acid is a cofactor in the normal production of NO. The recommended daily allowance is 400 mg. Omega-3 fatty acids, obtained from fatty fish, promote vascular health by inhibiting platelet aggregation and inflammation and by stimulating the release of NO [26]. As the American Heart Association and other professional organizations recommends one gram of omega-3s for individuals with cardiovascular disease, this is a logical recommendation for maintaining or improving both erectile and vascular health.

In men with ED, the intracellular levels of reduced glutathione are significantly lower compared with men with normal erectile function. Pomegranate, blueberries, chocolate, green tea, and red wine all contain high levels of polyphenols and have been shown to increase NO in various animal and human in vitro and in vivo studies [27]. Antioxidants promote NO synthesis and also protect it from degradation. Vitamins C and E have synergistic effects with regard to their serum levels achieved after ingestion, and may have additive or even synergistic effects on NO production. A reasonable dose of vitamin C is 500–1,000 mg. Vitamin E supplementation should be limited to <400 IU per day because of potential adverse long-term health effects of higher doses [26].

The effect of ginseng on male sexual function was investigated in several studies. Khera and Goldstein reviewed Panax ginseng data from six randomized trials conducted over a period of approximately 15 years that included a total of 349 men [28]. The investigators found that ginseng significantly improved erectile function compared with placebo over 4–12 weeks. Approximately 58 % of men experienced an improvement in some aspect of sexual function compared with 20 % of men who received the placebo.

There is much evidence for a causal relationship between salt intake and blood pressure. The current salt intake in many countries is between 9 and 12 g/day. A reduction in salt intake to the recommended level of 5 g/day lowers BP in both hypertensive and normotensive individuals [29]. Reducing sodium chloride intake

Table 17.1 Recommended lifestyle changes in ED and hypertension [12, 33]

Smoking cessation
Weight reduction and maintenance
Body mass index <25 kg/m^2
Waist circumference <102 cm for men and <88 cm for women
Regular physical exercise, i.e., at least 30 min of moderate intensity dynamic exercise (walking, jogging, cycling, or swimming) is recommended 5–7 days per week
Moderation of alcohol consumption to no more than 20–30 g ethanol per day for men and 10–20 g for women
Use of Mediterranean-type diet, which emphasizes fruits, vegetables, beans and legumes, whole grains, nuts, fish, poultry, lean red meat, cheese, and yogurt
Salt restriction to 5–6 g per day

by 4.7–5.8 g per day from an initial intake of around 10.5 g per day reduces blood pressure by an average of 5 mmHg [30]. The effect of sodium restriction is greater in blacks, older people, and patients with hypertension, diabetes, and chronic kidney disease. A further reduction to 3–4 g/day has a much greater effect. However, this is currently difficult to achieve and an achievable recommendation is less than 5 g/day sodium chloride. Prospective studies and outcome trials have demonstrated that a lower salt intake is associated with a decreased risk of cardiovascular disease [31].

17.7 Comprehensive Lifestyle Modification in the Management of Erectile Dysfunction and Hypertension

Comprehensive lifestyle modification is the cornerstone of the therapy for ED and hypertension [22]. Gupta et al. conducted a systematic review and meta-analysis of randomized controlled trials evaluating the effect of lifestyle interventions and pharmacotherapy for cardiovascular risk factors on the severity of ED [32]. Lifestyle modifications were associated with statistically significant improvement in sexual function ($n=597$): weighted mean difference 2.40 (95 % CI, 1.19–3.61). The lifestyle modification recommendations from 2013 ESH/ESC Guidelines for the Management of Arterial Hypertension and The Princeton III Consensus Recommendations for the Management of Erectile Dysfunction and Cardiovascular Disease are summarized in Table 17.1.

Conclusions

ED shares modifiable risk factors with hypertension. Randomized clinical trials have shown lifestyle modification to be of clinical benefit in improving ED. There is strong evidence that lifestyle modification for CV risk factors is effective in improving sexual function in men with ED. Improvement in sexual function is a strong motivator for male patients to adopt healthy lifestyle. Comprehensive lifestyle modification is the cornerstone of the therapy for ED and hypertension. Lifestyle changes are improving erectile function, lower elevated blood pressure, and reduce cardiovascular risk. Lifestyle measures to reduce the risk of SD, to reduce blood pressure, and to reduce the risk of blood pressure-related cardiovascular complications are: smoking cessation, weight reduction and maintenance, regular physical exercise, moderation of alcohol consumption, and dietary changes.

References

1. Javaroni V, Neves MF (2012) Erectile dysfunction and hypertension: impact on cardiovascular risk and treatment. Int J Hypertens 2012:627278
2. Hackett G, Kell P, Ralph D, Dean J et al (2008) British Society for Sexual Medicine guidelines on the management of erectile dysfunction. J Sex Med 5(8):1841–1865
3. Elmer PJ, Obarzanek E, Vollmer WM, Simons-Morton D et al (2006) Effects of comprehensive lifestyle modification on diet, weight, physical fitness, and blood pressure control: 18-month results of a randomized trial. Ann Intern Med 144:485–495
4. He J, Reynolds K, Chen J, Chen CS et al (2007) Cigarette smoking and erectile dysfunction among Chinese men without clinical vascular disease. Am J Epidemiol 166:803–809
5. Huisman M, Kunst AE, Mackenbach JP (2005) Inequalities in the prevalence of smoking in the European Union: comparing education and income. Prev Med 40(6):756–764
6. Pourmand G, Alidaee MR, Rasuli S, Maleki A et al (2004) Do cigarette smokers with erectile dysfunction benefit from stopping?: a prospective study. BJU Int 94:1310–1313
7. Sighinolfi MC, Mofferdin A, De Stefani S, Micali S et al (2007) Immediate improvement in penile hemodynamics after cessation of smoking: previous results. Urology 69:163–165
8. Harte CB, Meston CM (2012) Association between smoking cessation and sexual health in men. BJU Int 109(6):888–896
9. Hughes JR, Stead LF, Lancaster T (2007) Antidepressants for smoking cessation. Cochrane Database Syst Rev 1:CD000031
10. Zabelina DL, Erickson AL, Kolotkin RL, Crosby RD (2009) The effect of age on weight-related quality of life in overweight and obese individuals. Obesity (Silver Spring) 17:1410–1413
11. Neter JE, Stam BE, Kok FJ, Grobbee DE et al (2003) Influence of weight reduction on blood pressure: a meta-analysis of randomized controlled trials. Hypertension 42(5):878–884
12. Mancia G, Fagard R, Narkiewicz K, Redon J et al (2013) ESH/ESC guidelines for the management of arterial hypertension. J Hypertens 31(7):1281–1357
13. Esposito K, Giugliano F, Di Palo C, Giugliano G et al (2004) Effect of lifestyle changes on erectile dysfunction in obese men. JAMA 291:2978–2984
14. Derby CA, Mohr BA, Goldstein I, Feldman HA et al (2000) Modifiable risk factors and erectile dysfunction: can lifestyle changes modify risk? Urology 56:302–306
15. Dallal RM, Chernoff A, O'Leary MP, Smith JA et al (2008) Sexual dysfunction is common in the morbidly obese male and improves after gastric bypass surgery. J Am Coll Surg 207:859–864
16. Rosenblatt A, Faintuch J, Cecconello I (2013) Sexual hormones and erectile function more than 6 years after bariatric surgery. Surg Obes Relat Dis 9:636–640
17. La Vignera S, Condorelli R, Vicari E, D'Agata R et al (2012) Physical activity and erectile dysfunction in middle-aged men. J Androl 33:154–161
18. Selvin E, Burnett AL, Platz EA (2007) Prevalence and risk factors for erectile dysfunction in the US. Am J Med 120:151–157
19. Cornelissen VA, Fagard RH (2005) Effect of resistance training on resting blood pressure: a meta-analysis of randomized controlled trials. J Hypertens 23(2):251–259
20. Cheng JY, Ng EM, Ko JS, Chen RY (2007) Physical activity and erectile dysfunction: meta-analysis of population-based studies. Int J Impot Res 19:245–252
21. Lamina S, Okoye CG, Dagogo TT (2009) Therapeutic effect of an interval exercise training program in the management of erectile dysfunction in hypertensive patients. J Clin Hypertens (Greenwich) 11:125–129

22. Moyad MA, Park K (2012) What do most erectile dysfunction guidelines have in common? No evidence-based discussion or recommendation of heart-healthy lifestyle changes and/or Panax ginseng. Asian J Androl 14:830–841
23. Nicolosi A, Glasser DB, Moreira ED, Villa M (2003) Prevalence of erectile dysfunction and associated factors among men without concomitant diseases: a population study. Int J Impot Res 15:253–257
24. Cushman WC, Cutler JA, Hanna E, Bingham SF et al (1998) Prevention and Treatment of Hypertension Study (PATHS): effects of an alcohol treatment program on blood pressure. Arch Intern Med 158(11):1197–1207
25. Sofi F, Abbate R, Gensini GF, Casini A (2010) Accruing evidence on benefits of adherence to the Mediterranean diet on health: an updated systematic review and meta-analysis. Am J Clin Nutr 92(5):1189–1196
26. Meldrum DR, Gambone JC, Morris MA, Ignarro LJ (2010) Multifaceted approach to maximize erectile function and vascular health. Fertil Steril 94:2514–2520
27. Ignarro LJ, Byrns RE, Sumi D, de Nigris F et al (2006) Pomegranate juice protects nitric oxide against oxidative destruction and enhances the biologic actions of nitric oxide. Nitric Oxide 15:93–102
28. Khera M, Goldstein I (2011) Erectile dysfunction. Clin Evid (Online) pii:1803
29. Pimenta E, Gaddam KK, Oparil S, Aban I et al (2009) Effects of dietary sodium reduction on blood pressure in subjects with resistant hypertension: results from a randomized trial. Hypertension 54(3):475–481
30. He FJ, MacGregor GA (2011) Salt reduction lowers cardiovascular risk: meta-analysis of outcome trials. Lancet 378(9789):380–382
31. Taylor RS, Ashton KE, Moxham T, Hooper L et al (2011) Reduced dietary salt for the prevention of cardiovascular disease: a meta-analysis of randomized controlled trials (Cochrane review). Am J Hypertens 24(8):843–853
32. Gupta BP, Murad MH, Clifton MM, Prokop L et al (2011) The effect of lifestyle modification and cardiovascular risk factor reduction on erectile dysfunction. Arch Intern Med 171(20):1797–1803
33. Nehra A, Jackson G, Miner M, Billups K et al (2012) The Princeton III Consensus recommendations for the management of erectile dysfunction and cardiovascular disease. Mayo Clin Proc 87(8):766–778

Antihypertensive Drug Therapy and Erectile Dysfunction

18

Vasilios Papademetriou, Antonios Lazaridis, Eirini Papadopoulou, Theodosia Papadopoulou, and Michael Doumas

18.1 Introduction

Arterial hypertension represents a major cardiovascular risk factor and is associated with increased risk of myocardial infarction, congestive heart failure, left ventricular hypertrophy, stroke, transient ischemic attack, and end-stage renal disease [1]. Hypertension-induced vascular alterations are both structural and functional and are observed both in large vessels and the microvasculature [2, 3].

Antihypertensive therapy is associated with an impressive reduction of cardiovascular events [4, 5]. Several classes of antihypertensive drugs are currently available in our therapeutic armamentarium, including diuretics, calcium antagonists, angiotensin-converting enzyme (ACE) inhibitors, angiotensin receptor blockers (ARBs), beta-blockers, alpha-blockers, direct renin inhibitors, mineralocorticoid antagonists, centrally acting drugs, and direct vasodilators. In general, antihypertensive drugs exhibit similar blood pressure reduction without significant differences between drug categories [6]. Similarly, a large meta-analysis of the Blood

---

V. Papademetriou (✉)
Cardiology Department, VAMC Washington, DC
50 Irving Str., NW-151-E, Washington, DC 20422, USA
e-mail: vasilios.papademetriou@va.gov

A. Lazaridis • E. Papadopoulou • T. Papadopoulou
2nd Propedeutic Department of Internal Medicine, Aristotle University,
49, Konstantinoupoleos Street, Thessaloniki 54643, Greece
e-mail: spanbiol@hotmail.com; eirini.papadopoulou@yahoo.it; sissipapth@yahoo.gr

M. Doumas
2nd Propedeutic Department of Internal Medicine, Aristotle University,
126, Vas. Olgas Street, Thessaloniki 54645, Greece

George Washington University, Washington, DC, USA
e-mail: michalisdoumas@yahoo.co.uk

Pressure Lowering Treatment Trialists has shown that there are no substantial differences between the various drug categories in reducing the occurrence of cardiovascular events [7].

Erectile dysfunction is considered to be of vascular origin in the vast majority of cases, and the efficacy of PDE-5 inhibitors in patients with erectile dysfunction confirms this opinion [8–11]. Several lines of evidence have shown a close association between essential hypertension and erectile dysfunction [12, 13]. The prevalence of erectile dysfunction is higher in hypertensive compared with normotensive subjects [14, 15]. The mechanisms underlying this association are multiple and perplexed, with endothelial dysfunction, inflammation, testosterone, and vasoactive peptides being the major players [16–20].

Epidemiological data uncover another interesting finding: erectile dysfunction is more prevalent in treated than in untreated hypertensive patients [14, 21]. This association might be attributed to several causes: (a) drug-induced blood pressure reduction compromises penile blood supply and results in erectile dysfunction, (b) treated hypertensive patients might have more comorbidities than untreated patients and the increased erectile dysfunction prevalence is ought to the additional impact of comorbidities, and (c) antihypertensive drugs exert detrimental effects on erectile function and thus antihypertensive therapy is associated with increased prevalence of erectile dysfunction. Unfortunately, available data regarding the former two hypotheses are very limited and inconclusive, while data regarding the latter hypothesis is more robust.

Available data consistently point towards significant differences in the effects of different antihypertensive drug classes on erectile function. Data come from both experimental and clinical studies, observational and randomized. Therefore, existing data have been divided into five categories: (a) experimental studies, (b) observational studies, (c) small randomized studies, (d) large clinical trials, and (e) meta-analyses.

This chapter aims to summarize the effects of the various antihypertensive drug categories on erectile function, highlight the differences between drug categories, and discuss the effects of switching antihypertensive drug class on erectile function.

18.2 Experimental Studies

Experimental studies in rats indicate that hypertension results in structural and functional alterations in the cavernous tissue, just like in other vessels, and point towards significant between-class and in-class differences between antihypertensive drugs.

In a comparison study between normotensive Wistar-Kyoto (WKY) rats and spontaneously hypertensive rats (SHR) for 8 months, it was found that the cavernous smooth muscle proliferation score and the vascular smooth muscle proliferation score were significantly higher in hypertensive rats [22]. Similarly, the fibrosis score of cavernous tissue was higher in hypertensive than in normotensive rats. Another study evaluated the effects of candesartan, an ARB, on the structural alterations of cavernous tissue. Treatment with candesartan for 4 months attenuated the morphologic changes in the vessels and the cavernous spaces of erectile tissue, which were induced by hypertension, exhibiting a protective role in spontaneously hypertensive rats [23].

A disparity in the effects of different antihypertensive drugs was found in four experimental studies. The first study evaluated the effects of candesartan and atenolol for 6 months using untreated SHR and normotensive WKY rats as controls [24]. It was found that atenolol did not attenuate the structural alterations on erectile tissue associated with hypertension, while candesartan exhibited beneficial effects and the erectile morphology resembled the morphology of normotensive rats. The second study had a similar design and compared the effects of nebivolol with those of amlodipine for 6 months. It was found that amlodipine failed to attenuate the structural changes induced by hypertension in SHR, while nebivolol protected from the development of morphological alterations [25]. It was also found that nebivolol treatment enhanced the expression of endothelial nitric oxide synthase in erectile tissue reaching the levels observed in normotensive rats, while the expression was significantly lower in untreated and amlodipine-treated spontaneously hypertensive rats. In the third study, candesartan was compared with hydralazine for 4 months. The beneficial effects of candesartan on erectile structural and functional alterations were reconfirmed, while hydralazine failed to exert similar protective effects [26]. In the fourth study, losartan was compared with amlodipine for 6 months. Losartan exerted significant benefits on the morphology of erectile tissue, similar to the ones observed with candesartan in previous studies. In contrast, amlodipine therapy did not attenuate hypertension-induced structural alterations in erectile function [27]. It has to be noted that blood pressure reduction was similar between the two treatment drugs in all four experimental studies.

Taken together, the findings of experimental studies indicate that high blood pressure is associated with significant morphological and functional alterations in the erectile tissue. A large heterogeneity in the effects of antihypertensive therapy is observed. Some drugs (ARBs, nebivolol) seem to protect the erectile tissue, while other drugs (atenolol, amlodipine, hydralazine) do not have these protective properties. Therefore, the benefits of antihypertensive therapy seem to occur beyond blood pressure reduction, with significant differences not only between different drug classes (ARBs vs. calcium antagonists and hydralazine) but also within drug classes (nebivolol vs. atenolol).

The above mentioned differences between antihypertensive drugs were also observed in animals with chronic renal insufficiency via subtotal nephrectomy. It was found that RAS inhibitors (losartan and benazepril) exerted protective effects on penile structure, while amlodipine and atenolol failed to exert similar benefits [28].

Another significant set of information comes from studies that combined antihypertensive drugs with PDE-5 inhibitors. In one study, a combination therapy with losartan and sildenafil was compared to each monotherapy alone. It was found that the beneficial effects of combination therapy on penile structure and function were greater than the effects of each monotherapy alone [8]. The beneficial effects of combination therapy on the functional level were confirmed in human cavernosal with the combination of sildenafil and doxazosin [29].

18.3 Observational Studies

Data from observational studies suggest that there exist both between-class and within-class differences in the effects of antihypertensive therapy on erectile function.

A large, observational, cross-sectional study of 634 consecutive young and middle-aged (31–65 years) individuals assessed erectile function with different antihypertensive drug classes [21]. It was reported that erectile function scores were significantly lower with older antihypertensive drugs (diuretics and beta-blockers) than with newer-generation antihypertensive drugs (calcium antagonists, ACE inhibitors, ARBs). The higher erectile function score was observed in patients on ARBs. Of note, similar results were observed in females as well in another observational cross-sectional study of 417 women [30].

Another large, cross-sectional study evaluated the effects of beta-blockers on erectile function [31]. The study included 1,007 high-risk hypertensive patients (mean age 57.9 years) treated with beta-blockers for at least 6 months. The prevalence of erectile dysfunction was very high (71 %) in this group of patients and of relatively high severity (16.1 % severe; 16.8 % moderate; 38.1 % mild). Of major clinical significance, substantial differences between the various beta-blockers were reported. Specifically, nebivolol was associated with the lowest prevalence of erectile dysfunction, metoprolol and carvedilol were associated with the highest prevalence, and bisoprolol and atenolol lie in between.

18.4 Small Randomized Studies

Significant information about the effects of antihypertensive therapy on erectile function comes from clinical studies, which were specifically designed to address this issue.

A double-blind, randomized, crossover study of 90 hypertensive middle-aged men without sexual dysfunction evaluated the effects of lisinopril (20 mg) and atenolol (100 mg) for 16 weeks [32]. Sexual activity remained practically unaltered with lisinopril (from 7.1 to 7.7 sexual intercourses per month) but worsened significantly with atenolol (from 7.8 to 4.2 sexual intercourses per month), and the difference between the two groups was statistically significant ($p < 0.01$).

In a double-blind, randomized, crossover study of 160 newly diagnosed hypertensive males of middle age (40–49 years), free of sexual dysfunction, valsartan (80 mg) was compared to carvedilol (50 mg) for 16 weeks [33]. It was found that sexual activity was significantly improved with valsartan (from 8.2 to 10.2 sexual intercourses per month), while sexual activity deteriorated significantly with carvedilol (from 8.3 to 3.7 sexual intercourses per month). Erectile dysfunction was reported more frequently with carvedilol (13.5 %) than with valsartan (0.9 %).

Another double-blind, randomized study of 110 middle-aged hypertensive men naïve to antihypertensive therapy compared the effects of valsartan (80 mg) with those of atenolol (50 mg) for 16 weeks [34]. Sexual activity improved with valsartan (from 5.8 to 7.4 sexual intercourses per month) but deteriorated with atenolol (from 6.0 to 4.2 sexual intercourses per month), and the differences between the two groups were statistically significant ($p<0.05$). Testosterone levels remained unaffected with valsartan but were significantly reduced with atenolol. Of note, similar results were observed in hypertensive women as well. In a randomized study of 120 postmenopausal hypertensive women, sexual desire and sexual fantasy were significantly improved with valsartan and worsened with atenolol [35].

These studies were of high methodological standards and were designed to assess sexual function specifically and not as a secondary end point of a study designed to evaluate other topics. However, several limitations can be identified, including the relatively small patient population, the determination of sexual intercourses as an index of sexual activity instead of global erectile function, and the use of invalidated questionnaires. Despite these limitations, the importance of information derived from these studies remains substantial, since these small clinical studies are the only studies performed in untreated patients and specifically evaluating sexual function.

18.5 Large Clinical Trials

Several large multicenter trials reported the effects of antihypertensive therapy on erectile function during the last decades.

The Medical Research Council (MRC) trial for mild hypertension compared the effects of bendrofluazide and propranolol with those of placebo for 23.582 patient years of observation [36]. Withdrawal from the study due to impotence was twofold higher with diuretics than with beta blockers and substantially higher than with placebo ($p<0.001$ for all comparisons).

The Trial of Antihypertensive Interventions and Management (TAIM) was a multicenter, randomized, placebo-controlled study that included 697 overweight and obese patients with mild hypertension [37]. The study compared chlorthalidone and atenolol with placebo and evaluated the effects of diet. A worsening of erectile-related problems was significantly more common with chlorthalidone (28 %; 95 %CI: 15–41 %) compared with placebo (3 %; 95%CI: 0–9 %) and atenolol (11 %; 95%CI: 2–20 %). The detrimental effects of chlorthalidone on erectile function were attenuated by weight reduction.

The Treatment of Mild Hypertension Study (TOMHS) was a double-blind, randomized, placebo-controlled trial of 902 patients with mild hypertension [38]. Acebutolol, amlodipine, chlorthalidone, doxazosin, and enalapril were compared to placebo for 48 months. The incidence of erection problems was significantly higher with chlorthalidone (17.1 %) than with placebo (8.1 %; $p<0.03$) at 24 months posttherapy but the difference disappeared at 48 months. There were no significant differences between the remaining drugs and placebo both at 24 and 48 months. It has to be noted however that these older studies have significant limitations, including the exclusion of patients with more severe forms of hypertension and the assessment of erectile function with "primitive" methodology and not by validated questionnaires.

Two recently published trials overcome these obstacles. The Metoprolol vs. Nebivolol Study of Erectile Dysfunction (MR NOED) was a randomized double-blind study comparing nebivolol (5 mg) with metoprolol (95 mg) for 12 weeks in patients with mild hypertension [39]. Despite similar blood pressure reduction with both drugs, metoprolol was associated with detrimental effects on erectile function, while nebivolol use was associated with improvements on sexual activity scores and other subscores of erectile function. The MR NOED study is the only trial that was specifically designed to evaluate the effects of antihypertensive therapy on erectile function in hypertensive patients.

Erectile function was also evaluated in a pre-specified subgroup of patients participating in the ONTARGET/TRANSCEND Trial Programme [40]. The ONTARGET study compared ramipril and telmisartan with their combination, while the TRANSCEND study compared telmisartan with placebo in patients intolerant to ACE inhibitors. Erectile dysfunction was frequently encountered in this high-risk patient population (55 %). There were no significant differences on erectile function between the three arms of the ONTARGET study. Similarly, no significant difference between telmisartan and placebo was found in the TRANSCEND study. Therefore, telmisartan neither improved erectile function nor protected from incident erectile dysfunction. It has to be noted however that telmisartan was added on top of a multidrug regimen in a high-risk population, and thus, these studies were not appropriately designed to uncover the effects of ARBs on erectile function as monotherapy or in low-risk patients.

18.6 Meta-analyses

As depicted up to now, it is obvious that the number of high-quality, randomized studies evaluating the effects of antihypertensive therapy on erectile function is very limited and is not permitting the conduction of meta-analyses.

However, important information derives from the meta-analyses of adverse effects on antihypertensive drug therapy. Relevant data exist for older antihypertensive drugs, such as beta-blockers. A large meta-analysis of 15 randomized trials involving more than 35,000 patients revealed the negative effects of beta-blockers on sexual function [41]. The relative risk for sexual dysfunction with beta-blockers was increased by 10 % with marginal statistical significance (95 % CI: 0.96–1.25). Furthermore, a statistically significant increase on the incidence risk for sexual dysfunction was observed, with a difference of five cases/1,000 patients/year (95 % CI: 2–8). More importantly, the use of beta-blockers was associated with an almost fivefold increased risk of withdrawal due to sexual dysfunction (RR: 4.89; 95%CI: 2.98–8.03).

18.7 Change of Antihypertensive Class

The previously presented differences between antihypertensive drug classes suggest that hypertensive patients with erectile dysfunction while administering a drug with a detrimental effect might benefit from a change in therapeutic class with neutral or beneficial effects on erectile function. Indeed, some data point towards significant benefits of switching drug therapy to ARBs or nebivolol.

A large, open, prospective study evaluated the effects of valsartan monotherapy and in combination with a diuretic for 16 weeks in more than 2,000 hypertensive patients [42]. Sexual activity was significantly improved with valsartan monotherapy (from 1.0 to 1.6 sexual intercourses per week; $p<0.0001$), and the benefit was maintained even in the combination group (from 0.9 to 1.3 sexual intercourses per week; $p<0.0001$).

In another open, prospective study of 3.500 hypertensive patients, the effects of valsartan for 6 months on erectile function were evaluated by using appropriate methodology (the International Index of Erectile Function Questionnaire). Erectile function was significantly improved not only in previously untreated patients (from 65 % to 45 %; $p<0.0001$) but also in the total study population which was mostly treated with other drugs and switched to valsartan (from 75.4 % to 53 %; $p<0.0001$). Valsartan therapy was associated with significant improvements in sexual desire, orgasmic function, intercourse, and overall satisfaction [43]. Similar beneficial effects on erectile dysfunction (from 78.5 % to 63.7 %) were observed with irbesartan in a study of more than 1.000 patients with hypertension and metabolic syndrome [44].

Another open, prospective study of 44 hypertensive patients with erectile dysfunction while receiving beta-blockers evaluated the effects of switching prior therapy to nebivolol (5–10 mg) for 3 months. Erectile function was significantly improved in 68 % of the patients and was even normalized in more than half of patients experiencing improvement [45].

18.8 Further Gaps in Knowledge

A vivid discussion takes place regarding the effects of beta-blockade and combined antihypertensive therapy on erectile function.

The detrimental effects of beta-blockers on erectile function have been recently questioned. A study of 96 patients with recent cardiovascular disease evaluated the impact of the Hawthorne effect, the prejudice of erectile dysfunction occurrence with beta-blockers [46]. Indeed, erectile dysfunction was ten times more frequent in patients who received atenolol and were informed of its side effects on erectile function than in patients who were blinded on administered drug (31.2 % vs. 3.1 %; $p<0.01$). Patients who were informed on the drug given but not its side effects had intermediate occurrence of erectile dysfunction (15.6 %). Moreover, sildenafil and placebo were equally effective in patients reporting atenolol-induced erectile dysfunction. In our opinion, a certain degree of "placebo effect" is implicated in beta-blocker-induced erectile dysfunction; however, available data strongly suggest that beta-blockers exert detrimental effects on erectile function [47].

Monotherapy with any class of antihypertensive agents achieves blood pressure control in about one third of hypertensive patients, while the remaining two thirds require combination therapy to reach blood pressure targets [1, 6]. Therefore, the effects of combination antihypertensive therapy on erectile function are clinically meaningful. Unfortunately, relevant data are limited [48] and do not permit for definite conclusions, highlighting the need for further research in this field [49].

Conclusions

The prevalence of erectile dysfunction is higher in treated compared to untreated hypertensive patients, suggesting a detrimental effect of antihypertensive therapy on erectile function. Experimental data indicate that significant between-class and in-class differences exist regarding the effects of antihypertensive agents on erectile function. Data in humans come from observational and small randomized studies, large clinical trials, and meta-analyses and point towards the same direction. Diuretics and beta-blockers seem to be associated with incident erectile dysfunction, while ACE inhibitors and calcium antagonists seem to exert neutral effects on erectile function. ARBs and nebivolol seem to be associated with beneficial effects on erectile function; however, further studies are needed to confirm these benefits.

References

1. Mancia G, Fagard R, Narkiewicz K et al (2013) 2013 ESH/ESC guidelines for the management of arterial hypertension. J Hypertens 31:1281–1357
2. Laurent S, Briet M, Boutouyrie P (2009) Large and small artery cross-talk and recent morbidity-mortality trials in hypertension. Hypertension 54:388–392
3. Schifrin EL (2010) Circulatory therapeutics: use of antihypertensive agents and their effects on the vasculature. J Cell Mol Med 14:1018–1029
4. MacMahon S, Peto R, Cutler J et al (1990) Blood pressure, stroke, and coronary heart disease. Prolonged differences in blood pressure: prospective observational studies corrected for the regression dilution bias. Lancet 335:765–774
5. Lewington S, Clarke R, Qizilbash N et al (2002) Age-specific relevance of usual blood pressure to vascular mortality: a meta-analysis of individual data for one million adults in 61 prospective studies. Lancet 360:1903–1913
6. Law MR, Morris JK, Wald NJ (2009) Use of blood pressure lowering drugs in the prevention of cardiovascular disease: meta-analysis of 147 randomised trials in the context of expectations from prospective epidemiological studies. BMJ 338:b1665
7. Turnbull F, Blood Pressure Lowering Treatment Trialists' Collaboration (2003) Effects of different blood-pressure-lowering regimens on major cardiovascular events: results of prospectively-designed overviews of randomized trials. Lancet 362:1527–1535
8. Manolis A, Doumas M (2008) Sexual dysfunction: the 'prima ballerina' of hypertension-related quality-of-life complications. J Hypertens 26:2074–2084
9. Viigimaa M, Doumas M, Vlachopoulos C et al (2011) European Society of Hypertension Working Group on Sexual Dysfunction. Hypertension and sexual dysfunction: time to act. J Hypertens 29:403–407
10. Manolis A, Doumas M (2012) Antihypertensive treatment and sexual dysfunction. Curr Hypertens Rep 14:285–292
11. Doumas M, Douma S (2006) The effect of antihypertensive drugs on erectile function: a proposed management algorithm. J Clin Hypertens 8:359–364
12. Manolis A, Doumas M (2009) Hypertension and sexual dysfunction. Arch Med Sci 5:S337–S350
13. Douma S, Doumas M, Tsakiris A, Zamboulis C (2007) Male and female sexual dysfunction: is hypertension an innocent bystander or a major contributor? Rev Bras Hypertens 14:139–147

14. Doumas M, Douma S (2006) Sexual dysfunction in essential hypertension: myth or reality? J Clin Hypertens 8:269–274
15. Manolis AJ, Doumas M, Viigimaa M, Narkiewitz K (2011) Hypertension and sexual dysfunction. European Society of Hypertension Scientific Newsletter: Update on Hypertension Management 32
16. Vlachopoulos C, Rokkas K, Ioakeimidis N, Stefanadis C (2007) Inflammation, metabolic syndrome, erectile dysfunction, and coronary artery disease: common links. Eur Urol 52:1590–1600
17. Vlachopoulos C, Rokkas K, Ioakeimidis N et al (2005) Prevalence of asymptomatic coronary artery disease in men with vasculogenic erectile dysfunction: a prospective angiographic study. Eur Urol 48:996–1002
18. Vlachopoulos C, Ioakeimidis N, Terentes-Printzios D, Stefanadis C (2008) The triad: erectile dysfunction, endothelial dysfunction, cardiovascular disease. Curr Pharm Des 14:3700–3714
19. Vlachopoulos C, Jackson G, Stefanadis C, Montorsi P (2013) Erectile dysfunction in the cardiovascular patient. Eur Heart J 34:2034–2046
20. Vlachopoulos C, Ioakeimidis N, Terentes-Printzios D et al (2013) Plasma total testosterone and incident cardiovascular events in hypertensive patients. Am J Hypertens 26:373–381
21. Doumas M, Tsakiris A, Douma S et al (2006) Factors affecting the increased prevalence of erectile dysfunction in Greek hypertensive compared with normotensive subjects. J Androl 27:469–477
22. Toblli J, Stella I, Inserra F et al (2000) Morphological changes in cavernous tissue in spontaneously hypertensive rats. Am J Hypertens 13:686–692
23. Tobbli J, Stella I, Mazza ON et al (2004) Candesartan cilexetil protects cavernous tissue in spontaneously hypertensive rats. Int J Impot Res 16:305–312
24. Toblli J, Stella I, Mazza NO, Ferder L, Inserra F (2004) Protection of cavernous tissue in male spontaneously hypertensive rats. Beyond blood pressure control. Am J Hypertens 17:516–522
25. Toblli JE, Cao G, Casas G, Mazza ON (2006) In vivo and in vitro effects of nebivolol on penile structures in hypertensive rats. Am J Hypertens 19:1226–1232
26. Mazza ON, Angeros M, Becher E, Toblli JE (2006) Differences between candesartan and hydralazine in the protection of penile structures in spontaneously hypertensive rats. J Sex Med 3:604–611
27. Toblli JE, Stella I, Mazza ON ct al (2004) Different effect of losartan and amlodipine on penile structures in male spontaneously hypertensive rats. Am J Nephrol 24:614–623
28. Toblli JE, Stella I, Mazza ON et al (2006) The effect of different antihypertensive drugs on cavernous tissue in experimental chronic renal insufficiency. J Nephrol 19:419–428
29. Oger S, Behr-Roussel D, Gorny D et al (2009) Combination of doxazosin and sildenafil exerts an additive relaxing effect compared with each compound alone on human cavernosal and prostatic tissue. J Scx Med 6:836–847
30. Doumas M, Tsiodras S, Tsakiris A et al (2006) Female sexual dysfunction in essential hypertension: a common problem being uncovered. J Hypertens 24:2387–2392
31. Cordero A, Bertomeu-Martinez V, Mazon P et al (2010) Erectile dysfunction in high-risk hypertensive patients treated with beta-blockers agents. Cardiovasc Ther 28:15–22
32. Fogari R, Zoppi A, Corradi L et al (1998) Sexual function in hypertensive males treated with lisinopril or atenolol: a cross-over study. Am J Hypertens 11:1244–1247
33. Fogari R, Zoppi A, Poletti L et al (2001) Sexual activity in hypertensive men treated with valsartan or carvedilol: a crossover study. Am J Hypertens 14:27–31
34. Fogari R, Preti P, Derosa G et al (2002) Effect of antihypertensive treatment with valsartan or atenolol on sexual activity and plasma testosterone in hypertensive men. Eur J Clin Pharmacol 58:177–180
35. Fogari R, Preti P, Zoppi A et al (2004) Effect of valsartan and atenolol on sexual behavior in hypertensive postmenopausal women. Am J Hypertens 17:77–81
36. Medical Research Council Working Party on mild to moderate hypertension, report of 1981. Adverse reactions to bendrofluazide and propranolol for the treatment of mild hypertension. Lancet. 1981;2:539–543

37. Wassertheil-Smoller S, Blaufox MD, Oberman A et al (1991) Effect of antihypertensives on sexual function and quality of life: the TAIM study. Ann Intern Med 114:613–620
38. Grimm RH, Grandits GA, Prineas RJ et al (1997) Long-term effects on sexual function of five antihypertensive drugs and nutritional hygienic treatment in hypertensive men and women. Treatment of Mild Hypertension Study (TOMHS). Hypertension 29:8–14
39. Brixius K, Middeke M, Lichtenthal A, Jahn E, Schwinger RH (2007) Nitric oxide, erectile dysfunction and beta-blocker treatment (MR NOED study): benefit of nebivolol versus metoprolol in hypertensive men. Clin Exp Pharmacol Physiol 34:327–331
40. Böhm M, Baumhäkel M, Teo K (2010) ONTARGET/TRANSCEND Erectile Dysfunction Substudy Investigators. Erectile dysfunction predicts cardiovascular events in high-risk patients receiving telmisartan, ramipril, or both: the ongoing telmisartan alone and in combination with ramipril global endpoint trial/telmisartan randomized Assessment study in ACE intolerant subjects with cardiovascular disease (ONTARGET/TRANSCEND) trials. Circulation 121:1439–1446
41. Ko DT, Hebert PR, Coffey CS et al (2002) Beta-blocker therapy and symptoms of depression, fatigue, and sexual dysfunction. JAMA 288:351–357
42. Della Chiesa A, Pfifner D, Meier B et al (2003) Sexual activity in hypertensive men. J Hum Hypertens 17:515–521
43. Dusing R (2003) Effect of the angiotensin II antagonist valsartan on sexual function in hypertensive men. Blood Press 12:S29–S34
44. Baumhakel M, Schlimmer N, Bohm M (2008) Effect of irbesartan on erectile function in patients with hypertension and metabolic syndrome. Int J Impot Res 20:493–500
45. Doumas M, Tsakiris A, Douma S et al (2006) Beneficial effects of switching from beta-blockers to nebivolol on the erectile function of hypertensive patients. Asian J Androl 8:177–182
46. Silvestri A, Galetta P, Cerquetani E et al (2003) Report of erectile dysfunction after therapy with beta-blockers is related to patient knowledge of side effects and is reversed by placebo. Eur Heart J 24:1928–1932
47. Douma S, Doumas M, Petidis K, Triantafyllou A, Zamboulis C (2008) Beta blockers and sexual dysfunction: bad guys – good guys. In: Momoka Endo, Narami Matsumoto (eds) Beta blockers: new research. Nova Science Publishers Inc., Hauppauge, NY pp 1–13.
48. Yang L, Yu J, Ma R et al (2013) The effect of combined antihypertensive treatment (felodipine with either irbesartan or metoprolol) on erectile function: a randomized controlled trial. Cardiology 125:235–241
49. Doumas M, Viigimaa M, Papademetriou V (2013) Combined antihypertensive therapy and sexual dysfunction: terra incognita. Cardiology 125:232–234

PDE5 Inhibitors for the Treatment of Erectile Dysfunction in Patients with Hypertension

Peter Kokkinos, Apostolos Tsimploulis, and Charles Faselis

19.1 Introduction

Erectile dysfunction (ED) is defined as the inability to develop or maintain a penile erection during sexual performance. Its prevalence ranges from 25 % [1] to 52 % [2] among male adults aged 40–70 years. ED is an important risk factor for cardiovascular events [3, 4]. ED may also lower adherence to therapy in patients with chronic diseases, especially hypertension, since many antihypertensive medications have unfavorable effects on libido [5, 6].

In the past 15 years, phosphodiesterase 5 inhibitors (PDE5 inhibitors) have emerged as an efficacious therapy in the treatment of ED. The aim of the chapter is to discuss the use of PDE5 inhibitors in the treatment of ED in adult hypertensive patients.

Hypertension is an important contributor to ED. Its prevalence among hypertensive populations is approximately 46 % [7, 8]. There is concern that this prevalence may be accentuated by the unfavorable effects of antihypertensive medications [9]. Moreover, this may contribute to lower adherence rates to medication and thus poor control of blood pressure [6, 10, 11].

P. Kokkinos, PhD
Veteran Affairs Medical Center, 50 Irving Street NW, 20422 Washington, DC, USA

A. Tsimploulis, MD
Internal Medicine Department, Georgetown University Hospital/Washington Hospital Center, 110 Irving St NW, Washington, DC 20010, USA
e-mail: Apostolos.Tsimploulis@medstar.net

C. Faselis, MD (✉)
Veteran Affairs Medical Center, 50 Irving Street NW, 20422 Washington, DC, USA

Georgetown University, Washington, DC, USA
e-mail: Charles.Faselis@va.gov

Endothelial dysfunction is another important factor involved in the hypertension-ED association. Successful erection requires adequate function of local nerves, vessels, and muscles and the release of vasoactive factors (i.e., nitric oxide (NO)) [12, 13]. Consequently, we could confer that all comorbidities that deteriorate endothelial function, such as hypertension, diabetes, and dyslipidemia, could increase vascular cell contraction and lead to ED [14, 15]. PDE5 inhibitors could improve endothelial function through several mechanisms such as normalization of serum biomarkers, increased levels of endothelial progenitor cells, and ischemia-reperfusion protection mechanisms [16–18].

19.2 Patient Approach

A marked increase in patients discussing erectile function with their physician was noted following the introduction of PDE5 inhibitors [19]. However, most patients feel comfortable discussing ED only when the conversation is initiated by the clinician [20]. Thus, a careful and meticulous approach is fundamental. According to European Urology Association Guidelines [9], physicians should take the following approach: (1) conduct a detailed medical and psychosexual history with the partner present; (2) use credible questionnaires for assessing level of ED (e.g., IIEF, SEP 2 and 3); (3) proceed with a thorough physical examination and laboratory tests; and (4) assess self-esteem, partnership quality, and support. These assessments will assist the clinician in finding a common cause of ED, reversible or irreversible, including local defects such as penile deformities, prostate disease, neurologic decline, or systemic causes such as hypertension or cardiovascular problems. In addition, the patient's cardiac risk status during sexual activity should be considered prior to prescribing PDE5 inhibitors. Sexual activity increases myocardial oxygen demands by about three to five metabolic equivalents and augments the risk of myocardial infarction by two to four times in the 2 h after the intercourse [21, 22]. Accordingly, the Princeton III Consensus Recommendations [23] suggest that patients are stratified into three categories regarding their cardiovascular risk profile: low, intermediate, and high risk.

Upon completion of the aforementioned work-up, the physician will be in a better position to identify causes of ED (modifiable or not) and chart a more successful plan of treatment. Prescription of PDE5 inhibitors should also be accompanied with healthy lifestyle modifications, such as exercise and low fat diet [9]. Finally, establishing a trustful relationship and communication with the patient is paramount in increasing adherence.

19.3 PDE5 Inhibitors: Mechanism of Action

PDE5 inhibitors are considered the first-line treatment for ED and include some of the most widely prescribed medications. Drugs belonging to this family are sildenafil (Viagra, the older representative of this family), tadalafil (Cialis), and vardenafil (Levitra) which are approved for treating ED in the United States by Food and Drug Administration (FDA) and in Europe by the European Medicines Agency

(EMA). Some newer representatives are avanafil (Stendra) which has been recently approved by the FDA, udenafil (Zydena), and lodenafil (Helleva) whose distribution has so far been limited to a few countries. PDE5 inhibitors' main target is the enzyme phosphodiesterase 5 (PDE5).

PDE5 is found widely in platelets, veins, and arterial walls and in other tissues [24]. Although PDE5 inhibitors have an inhibitory effect on other enzymes [25], their affinity is substantially higher for PDE5. This accounts for their beneficial effects in ED. In this chapter, we will mainly refer to sildenafil, tadalafil, and vardenafil, the most widely used agents in this category.

PDE5 inhibitors' mechanism of action is well understood. The normal erection reflex requires the cooperation of nerves, vessels, and smooth muscles. After the appropriate sexual perception, the brain (central) exerts its exhibitory stimulus causing the activation of a spinal reflex by spinal nerves (peripheral). Following this, NO is released by the nitrinergic nerves and endothelial cells to the penis, leading to the activation of the enzyme guanyl cyclase which causes production of cyclic guanosine monophosphate (cGMP) [26]. The final result is the sequestration of Ca++ from cytosol to the endoplasmic reticulum, arterial and trabecular smooth muscle relaxation, arterial dilation, and venous constriction [15, 27]. PDE5, which is widely distributed in the corpus cavernosum, hydrolyses cGMP leading to penis relaxation. PDE5 inhibitors exert their action at this step by competitively inhibiting PDE5 and causing preservation of erection [26].

It is apparent that the importance of normal NO release is paramount for erectile function. Several comorbidities such as hypertension, diabetes, and aging affect nerves and endothelial function adversely and cause decline in NO formation and release necessary for erection [27, 28].

Since PDE5 inhibitors' main action is to inhibit NO degradation and preserve preexisting levels, conditions that interfere with NO release may hinder the efficacy of PDE5 inhibitors. This mechanism is considered one of the reasons of poor response to these medications.

19.4 PDE5 Inhibitors: Pharmacokinetics

PDE5 inhibitors share similar characteristics regarding their pharmacokinetics.

Sildenafil, the pioneer of this class, was approved for prescription in 1998. It is available in oral doses of 25, 50, and 100 mg. The recommended initial dose is 50 mg, unless certain comorbidities exist [9]. Sildenafil should be taken 30–60 min prior to intercourse and it should not be combined with fatty meals, for they may reduce its absorption [25]. Its duration of action may last up to 8–12 h [29, 30]. The pharmacokinetics of sildenafil, as well as some special considerations requiring dose adjustments, are included in Table 19.1.

Vardenafil, introduced in 2003, is available in oral doses of 2.5, 5, 10, and 20 mg, while the recommended starting dose is 10 mg [9]. The medication should be taken 30 min prior to intercourse in a fasting state, as it is also affected by fatty meals. It has a higher affinity to PDE5 than sildenafil which makes it more potent and extends its duration of efficacy up to 10 h [33]. It may cause QT prolongation;

Table 19.1 Pharmacokinetics

Variables	Sildenafil	Vardenafil	Tadalafil
Tmax con	60 min	60 min	2 h
T 1/2	4 h	4 h	17.5 h
Protein binding	96 %	95 %	94 %
Bioavailability	41 %	15 %	Not determined
Metabolism	CYP3A4 (major route)	CYP2A4 (predominantly)	CYP3A4
	CYP2C9 (minor route)	CYP3A5, CYP2C (minor)	
Excretion after oral dose	Feces (80 %)	Feces (91–95 %)	Feces (61 %)
	Urine (13 %)	Urine (2–6 %)	Urine (36 %)
Dose adjustment			
Hepatic failure	25 mg	5 mg	<10 mg
Renal failure	Dose adjustment 25mg only in patients with GFR <30 ml/min	No dose adjustment is needed for Vardenafil in patients with renal failure	5 mg
Age >65 years	25 mg	5 mg	No adjustment

Information on table is derived from references [25, 31, 32]

thus caution should be taken when it is administered with drugs that prolong QT interval such as type 1A and type 3 antiarrhythmics or in patients with a congenitally prolonged QT syndrome [34]. A new orodispersible tablet is available which appears to have the same efficacy as the traditional tablet, but is not affected by meals [35, 36]. The pharmacokinetic characteristics of vardenafil are presented in Table 19.1.

Tadalafil was also introduced in 2003. The available oral doses are 2.5, 5, 10, and 20 mg and recommended starting dose of 10 mg [9]. It should be taken approximately 30 min before intercourse. Its unique characteristic is its extended duration of action up to 36 h and it is not affected by food [31]. A daily treatment of 2.5 or 5 mg has been approved for ED for a more spontaneous intercourse [9, 37, 38]. Pharmacokinetic data regarding tadalafil are presented in Table 19.1.

The effect of PDE5 inhibitors on blood pressure and heart rate is minimal when prescribed alone. The main metabolic pathway of PDE5 inhibitors is via cytochrome P450, specifically CYP3A4 (Table 19.1). In this regard, any inhibitors or inducers of these enzymes will influence the drugs' concentration and dose adjustment may be needed. Therefore, caution should be taken when cytochrome P450 inhibitors are concomitantly prescribed with erythromycin, ketoconazole, itraconazole, clarithromycin, HIV protease inhibitors, or grapefruit juice [39]. Dose adjustment is necessary for ritonavir because it markedly increases PDE5 inhibitor concentrations [40]. Conversely, inducers of cytochrome P450, including carbamazepine, phenytoin, and phenobarbital, likely decrease PDE5 inhibitor levels. No notable interactions with widely prescribed medications such as warfarin, azithromycin, selective serotonin reuptake inhibitors, thiazides, angiotensin-converting enzyme inhibitors, calcium channel blockers, antacids, glyburide, digoxin, ranitidine, midazolam, lovastatin, or theophylline have been noted [40].

19.5 PDE5 Inhibitors: Safety and Efficacy

PDE5 inhibitors are safe when used with common antihypertensive medications (angiotensin-converting enzyme inhibitors, angiotensin-receptor blockers, calcium channel blockers, β-blockers, and diuretics) [41, 42]. A slight pressure decrease may be observed as a result of additional vasodilatory characteristics of PDE5 inhibitors [43, 44]. On the other hand, better management of systolic blood pressure was observed in hypertensive population with ED who were administered PDE5 inhibitors [45, 46], leading to a possible application of this drug in the resistant hypertensive population [47].

The use of PDE5 inhibitors improves adherence to antihypertensive therapy. The percentage of hypertensive patients who became adherent to treatment after sildenafil use increased from 22 to 36 % [48]. Newer long-acting PDE5 inhibitors are now being tested in pivotal clinical studies for the treatment of mild to moderate arterial hypertension [49]. In addition, experimental data indicates that chronic PDE5 inhibition might be associated with significant regression of left ventricular hypertrophy [50].

The co-administration of PDE5 inhibitors and α-blockers is not contraindicated. However, the combination could potentially cause symptomatic hypotension due to shared vasodilatory characteristics [34, 51]. Differences regarding the degree of interaction among the PDE5 inhibitors with different α-blockers (uroselective such as tamsulosin and alfuzosin and less selective such as terazosin and doxazosin) have also been described [40, 52, 53]. Thus, PDE5 inhibitors should only be prescribed to patients who take α-blockers chronically, without presenting blood pressure variations or symptoms of hypotension. They should be prescribed at the lowest dose and the two drugs should preferably be administered several hours apart.

The efficacy of PDE5 inhibitors in treating ED in general population is well established [54]. The success rates may approach 78 % regardless of comorbidities such as hypertension and diabetes [55]. In the REALIZE trial ($n=73,946$), erectile function was markedly improved in 93.6 % of hypertensive patients treated with vardenafil [56], regardless of baseline severity. Similar but less impressive results were reported in a meta-analysis of hypertensive patients [57]. An improvement of 8.9 points in the International Index of Erectile Function (IIEF) questionnaire was noted as well as 32.9 % in the ability to obtain erections (SEP 2) and 38 % to maintain erections (SEP 3) compared to placebo. Successful results in hypertensive patients were observed from the first dose of tadalafil with improvement in SEP 2 and SEP 3 scores. Improvement of ED was observed in patients taking tadalafil and thiazides [58]. Patients using sildenafil while on multiple antihypertensive medications reported success rates of above 80 % in a 12-week time frame [42].

PDE5 inhibitors are well tolerated and are considered relatively safe medications. Patients taking PDE5 inhibitors did not present an increase in the rates and mortality of serious cardiovascular events, such as myocardial infarction, cardiovascular death, or cerebrovascular death, compared to placebo [59, 60]. In contrast, a trend towards improved survival with PDE5 inhibitors has been observed in diabetic patients [61], highlighting the need for relevant studies in patients with hypertension and other cardiovascular disease conditions.

However, in hypertensive patients treated with nitrates, PDE5 inhibitors can decrease systolic and diastolic blood pressure [25, 31, 32, 62]. When PDE5 inhibitors are co-administered with organic nitrates (NO donors) such as nitroglycerine, isosorbide mononitrate, and isosorbide dinitrate as well as amyl nitrite or amyl nitrate ("poppers"), an unpredictable vasodilatory and hypotensive effect may be observed [34, 40]. A significant drop of 85 mmHg in standing and supine systolic blood pressure was observed in patients taking sildenafil or tadalafil compared to placebo [63]. In this context, the co-administration of PDE5 inhibitors and nitrates is contraindicated. Nitrates should not be taken in the 24 h preceding the administration of sildenafil and vardenafil and for 48 h before the use of tadalafil [9, 34]. The marked hypotensive effect of this combination might be beneficial in patients with resistant hypertension [64]; however, close monitoring and extreme care is needed to avoid significant adverse effects.

References

1. National Institutes of Health Consensus Development Statement (1992) Impotence. 10(4):1–31
2. Feldman HA, Goldstein I, Hatzichristou DG, Krane RJ, McKinlay JB (1994) Impotence and its medical and psychosocial correlates: results of the Massachusetts male aging study. J Urol 151(1):54–61
3. Jackson G, Boon N, Eardley I, Kirby M, Dean J, Hackett G, Montorsi P, Montorsi F, Vlachopoulos C, Kloner R, Sharlip I, Miner M (2010) Erectile dysfunction and coronary artery disease prediction: evidence-based guidance and consensus. Int J Clin Pract 64(7):848–857
4. Nehra A, Jackson G, Miner M, Billups KL, Burnett AL, Buvat J, Carson CC, Cunningham GR, Goldstein I, Guay AT, Hackett G, Kloner RA, Kostis J, Montorsi P, Ramsey M, Rosen RC, Sadovsky R, Seftel AD, Vlachopoulos C, Wu FC (2013) Diagnosis and treatment of erectile dysfunction for reduction of cardiovascular risk. J Urol 189(6):2031–2038
5. Scranton RE, Goldstein I, Stecher VJ (2013) Erectile dysfunction diagnosis and treatment as a means to improve medication adherence and optimize comorbidity management. J Sex Med 10(2):551–561
6. Doumas M, Douma S (2006) The effect of antihypertensive drugs on erectile function: a proposed management algorithm. J Clin Hypertens (Greenwich) 8(5):359–364
7. Seftel AD, Sun P, Swindle R (2004) The prevalence of hypertension, hyperlipidemia, diabetes mellitus and depression in men with erectile dysfunction. J Urol 171(6 Pt 1):2341–2345
8. Aranda P, Ruilope LM, Calvo C, Luque M, Coca A, Gil de Miguel A (2004) Erectile dysfunction in essential arterial hypertension and effects of sildenafil: results of a Spanish national study. Am J Hypertens 17(2):139–145
9. European Urology Association Guidelines for Male Sexual Dysfunction (2013)
10. Manolis A, Doumas M (2012) Antihypertensive treatment and sexual dysfunction. Curr Hypertens Rep 14(4):285–292
11. Silvestri A, Galetta P, Cerquetani E, Marazzi G, Patrizi R, Fini M, Rosano GM (2003) Report of erectile dysfunction after therapy with beta-blockers is related to patient knowledge of side effects and is reversed by placebo. Eur Heart J 24(21):1928–1932
12. Meldrum DR, Gambone JC, Morris MA, Meldrum DA, Esposito K, Ignarro LJ (2011) The link between erectile and cardiovascular health: the canary in the coal mine. Am J Cardiol 108(4):599–606
13. Corbin JD (2004) Mechanisms of action of PDE5 inhibition in erectile dysfunction. Int J Impot Res 16(Suppl 1):S4–S7

14. Nunes KP, Labazi H, Webb RC (2012) New insights into hypertension-associated erectile dysfunction. Curr Opin Nephrol Hypertens 21(2):163–170
15. Cheitlin MD (2004) Erectile dysfunction: the earliest sign of generalized vascular disease? J Am Coll Cardiol 43:185–186
16. Schwartz BG, Jackson G, Stecher VJ, Campoli-Richards DM, Kloner RA (2013) Phosphodiesterase type 5 inhibitors improve endothelial function and may benefit cardiovascular conditions. Am J Med 126(3):192–199
17. Balarini CM, Leal MA, Gomes IB, Pereira TM, Gava AL, Meyrelles SS, Vasquez EC (2013) Sildenafil restores endothelial function in the apolipoprotein E knockout mouse. J Transl Med 11:3
18. La Vignera S, Condorelli R, Vicari E, D'Agata R, Calogero AE (2012) Circulating endothelial progenitor cells and endothelial microparticles in patients with arterial erectile dysfunction and metabolic syndrome. J Androl 33(2):202–209
19. Wilson EC, McKeen ES, Scuffham PA, Brown MC, Wylie K, Hackett G (2002) The cost to the United Kingdom National Health Service of managing erectile dysfunction: the impact of sildenafil and prescribing restrictions. Pharmacoeconomics 20(13):879–889
20. Bedell SE, Graboys TB, Duperval M, Goldberg R (2002) Sildenafil in the cardiologist's office: patients' attitudes and physicians' practices toward discussions about sexual functioning. Cardiology 97(2):79–82
21. Cheitlin MD (2005) Sexual activity and cardiac risk. Am J Cardiol 96(12B):24M–28M
22. Mittleman MA, Maclure M, Glasser DB (2005) Evaluation of acute risk for myocardial infarction in men treated with sildenafil citrate. Am J Cardiol 96(3):443–446
23. Nehra A, Jackson G, Miner M, Billups KL, Burnett AL, Buvat J, Carson CC, Cunningham GR, Ganz P, Goldstein I, Guay AT, Hackett G, Kloner RA, Kostis J, Montorsi P, Ramsey M, Rosen R, Sadovsky R, Seftel AD, Shabsigh R, Vlachopoulos C, Wu FC (2012) The Princeton III Consensus recommendations for the management of erectile dysfunction and cardiovascular disease. Mayo Clin Proc 87(8):766–778
24. Wallis RM, Corbin JD, Francis SH, Ellis P (1999) Tissue distribution of phosphodiesterase families and the effects of sildenafil on tissue cyclic nucleotides, platelet function, and the contractile responses of trabeculae carneae and aortic rings in vitro. Am J Cardiol 83(5A):3C–12C
25. Pfizer. VIAGRA (sildenafil citrate) prescribing information. Available at: http://www.pfizer.com/files/products/uspi_viagra.pdf. Accessed 29 Mar 2014
26. Francis SH, Corbin JD (2005) Phosphodiesterase-5 inhibition: the molecular biology of erectile function and dysfunction. Urol Clin North Am 32(4):419–429
27. Gur S, Kadowitz PJ, Hellstrom WJ (2010) Exploring the potential of NO-independent stimulators and activators of soluble guanylate cyclase for the medical treatment of erectile dysfunction. Curr Pharm Des 16(14):1619–1633
28. Condorelli RA, Calogero AE, Favilla V, Morgia G, Johnson EO, Castiglione R, Salemi M, Mongioí L, Nicoletti C, Duca Y, Di Mauro M, Vicari E, La Vignera S (2013) Arterial erectile dysfunction: different severities of endothelial apoptosis between diabetic patients "responders" and "non responders" to sildenafil. Eur J Intern Med 24(3):234–240
29. McCullough AR, Steidle CP, Kaufman J, Goldfischer ER, Klee B, Carlsson M (2008) Sildenafil citrate efficacy 8 h postdose in men with mild to moderate erectile dysfunction. Int J Impot Res 20(4):388–395
30. Moncada I, Jara J, Subirá D, Castaño I, Hernández C (2004) Efficacy of sildenafil citrate at 12 hours after dosing: re-exploring the therapeutic window. Eur Urol 46(3):357–360
31. Eli Lilly and Co. CIALIS (tadalafil) prescribing information. Available at: http://pi.lilly.com/us/cialis-pi.pdf. Accessed 29 Mar 2014
32. Bayer Health Care Pharmaceuticals. Product monograph for LEVITRA (vardenafil HCL)
33. Porst H, Sharlip ID, Hatzichristou D, Rubio-Aurioles E, Gittelman M, Stancil BN, Smith PM, Wilkins HJ, Pommerville P, Vardenafil Study Group (2006) Extended duration of efficacy of vardenafil when taken 8 hours before intercourse: a randomized, double-blind, placebo-controlled study. Eur Urol 50(5):1086–1094
34. Jackson G, Rosen RC, Kloner RA, Kostis JB (2006) The second Princeton consensus on sexual dysfunction and cardiac risk: new guidelines for sexual medicine. J Sex Med 3(1):28–36

35. Sperling H, Debruyne F, Boermans A, Beneke M, Ulbrich E, Ewald S (2010) The POTENT I randomized trial: efficacy and safety of an orodispersible vardenafil formulation for the treatment of erectile dysfunction. J Sex Med 7(4 Pt 1):1497–1507
36. Gittelman M, McMahon CG, Rodríguez-Rivera JA, Beneke M, Ulbrich E, Ewald S (2010) The POTENT II randomised trial: efficacy and safety of an orodispersible vardenafil formulation for the treatment of erectile dysfunction. Int J Clin Pract 64(5):594–603
37. Washington SL 3rd, Shindel AW (2010) A once-daily dose of tadalafil for erectile dysfunction: compliance and efficacy. Drug Des Devel Ther 4:159–171
38. Porst H, Rajfer J, Casabé A, Feldman R, Ralph D, Vieiralves LF, Esler A, Wolka AM, Klise SR (2008) Long-term safety and efficacy of tadalafil 5 mg dosed once daily in men with erectile dysfunction. J Sex Med 5(9):2160–2169
39. Gur S, Kadowitz PJ, Gokce A, Sikka SC, Lokman U, Hellstrom WJ (2013) Update on drug interactions with phosphodiesterase-5 inhibitors prescribed as first-line therapy for patients with erectile dysfunction or pulmonary hypertension. Curr Drug Metab 14(2):265–269
40. Schwartz BG, Kloner RA (2010) Drug interactions with phosphodiesterase-5 inhibitors used for the treatment of erectile dysfunction or pulmonary hypertension. Circulation 122(1):88–95
41. Böhm M, Burkart M, Baumann G (2007) Sildenafil is well tolerated by erectile dysfunction patients taking antihypertensive medications, including those on multidrug regimens. Curr Drug Saf 2(1):5–8
42. Pickering TG, Shepherd AM, Puddey I, Glasser DB, Orazem J, Sherman N, Mancia (2004) Sildenafil citrate for erectile dysfunction in men receiving multiple antihypertensive agents: a randomized controlled trial. Am J Hypertens 17(12 Pt 1):1135–1142
43. Kloner RA, Mitchell M, Emmick JT (2003) Cardiovascular effects of tadalafil in patients on common antihypertensive therapies. Am J Cardiol 92(9A):47M–57M
44. Zusman RM, Prisant LM, Brown MJ (2000) Effect of sildenafil citrate on blood pressure and heart rate in men with erectile dysfunction taking concomitant antihypertensive medication. Sildenafil study group. Hypertens 18(12):1865–1869
45. Ghiadoni L, Versari D, Taddei S (2008) Phosphodiesterase 5 inhibition in essential hypertension. Curr Hypertens Rep 10(1):52–57
46. Scranton RE, Lawler E, Botteman M, Chittamooru S, Gagnon D, Lew R, Harnett J, Gaziano JM (2007) Effect of treating erectile dysfunction on management of systolic hypertension. Am J Cardiol 100(3):459–463
47. Quinaglia T, de Faria AP, Fontana V, Barbaro NR, Sabbatini AR, Sertório JT, Demacq C, Tanus-Santos JE, Moreno H (2013) Acute cardiac and hemodynamic effects of sildenafil on resistant hypertension. Eur J Clin Pharmacol 69(12):2027–2036
48. McLaughlin T, Harnett J, Burhani S, Scott B (2005) Evaluation of erectile dysfunction therapy in patients previously nonadherent to long-term medications: a retrospective analysis of prescription claims. Am J Ther 12:605–611
49. Wolk R, Smith WB, Neutel JM et al (2009) Blood pressure lowering effects of a new long-acting inhibitor of phosphodiesterase 5 in patients with mild to moderate hypertension. Hypertension 53:1091–1097
50. Takimoto E, Champion HC, Li M et al (2005) Chronic inhibition of cyclic GMP phosphodiesterase 5° prevents and reverses cardiac hypertrophy. Nat Med 11:214–222
51. Reffelmann T, Kloner RA (2006) Sexual function in hypertensive patients receiving treatment. Vasc Health Risk Manag 2(4):447–455
52. Kloner RA, Jackson G, Emmick JT, Mitchell MI, Bedding A, Warner MR, Pereira A (2004) Interaction between the phosphodiesterase 5 inhibitor, tadalafil and 2 alpha-blockers, doxazosin and tamsulosin in healthy normotensive men. J Urol 172(5 Pt 1):1935–1940
53. Auerbach SM, Gittelman M, Mazzu A, Cihon F, Sundaresan P, White WB (2004) Simultaneous administration of vardenafil and tamsulosin does not induce clinically significant hypotension in patients with benign prostatic hyperplasia. Urology 64(5):998–1003
54. Yuan J, Zhang R, Yang Z, Lee J, Liu Y, Tian J, Qin X, Ren Z, Ding H, Chen Q, Mao C, Tang J (2013) Comparative effectiveness and safety of oral phosphodiesterase type 5 inhibitors for erectile dysfunction: a systematic review and network meta-analysis. Eur Urol 63(5):902–912

55. Cheng E (2007) Real-life safety and efficacy of vardenafil in the treatment of erectile dysfunction-results from 30,010 U.S. patients. J Sex Med 4(2):432–439
56. Van Ahlen H, Zumbé J, Stauch K, Hanisch JU (2010) The Real-Life Safety and Efficacy of vardenafil (REALISE) study: results in men from Europe and overseas with erectile dysfunction and cardiovascular or metabolic conditions. J Sex Med 7(9):3161–3169
57. Shabsigh R, Duval S, Shah M, Regan TS, Juhasz M, Veltry LG (2007) Efficacy of vardenafil for the treatment of erectile dysfunction in men with hypertension: a meta-analysis of clinical trial data. Curr Med Res Opin 23(10):2453–2460
58. Kloner RA, Sadovsky R, Johnson EG, Mo D, Ahuja S (2005) Efficacy of tadalafil in the treatment of erectile dysfunction in hypertensive men on concomitant thiazide diuretic therapy. Int J Impot Res 17(5):450–454
59. Kloner RA, Jackson G, Hutter AM, Mittleman MA, Chan M, Warner MR, Costigan TM, Vail GM (2006) Cardiovascular safety update of Tadalafil: retrospective analysis of data from placebo-controlled and open-label clinical trials of Tadalafil with as needed, three times-per-week or once-a-day dosing. Am J Cardiol 97(12):1778–1784
60. Jackson G, Kloner RA, Costigan TM, Warner MR, Emmick JT (2004) Update on clinical trials of tadalafil demonstrates no increased risk of cardiovascular adverse events. J Sex Med 1(2):161–167
61. Gazzaruso C, Solerte SB, Pujia A et al (2008) Erectile dysfunction as a predictor of cardiovascular events and death in diabetic patients with angiographically proven asymptomatic coronary artery disease: a potential protective role for statins and 5-phosphodiesterase inhibitors. J Am Coll Cardiol 51:2040–2044
62. Prisant LM (2006) Phosphodiesterase-5 inhibitors and their hemodynamic effects. Curr Hypertens Rep 8(4):345–351
63. Emmick JT, Stuewe SR, Mitchell M (2002) Overview of the cardiovascular effects of tadalafil. Eur Heart J Suppl 4:H32–H47
64. Oliver JJ, Hughes VE, Dear JW, Webb DJ (2010) Clinical potential of combined organic nitrate and phosphodiesterase type 5 inhibitor in treatment-resistant hypertension. Hypertension 56:62–67

Management of Erectile Dysfunction Beyond PDE-5 Inhibitors

20

Konstantinos Rokkas

20.1 Introduction

Although phosphodiesterase type 5 (PDE5) inhibition is the recommended first-line treatment, up to 35 % of patients with erectile dysfunction (ED) are nonresponders to this therapy. Common etiologies of this response failure are comorbidities such as diabetes and severe neurological or vascular diseases. Although there is no consensus on how to define the failure of PDE5 inhibitors, the inability to attain or maintain adequate penile erection during sexual intercourse on at least four consecutive occasions, in spite of optimum drug dosing, is an acceptable definition. Patients who have failed a trial with PDE5 inhibitor therapy should be informed of the benefits and risks of other pharmacological or non-pharmacological interventions. Management of ED beyond PDE5 inhibitor consists mainly of three therapeutical categories:

- Intracavernosal injections
- Penile implants
- Shock wave therapy for penile revascularization

20.2 Intracavernosal Injections

The era of the intracavernosal injections starts in 1982 [1] with the first totally induced erection with intracavernosal autoinjection of phenoxybenzamine from Brindley [1–3]. After this Virag has used papaverine as a substance for injection use [4]. From that point many substances are proposed for this use like phentolamine, prostaglandin E1 (PGE1), vasoactive intestinal peptide, NO donors etc. with proven results. Nowadays three are the main substances used for this kind of treatment, papaverine, phentolamine, and prostaglandin E1.

Nowadays there are more than 500 publication for the injection therapy, and the success rate is variable from 54 % for papaverine, 71 % for the combination of papaverine and phentolamine, 73 % for PGE1, and 75 % for the mixture of the three substances [5–7].

The first injection should always be administered by a medical doctor, and then when the accurate dosage is determined, the patient is trained to autoinject himself sometimes using injection devices for easier usage. The injection should be done in the dorsolateral and proximal part of the penis in aseptic conditions changing every time the site of the injection. Also the patient has to learn to avoid the urethral part of the penis when autoinjecting because this will cause a lot of pain and no erectile result. When deterring the dosage normally the doctor starts with 10 μg of PGE1 or in patients with neurological cause with 5 μg of PGE1 increasing until reaching the desirable effect until a maximum of 40 μg of PGE1. Alternatively can be used a mixture of papaverine and phentolamine (15 mg/ml of papaverine and 0.5 mg/ml of phentolamine) starting from 0.5 ml and reaching in maximum 3 ml.

20.2.1 Types of Substances

Papaverine
It was the first substance used for this purpose and it is provided by the Papaver somniferum that provides an alkaloid of the opium without any narcotic effect. It was first used by Virag [5] and within 2 years was the most common substance used for this purpose. Studies were executed with dosages from 5 to 160 mg [8]. The most common side effects are prolonged erection found in 5.1 % of the patients during the treatment period [9–11] and intracavernosal fibrosis in 6 % of the patients [8]. Painful erections are very rare; the rate of the patients that stop the treatment is 31.3 %.

Phentolamine
Phentolamine is a selective antagonist of the alpha adrenoreceptors and it stops the contractions of the muscular cells. In 1978 Domer proposed the use of phentolamine and in 1982 Zorgniotti and Lefleurs have injected 30 mg of papaverine and 1 mg of phentolamine. Prolonged erection using the mixture of papaverine-phentolamine is reported in 7.5 % of the patients and penile fibrosis in 6 % of them [12].

Prostaglandin E1 (PGE1)

It is a prostanoid that has effect in various organs relaxing the arterioles with positive effect on the arterial circulation increasing the cAMP. It was first presented by Sidi et al. in 1986 [12] and the first clinical results were presented by Stackl et al. [13] and Porst [9]. The dosage is variable from 5 to 40 µg and the success rate is elevated to 73 %. The main side effect is painful erection present in 15 % of the patients during treatment period [14]. Prolonged erections are very rare around 1 % [11] and penile fibrosis arrives to 2.7 % [11]. The PGE 1 is the most common commercially used substance and it is the gold standard for the intracavernosal injection.

Combination Therapy

The combination of the three drugs is called Trimix and it is a mixture of papaverine/phentolamine/PGE1 with success rate of 75.5 %. Painful erection is reported in the 2.9 % of the patients, whereas penile fibrosis in 2.3 % of the patients. Combination therapy is used as a last solution when monotherapy with PGE1 is not successful.

In conclusion the long-term treatment with intracavernosal injections in terms of success is very good. The drugs are easy to use and disposable at the patients, and most of them learn very easily how to autoinject themselves and maintain a very hard erection without notable side effects providing that the patient training and the dosage determination are made in a very organized way.

20.3 Penile Implants

Also urologists were not highly interested in the treatment of ED until the inflatable penile prosthesis was introduced in 1973. For the next 10 years, there were two solutions: sex therapy for potentially reversible ED and penile prosthesis implantation for the other forms. Nowadays, many possibilities are available for ED, that is, systematic therapy, sex therapy, vacuum erection devices, intraurethral medication, penile injection therapy, penile revascularization, and penile prosthesis implantation [15].

20.3.1 Prosthesis Types

Rod prostheses are paired solid devices implanted in the corpora cavernosa that produce constant penile rigidity. The advantage of these devices is that they are designed to be *easy* to *implant* and relative freedom from medical failure. Disadvantages are a constant rigidity of the penis like neither normal erection nor flaccidity, difficulties with concealment, and a higher risk of erosion for device.

There are three companies: American Medical Systems (AMS, Minnetonka, MN) for a malleable penile prosthesis, the AMS Malleable 650 and Mentor (Santa Barbara CA) for the semirigid rod prostheses, the Mentor Malleable and the Acu-Form prosthesis. Timm Medical Technologies (Eden Prairie, MN) manufacturers the Dura-II prosthesis, which has a central cable running through articulated polysulfone segments. At the end of the cable, there is a spring that allows the device to have better position ability than the other rod prostheses [16].

20.3.2 Inflatable Prostheses

One-Piece Inflatable Devices
These devices are no more produced in the United States; they were paired hydraulic devices inflated into the corpora that created penile rigidity similar to the one produced by rod prostheses but without girth expansion. When deflated, these devices lost a part of their rigidity giving a more natural look on palpation than solid rod implants. They were manufactured by Surgitek (Racine, WI) and the Hydroflex and Dynaflex devices by AMS. They did not satisfy completely the expectations and are no longer implanted [17].

Two-Piece Inflated Devices
These devices are paired cylinders connected by tubing to a scrotal component. They are manufactured by AMS. A small scrotal pump transfers fluid from the proximal portion of the cylinders to the distal portion, resulting in rigidity without girth expansion. Mentor manufacturers the Mark II prosthesis. The paired cylinders of this device are connected to a 25-ml scrotal component that serves as a pump and reservoir [17].

Three-Piece Inflatable Device
These devices have paired cylinders, a small scrotal pump, and a large-volume abdominal fluid reservoir (Fig. 20.1). AMS manufacturers three types: AMS 700CX introduced in 1987 has cylinders that produce controlled girth expansion and rigidity. The AMS 700CXM is similar to the AMS 700CX but with smaller cylinders, pump, and reservoir. The AMS 700cxmfirst, created for men with small penises, now is used for men with fibrotic corpora. In 1990 AMS introduced the Ultrex inflatable penile prosthesis. In this model the three-piece device provides girth and length expansion. After some time, it was proved that the ability of the cylinders to lengthen was obtained at the expense of decreased cylinder duration. In 1993 the Ultrex cylinders were changed to provide a stronger middle layer. Since then only 142 Ultrex were implanted with only three cylinder failures. However, more follow-up is requested to determine if the improved cylinders are reliable.

Mentor manufacturers two to three-piece inflatable prostheses: the Alpha I and the Alpha I Narrow Back, a small-diameter version for men with fibrotic penises [17].

Nowadays in extended use is the AMS INIBHIZONE already embedded in antibiotic (solution) and the COLOPLAST TITAN OTR embedded in antibiotic solution during the surgical procedure.

20.3.3 Preparing to the Surgery

The patient must be prepared for the surgery to decrease the risk of infections. Some general rules are to start scrubbing the external genitalia with povidone solution a week

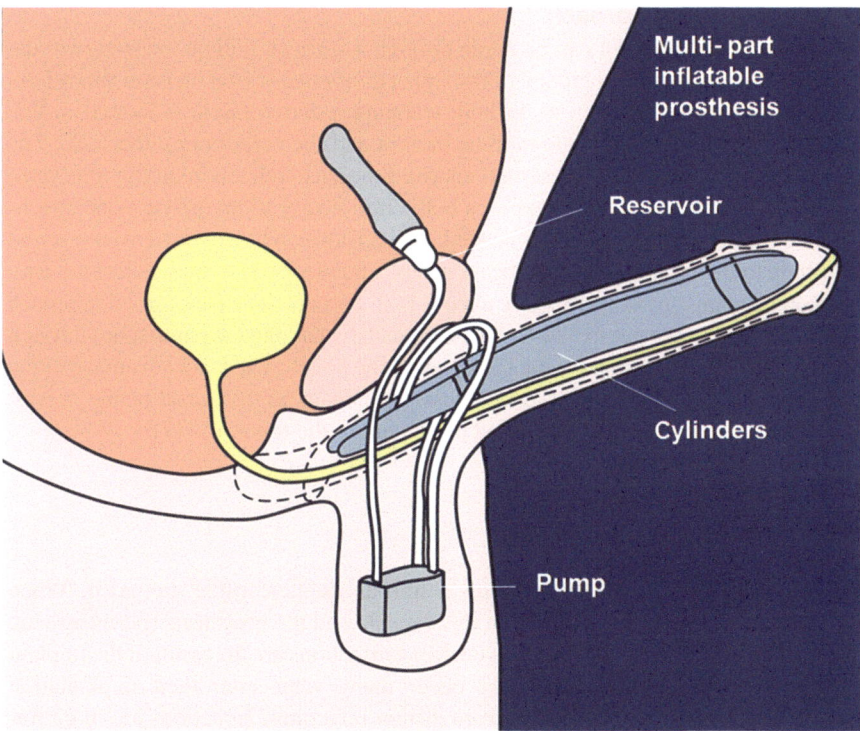

Fig. 20.1 The three-piece inflatable penile prosthesis creates a firmer erection than its two-piece counterpart. This fluid-filled implant features two inflatable cylinders implanted in the penis, a pump placed in the scrotum, and a reservoir implanted in the lower abdomen. When you are ready to have sex, you pump the fluid from the reservoir into the cylinders to create a rigid erection. After sexual intercourse, you release the valve inside of the scrotum to drain the fluid back into the reservoir to return to flaccidity

before the procedure. Some authors suggest to sterilize the urine with ofloxacin 5 days before the surgery. The standard procedure is the combination of gentamycin (80 mg tid) and vancomycin (1 g bid) starting the day of the surgery and for 2 days after.

Some authors are used to irrigate the surgery field with a solution of vancomycin (2 g) and protamine that allows the antibiotics to enter through the bacterial shields [18].

20.3.4 Surgical Approaches

The Infrapubic Approach
This approach that consists of a small vertical or transverse incision is made below the pubis just above the penis. The main advantage of this method is the possibility to place the reservoir under direct vision. Disadvantages: limit of corporeal exposure, impossibility to anchor the pump in the scrotum, and possible damage to the dorsal nerves of the penis.

The Penoscrotal Approach

The penoscrotal approach can be made through a vertical midline incision over the urethra at the penoscrotal junction or through a transverse scrotal incision about 1 cm below the penoscrotal junction. In both techniques dartos fascia is incised in line with the incision, exposing the midline urethra and the corpora or either side. The surgeons prefer the transverse scrotal approach because retraction on the transverse lower flap of the dartos fascia exposes both crura nearly to the pelvic bone attachments. If further distal exposure is needed, the incision can be extended in an inverted T-fashion to the frenular area. To the surgeons' knowledge, this approach is the only incision that can almost completely expose both corpora. The penoscrotal approach also permits to fix the pump in its subdartos pouch by passing the pump tubes through three separate stab incisions in the back wall of the pouch. The main advantage of the penoscrotal approach is that it avoids possible damage to the dorsal penile nerves. The disadvantage is that it needs blind placement of the reservoir [17].

20.3.5 Infection

When using silicone, our body forms a fibrous pseudocapsule around it. When infections arise in the space between this capsule and the prosthesis (periprosthetic infections), the device must be removed. Most infections are the result of the implant procedure; however, infections may occur many years after their implantation because of blood-borne organisms from distant infections. Infections are more frequent in secondary implants or procedures associated with reconstruction. Jarow reported a 1.8 % infection rate in 114 primary procedures, a 13.3 % infection rate in 30 secondary procedures, and a 21.7 % infection rate in 23 implants connected with reconstructive procedures.

It is not clear whether diabetes increases the risk for periprosthetic infection. In a study a higher risk was proved in diabetics with glucosylated hemoglobin around 11.5 %. In another study no correlation was found between infections and glucosylated hemoglobin. In two other studies there were no significant differences between diabetic and nondiabetic patients.

When a periprosthetic infection occurs, it is necessary to remove the entire prosthesis because there are bacteria in a biofilm that is adherent to the device. For many years, the reimplantation of the device was delayed for 6–12 months. Infection destroys some or all of the corpora cavernosa, and a scar occurs. With time, this scar contracts and the penis becomes smaller and creates difficulties in placing the cylinder during the implantation.

In case of infective penile prosthesis, current practice tends to device salvage or device removal with early reimplantation [18, 19].

20.3.6 Mechanical Reliability and Patient Satisfaction

In a long-term (median follow-up 47.7 months) multicenter study made in the United States, AMS 700CX inflatable prosthesis was evaluated for longevity, morbidity, and patient satisfaction rates. The control was carried out in two phases. Phase 1 was a medical record review of 372 patients who had implantation with the AMS 700CX penile prosthesis from 1987 to 1996 by seven frequent penile prosthesis implanters. Phase 2 was a telephone interview of 207 men by a neutral observer. For the 372 men in phase 1, mean device mechanical reliability was 92.1 ± 3.3 % after 3 years and 86.2 ± 4.6 % after 5 years. 3.2 and 17.5 % of the cases, respectively, developed postoperative infection and device malfunction. In phase 2, of the 207 patients called, 86.2 % still had an AMS 700CX penile prosthesis implanted and 87.1 % with erection suitable for coitus; 88.2 % would suggest an implant to a relative or a friend [20, 21].

20.4 Low-Intensity Shock Wave Therapy

The most recent treatment for ED is the shock wave therapy for the revascularization of the corpus cavernosum in cases of vascular ED [22]. The treatment can be done using either electrohydraulic or electromagnetic sources of producing shock waves. In the first animal study, the researchers demonstrated that low-intensity shock wave therapy (Li-SWT) promotes regeneration of nNOS-positive penile dorsal nerve, penile dorsal artery, and penile sinusoids [23]. Tom Lue's team also found out that Li-SWT promotes the re-endothelialization of the penile sinusoids and arteries and penile smooth muscle content [24]. These beneficial effects are possibly mediated by increased recruitment of mesenchymal stem cells (MSCs) that promote the regeneration of diabetes mellitus-damaged erectile tissues (Fig. 20.2). This group demonstrated upregulation of the expression of α-SMA, vWF, nNOS, and VEGF. They also demonstrated that the therapeutic effect might relate to the treatment dose positively

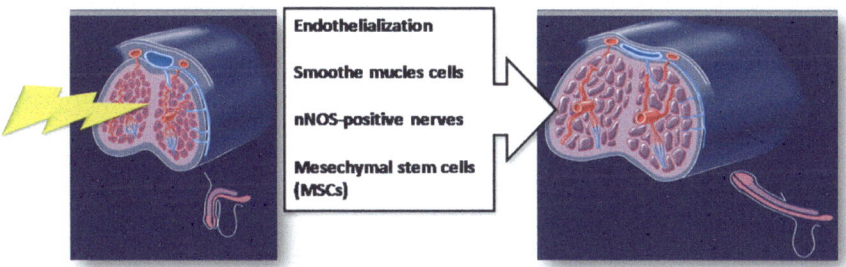

Fig. 20.2 Potential mechanisms for the effects of low-intensity shock wave therapy on erectile function in diabetic animal models. Low-intensity shock wave therapy could partially ameliorate diabetes mellitus-associated ED by promoting regeneration of smooth muscle, endothelium, and nNOS-positive nerves, and low-intensity shock wave therapy appeared to be able to recruit endogenous mesenchymal stem cells, which had beneficial effects for the repair of damaged tissue

1000 – Meta Analysis*

N=191 (TRT-155, PLC-36)

Median age = 59

ED duration 65.1 months

Diabetics – 61 patients (40%)

Change in the IIEF-ED domain scores before and after treatment: Comparison to Sham

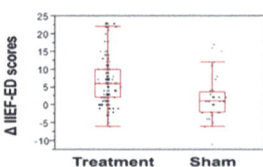

Treated (n=155) - Median score change 6, mean change 6.44
Placebo (n=36) – Median score change 1, mean change 1.77 (P< 0.0001)

	No response	Partial response	Good response	
Treated (%)	34.19	25.16	40.65	100% (n=155)
Placebo (%)	75.00	8.33	16.67	100% (n=36)

Fig. 20.3 Effect of low-intensity shock wave therapy on erectile function at 6 months follow-up

and the maximal therapeutic effect was achieved in Li-SWT of 300 shocks per treatment site and energy of 7.33 MPa [25]. After that, they decided to apply this animal model to human corpora cavernosum. The first double-blinded placebo control showed that 68 % of the patients went from Erection Hardness Score (EHS) 1 and 2 to EHS 3 and 4 involving patients responding to PDE5 Inhibitors. Another study demonstrated that the patients at baseline did not respond to PDE5 inhibitors but with the shock waves treatment, they regained their ability to respond to PDE5 inhibitors and to have sex life. It is possible that with further treatments, these patients will not require PDE5 inhibitors [25]. Also 6 months after the treatment, a significant number of patients maintain their good result [26, 27] (Fig. 20.3).

Conclusions

Regarded as a second-line treatment for ED, the main advantage of therapy with intracavernosal injections is that the erection achieved is predictable and occurs rapidly. Penile prosthesis implantation, the third-line treatment for ED, is one of the few successful surgical treatments for ED. Implantation of a penile prosthesis is usually the last resort for treatment of ED, when other modalities have failed or are not preferred by the patient. Low-intensity shock wave therapy is a noninvasive treatment for ED with significant results and with no side effects offering to the patient a more permanent solution.

References

1. Brindley GS (1983) Cavernosal alpha blockage: a new technique for investigating and treating impotence. Br J Psychiatry 143:332–337
2. Brindley GS (1986) Pilot experiments to drugs injected to the human corpus cavernosum penis. Br J Pharmacol 87:495–500

3. Brindley GS (1986) Maintenance treatment of erectile impotence by cavernosal unstriated muscle relaxant injection. Br J Psychiatry 149:210–215
4. Virag R (1982) Intracavernous injection of papaverine for erectile failure. Lancet 2:938
5. Porst H (1994) Ten years of experience with various vasoactive drugs – comparative studies in over 4000 patient. Int J Impot Res 6(Suppl 1):D149
6. Keogh EJ, Watters GR, Earle CM et al (1989) Treatment of impotence by intrapenile injections: a comparison study papaverine versus papaverine and phentolamine: a double blind crossover trial. J Urol 142:726–728
7. Liu LC, Wu CC, Liu LH et al (1991) Comparison of the effects of papaverine versus prostaglandin E1 on penile blood flow by color duplex sonography. Eur Urol 19:49–53
8. Padma-Nathan H, Goldstein I (1987) Intracavernosal pharmacotherapy the pharmacological erection program. World J Urol 5:160–165
9. Porst H (1993) Effektivitat und Haemodynamik von SIN-I versus prostagladine E1. Urologe A 32(Suppl):A9, Lecture XLV DGU Congress 1993, Wiesbaden
10. Ishii N, Watanabe H, Irisawa C et al (1986) Therapeutic trial with prostaglandin E1 for organic impotence In: Proceedings of the Fifth Conference on Vasculogenic Impotence and Corpus Cavernosum Revascularization. Second World Meeting on Impotence. Prague: ISSIR; 11:2
11. Buvat J, Lemaire A, Herbaut-Buvat M (1994) Comparison of the two second generation drugs for intracavernosal injection. Int J Impot Res 6(Suppl 1):P39
12. Sidi AA, Cameron JS, Duffy LM et al (1986) Intracavernous drug-induced erections in the management of male erectile dysfunction. J Urol 135:7004–7006
13. Stackl W, Hasun R, Marberger M (1988) Intracavernous injection of prostaglandin E1 in impotent men. J Urol 140:66–68
14. Buvat J (1990) Reduced rate of fibrotic nodules of the cavernous bodies following auto-intracavernous injections of moxisylyte compared to papaverine. Int J Impot Res 2(Suppl 2):299–300
15. Shabsigh R (1998) Penile prostheses toward the end of the millennium. J Urol 159:819
16. Anastasiadis AG, Wilson SK, Burchardt M et al (2001) Long-term outcomes of inflatable penile implants: reliability, patient satisfaction and complication management. Curr Opin Urol 11:619–623
17. Montague DK, Angermeier KW (2001) Penile prosthesis implantation. Urol Clin North Am 8(2):355–361
18. Wilson SK, Delk JR II (1995) Inflatable penile implant infection: predisposing factors and treatment suggestions. J Urol 153:659–661
19. Derouet H, Michael U, Freyfogle EB et al (2002) Successful conservative treatment of infected penile prostheses. Eur Urol 41:66–70
20. Wilson SK, Cleves MA, Delk JR II (1999) Comparison of mechanical reliability of original and enhanced Mentor Alpha I penile prosthesis. J Urol 162:715–718
21. Levine LA, Estrada CR, Morgentaler A (2001) Mechanical reliability and patient satisfaction with the Ambicor inflatable penile prosthesis: results of a 2 center study. J Urol 166:932–937
22. Vardi B, Appel A, Kilchevsky I et al (2012) Does low intensity extracorporeal shock wave therapy have a physiological effect on erectile function? Short-term results of a randomized, double-blind, sham controlled study. J Urol 187:1769–1775
23. Liu J, Zhou F, Li GY et al (2013) Evaluation of the effect of different doses of low energy shock wave therapy on the erectile function of streptozotocin (STZ)-induced diabetic rats. Int J Mol Sci 14:10661–10673
24. Qiu X, Lin G, Xin Z et al (2013) Effects of low-energy shockwave therapy on the erectile function and tissue of a diabetic rat model. J Sex Med 10(3):738–746
25. Gruenwald I, Appel B, Vardi Y (2012) Low-intensity extracorporeal shock wave therapy–a novel effective treatment for erectile dysfunction in severe ED patients who respond poorly to PDE5 inhibitor therapy. J Sex Med 9:259–264
26. Vardi Y, Appel B, Jacob G et al (2010) Can low-intensity extracorporeal shockwave therapy improve erectile function? A 6-month follow-up pilot study in patients with organic erectile dysfunction. Eur Urol 58(2):243–248
27. Vardi Y, Appel B, Gruenwald I (2012) The effect of low intensity shock waves on erectile dysfunction: 6-month follow up, ISSM, 2012

Cognitive Behavioral Therapy in Sexual Dysfunction

21

Penelope-Alexia Avagianou

21.1 Introduction

Sexual dysfunction is characterized by disturbances in sexual desire and in the psycho-physiological changes associated with the sexual response cycle in men and women [1]. Sexual dysfunction is highly prevalent in the general population and associated with psychological distress. It seems obvious that psychological factors play an important role in the etiology and maintenance of sexual problems. When we refer to psychological factors, we have to consider the impact of family origin, traumatic sexual experiences, religious and cultural beliefs, as well as personality characteristics. Sexual dysfunction is very common and seems to affect up to 46 % of the general population [2]. It is influenced by a variety of predisposing, precipitating, maintaining, and contextual factors [3]. Predisposing factors include constitutional and prior life experiences, precipitating factors trigger sexual problems, maintaining factors include psychological problems such as low self-esteem or guilt, and finally contextual factors encompass the present-day stresses [4]. Sexual dysfunction may impair the whole life of affected persons. The literature shows that women with sexual problems report lower quality of life and less satisfaction [5]. Moreover, a high risk of female sexual dysfunction is related to depressive symptoms [6].

Male sexual dysfunction (MSD) symptoms are highly prevalent and must be considered among the most frequently reported health complaints [7]. For all MSD's, the negative impact on quality of life and satisfaction with sexual life and their connection with psychosocial factors are documented in a number of studies [8].

P.-A. Avagianou
Pre-School Education Department, University of Thessaly,
Fillelinon & Argonafton, Volos 38221, Greece
e-mail: penavagia@yahoo.gr

Sexual dysfunction is more prevalent for women (43 %) than men (31 %) and is associated with various demographic characteristics, including age and educational attainment. Women of different racial groups demonstrate different patterns of sexual dysfunction. Differences among men are not as marked but generally consistent with women. Experience of sexual dysfunction is more likely among women and men with poor physical and emotional health. Moreover, sexual dysfunction is highly associated with negative experiences in sexual relationships and overall well-being [7].

21.2 Cognitive Behavioral Therapy

Cognitive behavior therapy (CBT) is a type of psychotherapeutic treatment that helps patients understand the thoughts and feelings that influence behaviors. CBT is commonly used to treat a wide range of disorders and is generally short term focusing on helping clients deal with a very specific problem. During the course of treatment, people learn how to identify and change destructive or disturbing thought patterns that have a negative influence on behavior. Cognitive behavioral therapy (CBT) refers to interventions that share the basic idea that mental disorders and psychological distress are maintained by cognitive factors. The core concept of this treatment approach, as pioneered by Beck [9], suggests that maladaptive cognitions contribute to the maintenance of emotional distress and behavioral problems. According to Beck's model, these maladaptive cognitions include general beliefs, or schemas, about the world, the self, and the future, giving rise to specific and automatic thoughts in particular situations. The basic model posits that therapeutic strategies to change these maladaptive cognitions lead to changes in emotional distress and problematic behaviors.

Consistent with the medical model of psychiatry, the overall goal of treatment is symptom reduction, improvement in functioning, and remission of the disorder. In order to achieve this goal, the patient becomes an active participant in a collaborative problem-solving process to test and challenge the validity of maladaptive cognitions and to modify maladaptive behavioral patterns [10].

21.3 The Idea of Cognitive Schemas in Sexual Functioning

By definition cognitive schemas are responsible for the way people interpret and give meaning to all sorts of different experiences. When a negative sexual event takes place, schemas generate negative thoughts (demand for performance, anticipation) and emotions (sadness, fear), interfering with sexual arousal. As a result of all the above, a negative cycle could be established maintaining an individual's poor sexual performance [11].

Few studies have explored the role of cognitive schemas on sexual functioning. The application of the schema concept to the domain of sexual dysfunctions has only recently begun to be noted. Cognitive schemas are ideas we have about ourselves, others, and the future that guide the way we give meaning to a particular event or situation. When the meaning is biased or inadequate, this may result in a dysfunctional emotional and behavior response. According to Alford and Beck [12], individuals may develop specific maladaptive schemas that can lead to the development of different psychopathologies. Beck [13] refers to two categories of negative schemas related to psychopathology: helpless schemas related to the idea that one is powerless or incompetent and unlovable schemas related to the idea of not being loved by others. In an attempt to connect this evidence with sexual dysfunction, it is interesting to refer to some clinical studies. Most studies suggest that men interpret sexual dysfunction as personal weakness and incompetence, better explained by the "helpless domain" [14]. On the contrary, for women most clinical evidence suggests that mainly social and interpersonal issues are involved in sexual dysfunctions, better explained by the "unlovability domain."

Clinical observation and theoretical models emphasize the importance of core cognitive structures (schemas or core beliefs) on sexual dysfunctional processes [15, 16]. Barlow has worked on the study of cognitive factors underlying sexual dysfunctional behaviors. Barlow's [17] cognitive-affective model postulated that the interaction between autonomic arousal (sympathetic activation) and cognitive interference plays a central role in determining sexually functional and dysfunctional responses. More recently, Sbrocco and Barlow [14] and Wiegel et al. [18] further developed the original model, indicating that schematic vulnerability is one of the main components implicated in sexual dysfunction. They suggested that the schema concept consists of ideas people have about sexuality and themselves as sexual beings and includes a set of standards and expectations regarding sexual issues. They assumed that individuals with sexual dysfunction have a set of sexual beliefs that are most of the times unrealistic and inflexible. Usually, these beliefs facilitate the development of negative self-schemas and may contribute to the development or maintenance of sexual difficulties.

Studies about male and female versions of sexual self-schema [19, 20] have shown that women with negative sexual self-schemas present lower affective involvement with partner, higher avoidance of intimacy, and higher anxiety levels of being unloved or abandoned. Furthermore, these studies have shown that [19, 20] both men and women with negative sexual self-schemas report lower frequency of sexual activity and fewer sexual partners. Studies concerning the influence of sexual self-schemas on sexual functioning have produced mixed results. In particular Andersen and Cyranowski [21] indicate that women with negative sexual self-schemas report less interest in sexual activity and less frequency of sexual thoughts. Studies with men indicate that negative sexual self-schemas correlate with lower arousability levels [20]. Moreover, Cyranowski [21] noted that low interest for sex in women with negative sexual self-schemas does not mean that there is a sexual desire disorder. It therefore seems that the ability of the concept of sexual self-schema to predict sexual dysfunction has not received conclusive empirical support.

21.4 Biopsychosocial Model: Integrated Treatment

The advancement of sexual medicine, as suggested by Berry and Berry [22], embodied particularly in the revolutionary advances of pharmacotherapy. However, pharmacotherapy as a stand-alone treatment option has been criticized as incomplete. It is widely argued that drug treatment alone often does not meet the standards of biopsychosocial therapy. This model of treatment appears to have an obvious meaning (treatment of three facets of the patients' biological, psychological, and social condition). However, research suggests that clear treatment algorithms are still in development [22].

The term integrated is referred to the combination of psychological and medical interventions. Often medical treatments are directed at specific sexual dysfunctions and fail to address the psychological issues. Although medical treatments usually work, most of the individuals fail to continue treatment. Research suggests that this is a result of clinicians failing to address the relevant psychological and interpersonal issues [23].

A meta-analysis study by Fruhauf and his colleagues [1] found evidence that psychological interventions are effective in improving both symptom severity and sexual satisfaction in patients with certain types of sexual dysfunction. The lack of treatment efficacy studies for particular types of sexual dysfunction and pronounced use of particular intervention strategies have been reported in a number of review studies [24, 25]. In Frauhauf's study [1], the evidence for the efficacy of psychological interventions differed across the target sexual dysfunctions. Significant effects on symptom severity were found for patients with female hypoactive sexual desire disorder (FHSDD) and female orgasmic disorder (FOD). Frauhauf's study also showed that well-established psychological interventions exist for FHSDD.

21.5 Cognitive Behavioral Therapy for Sexual Dysfunctions

One of the most promising methods of treatment and one that has received some empirical support is cognitive behavioral therapy (CBT). CBT for impaired sexual desire, arousal, and orgasm is generally aimed at influencing maintaining factors [26]. CBT in sexual dysfunctions is based upon Masters and Johnson [27] work and Barlow's model of sexual dysfunction [17]. Both models focus on the importance of attention in facilitating or hampering levels of sexual arousal. The goals of CBT for female sexual dysfunction are to help the individual refocus her attention on pleasurable sexual stimuli and to reduce levels of anxiety surrounding sexual activity through a combination of sensate focus exercises, exposure work, and cognitive restructuring [28].

Considering the fact that hypoactive sexual desire disorder (HSDD) is the most prevalent female sexual complaint [4], it is of great interest to see the results of CBT in this particular disorder. The efficacy of CBT for women with HSDD has been reported in a number of studies. In particular, McCabe [4] found that women who followed ten sessions of CBT (focusing on communication between partners, increasing sexual skills, and reducing anxiety) reported improvement (44 %). In another study conducted by Trudel et al. [29], it was reported that only 26 % of low desire women continued to report problems after undergoing CBT. Moreover, compared to the control group, CBT resulted in a significant improvement in the quality of sexual and marital life, sexual satisfaction, perception of sexual arousal, and sexual self-esteem. Hurlbert et al. [30] found that at 6-month follow-up women who participated in CBT group therapy sessions with their partner reported higher degree of sexual desire compared with women who participated alone.

As far as orgasmic disorders in women are concerned, Gunzler and Berner [31] suggest that behavioral approaches and sex therapy seem to have at least a short-term efficacy. CBT (especially dilator exercises) was also found to be somewhat effective in women with vaginismus in some studies [32]. Cognitive behavioral couple therapy seems to improve the sexual function of women but not men. In particular it seems to be effective in vaginismus but not indicated in dyspareunia [33].

As already mentioned above, studies concerning cognitive schemas suggest that specific faulty cognitive constructions underlying sexual dysfunctions and encourage the development of models and treatment approaches based on cognitive therapy [11]. Studies suggest that men with sexual problems attribute negative sexual events to a personal incompetence, interpreting those situations as a sign of personal failure, along with beliefs of being different, powerless, and weak [34]. Moreover, Quinta Gomes and Nobre [35] refer that differences between men with and without sexual dysfunction were observed for difference, helpless, and incompetence schemas, and the highest level of schema activation in the clinical group was observed for the incompetence domain. These findings have some clinical implications for the assessment and treatment of sexual dysfunction. As Quinta Gomes and Nobre [35] suggest, the evaluation of individual's core beliefs should be integrated into assessment protocols in sex therapy. Furthermore, individuals with sexual difficulties would benefit from cognitive techniques focused on restructuring maladaptive beliefs and behavior patterns involved in the maintenance of sexual problems.

21.6 Conclusions and Recommendations

Advances in medical and psychological therapies for sexual dysfunctions must take into account the biopsychosocial influences of the patient, the partner, and the couple. Research on this field is extremely limited and mainly based upon female sexual dysfunctions. One can say that psychological interventions can be recommended as effective treatment options for particular types of sexual dysfunction since they have been shown to improve both symptom severity and sexual satisfaction. When assessing the outcome of treatment for sexual dysfunctions, researchers often focus on sexual functioning only or combine measures of sexual functioning, sexual satisfaction, and sexual distress into a single outcome. Failing to identify and analyze these distinct outcomes may affect important findings.

In summary, findings suggest that cognitive schemas associated with sexual events are closely related to sexual dysfunctions emphasizing the need for evaluating cognitive structures and including cognitive therapy approaches. It would be of great interest—since early maladaptive schemas are created during the first years of our lives—to research upon the factors that influence our cognitive schemas that are related to sexuality in general. Especially the family role and parental bonding might act as a predisposing or as a preventing factor towards sexual dysfunctions. However, there is a need for further psychotherapy research into these conditions. Research on future psychological interventions might address a systemic perspective beside disorder specificity.

References

1. Fruhauf S, Gerger H, Schmidt HM, Munden T, Barth J (2013) Efficacy of psychological interventions for sexual dysfunction: a systematic review and meta-analysis. Arch Sex Behav 42:915–933
2. Simons JS, Carey MP (2001) Prevalence of sexual dysfunctions: results from a decade of research. Arch Sex Behav 30:177–219
3. Hawton K, Catalan J (1986) Prognostic factors in sex therapy. Behav Res Ther 24:377–385
4. McCabe M, Althof SE, Assalian P, Chevret-Measson M, Leiblum SR, Simonelli C, Wylie K (2010) Psychological and interpersonal dimensions of sexual function and dysfunction. J Sex Med 7:327–336
5. Christensen BS, Gronbaek M, Osler M, Pedersen BV, Graugaard C, Frisch M (2011) Associations between physical and mental health problems and sexual dysfunctions in sexually active Danes. J Sex Med 8(1890):902
6. Shindel AW, Eisenberg ML, Breyer BN, Sharlip ID, Smith JF (2011) Sexual function and depressive symptoms among female North American medical students. J Sex Med 28:391–399
7. Lauman EO, Paik A, Rosen RC (1999) Sexual dysfunctions in the United States. Prevalence and predictors. JAMA 281:537–544
8. Latini DM, Penson DF, Allace KL, Lubeck DP, Lue TF (2006) Clinical and psychosocial characteristics of men with erectile dysfunction: baseline data from ExCEED. J Sex Med 3:1059–1067
9. Beck AT (1970) Cognitive therapy: nature and relation to behavior therapy. Behav Ther 1:184–200
10. Hofmann SG, Asnaani A, Vonk IJ, Sawyer AT, Fang A (2012) The efficacy of cognitive behavioral therapy: a review of meta-analyses. Cogn Ther Res 13:12–2
11. Nobre PJ (2010) Psychological determinants of erectile dysfunction: testing a cognitive emotional model. J Sex Med 7:1429–1437
12. Alford BA, Beck AT (1997) The integrative power of cognitive therapy. Guilford Press, New York
13. Beck AT (1996) Beyond belief: a theory of modes, personality and psychopathology. In: Salkovskis PM (ed) Frontiers of cognitive therapy. Guilford Press, New York, pp 1–25
14. Sbrocco T, Barlow DH (1996) Conceptualizing the cognitive component of sexual arousal: implications for sexuality research and treatment. In: Salkovskis PM (ed) Frontiers of cognitive therapy. Guilford Press, New York, pp 419–449
15. Carey MP, Wincze JP, Meisler AW (1993) Sexual dysfunction: male erectile disorder. In: Barlow DH (ed) Clinical handbook of psychological disorders: a step by step treatment manual. Guilford Press, New York, pp 442–480
16. Rosen RC, Leiblum SR, Spector I (1994) Psychologically based treatment for male erectile disorder: a cognitive-interpersonal model. J Sex Marital Ther 20:67–85
17. Barlow DH (1986) Causes of sexual dysfunction: the role of anxiety and cognitive interference. J Consult Clin Psychol 54:140–148

18. Wiegel M, Scepkowski L, Barlow D (2007) Cognitive-affective processes in sexual arousal and sexual dysfunction. In: Janssen E (ed) The psychophysiology of sex. Indiana University Press, Bloomington, pp 143–165
19. Andersen BL, Cyranowski JM (1994) Women's sexual self schema. J Pers Soc Psychol 67:1079–1100
20. Andersen BL, Cyranowski JM, Espindle D (1999) Men's sexual self-schema. J Pers Soc Psychol 76:645–661
21. Cyranowski JM, Aarestad SL, Andersen BL (1999) The role of sexual-schema in a diathesis-stress model of sexual dysfunction. Appl Prev Psychol 8:217–228
22. Berry MD, Berry PD (2013) Contemporary treatment of sexual dysfunction: reexamining the biopsychocosial model. J Sex Med 10:2627–2643
23. Althof S (2002) When an erection alone is not enough: biopsychosocial obstacles to lovemaking. Int J Impot Res 14:99–104
24. McGuire H, Hawton K (2003) Interventions for vaginismus. Cochrane Database Syst Rev (1):CD001760
25. O'Donohue WT, Swingen DN, Dopke CA, Regev LG (1999) Psychotherapy for male sexual dysfunction: a review. Clin Psychol Rev 19:591–630
26. Stephenson KR, Rellini AH, Meston CM (2013) Relationship satisfaction as a predictor of treatment response during cognitive behavioral sex therapy. Arch Sex Behav 42:143–152
27. Masters WH, Johnson VE (1970) Human sexual inadequacy. Bantam Books, New York
28. Stinson RD (2009) The behavioral and cognitive-behavioral treatment of female sexual dysfunction: how far we have come and the path left to go. Sex Relationsh Ther 24:271–285
29. Trudel G, Laurin F (1988) The effects of bibliotherapy on orgasmic dysfunction and couple interactions: an experimental study. Sex Marital Ther 3:223–228
30. Hurlbert D, White L, Powell R, Apt C (1993) Orgasm consistency training in the treatment of women reporting hypoactive sexual desire: an outcome comparison of women-only groups and couples-only groups. J Behav Ther Exp Psychiatry 24:3–13
31. Gunzler C, Berner MM (2012) Efficacy of psychosocial interventions in men and women with sexual dysfunctions. A systematic review of controlled clinical trials. J Sex Med 9:3108–3125
32. van Lankveld JJ, Everaerd W, Grotjohann Y (2001) Cognitive behavioral bibliotherapy for sexual dysfunctions in hetero- sexual couples: a randomized waiting list controlled clinical trials in the Netherlands. J Sex Res 45:359–373
33. LoPiccolo J, Heiman JR, Hogan DR, Roberts CW (1985) Effectiveness of single therapists versus cotherapy teams in sex therapy. J Consult Clin Psychol 53:287–294
34. Nobre PJ, Pinto-Gouveia J (2009) Cognitive schemas associated with negative sexual events: a comparison of men and women with and without sexual dysfunction. Arch Sex Behav 38:842–851
35. Quinta Gomes AL, Nobre P (2012) Early maladaptive schemas and sexual dysfunction in men. Arch Sex Behav 41:311–320

Basic Principles of the Princeton Recommendations

22

Patrick S. Whelan and Ajay Nehra

22.1 Introduction

The Princeton Consensus Conference, an international, multidisciplinary collaboration, designed to optimize the treatment of sexual dysfunction while preserving cardiovascular health, released their most recent recommendations in 2012. Initially convened in 1999 for the management of sexual dysfunction in men and women with known CVD, the Conference assigned risk stratification to low- and high-risk patients based on existing CVD [1]. Low-risk patients could resume sexual activity with recommended treatment. Those in the high-risk group were recommended to stop sexual activity until proper treatment of CVD was initiated and disease stabilized.

New recommendations were released in 2005 from the second Conference with the inclusion of risk factor evaluations and lifestyle management in men with ED [2]. Additionally, recommendations of appropriate phosphodiesterase type 5 (PDE5) inhibitors in men with ED and CVD were first included [2].

The 2012 recommendations updated the 2005 recommendations for cardiovascular risk with sexual activity in men with known CVD and included predictive value of vasculogenic ED by assigning risk to men of all ages [3]. The main objective developed an approach to cardiovascular evaluation in men with ED, but no

P.S. Whelan
Department of Urology, Rush Medical College, Rush University Medical Center,
600 S Paulina St., Chicago, IL 60612, USA
e-mail: patrick_s_whelan@rush.edu

A. Nehra (✉)
Department of Urology, Rush University Medical Center,
1725 W Harrison St Suite 762, Chicago, IL 60612, USA
e-mail: Ajay_Nehra@rush.edu

known CVD [3]. Additionally, testosterone's role in erectile function and cardiovascular health were first included in the recommendations. A thorough review of the epidemiology and physiology of ED, CVD, hypogonadism, the use of testosterone, and emerging risk factors based on current scientific evidence led to the most recent recommendations from the third Princeton Consensus Conference [3].

22.2 Evaluation and Management of CV Risk in Patients with ED and No Known CVD

Cardiovascular risk is defined as the risk of morbid events over a 3- to 5-year interval from the onset of ED [4, 5]. The Panel broadened the current 2010 American College of Cardiology Foundation/American Heart Association (ACCF/AHA) guidelines [6] for the assessment of cardiovascular risk to include cardiovascular risk assessment in asymptomatic men with ED.

ED should be used as an opportunity to evaluate CVD risk reduction [7]. This recommendation is based on studies that show that ED provides significant predictive value for cardiovascular events on par with traditional risk factors (such as family history of myocardial infarction (MI), smoking, and hyperlipidemia) [8, 9]. Additionally, ED is predictive of silent coronary artery disease (CAD) [3, 10–12] with a 2–5-year time window (class Ia) [4, 5, 13] before the onset of symptomatic CAD. ED shares several risk factors with CVD [14, 15] and evidence (class Ia) shows that it is an independent marker of increased CVD risk [16–22], CAD, peripheral arterial disease (PAD), stroke, and all-cause mortality [3, 23, 24]. When added to the Framingham Risk Score (FRS), 6.4 % of patients were reassigned from low risk to intermediate risk, nearly doubling their cardiovascular event probability [16]. Furthermore, ED appears to be more predictive of CAD in men aged 40–49 as shown in the Olmsted County Study [25]. Epidemiologic data from Western Australia suggests that atherosclerotic cardiovascular events are seven times more likely in men <40 years old with ED [26]. Therefore, ED may be particularly beneficial in assessing cardiovascular risk in younger patients and minorities whose cardiovascular risk may be underestimated by the FRS [27, 28].

Additionally, degree of ED severity must be assessed [3]. More severe ED has been associated with greater risk of cardiovascular events [29], CAD [24, 30], extent of CAD [11, 13, 31], and risk of PAD [23] (ACCF/AHA class Ia). This has been further supported in a recent meta-analysis of 36,744 men as displayed in Table 22.1 [22]. ED was shown to be an independent marker of cardiovascular

Table 22.1 Relative cardiovascular risks for men with ED [22]

	Relative risk	95 % Confidence interval	P value
Overall	1.48	1.25–1.74	<0.001
CAD	1.46	1.31–1.63	<0.001
Stroke	1.35	1.19–1.54	<0.001
All-cause mortality	1.19	1.05–1.34	0.005

events and all-cause mortality in addition to conventional risk factors (i.e., age, weight, hypertension, diabetes (DM), hyperlipidemia, and smoking).

The FRS is a very useful tool to estimate the 10-year cardiac event risk in patients and is supported by the 2010 ACCF/AHA guideline [6] for assessment of cardiovascular risk in asymptomatic adults (ACCF/AHA class I, LOE B) by incorporating age, sex, total cholesterol, high-density lipoprotein (HDL), and use of antihypertensive medications to stratify CVD risk [32]. However, there is little data in patients less than 40 years old suggesting that FRS does not appropriately assess risk in younger patients, especially those with ED. It also lacks family history, fasting glucose level, serum creatinine, urinary albumin to creatinine ratio, and potentially, testosterone level that should be considered to estimate cardiovascular risk in men with ED. The Consensus continues to recommend the FRS as a useful starting tool to estimate subclinical atherosclerosis in men with ED [3]. However, it cautions the use of the FRS alone in men with ED aged 30–60 years without further investigation to other CVD risk factors [3]. ED should alert the physician to increased CVD risk.

The Consensus recommends risk assessments to all men who present with ED regardless of other symptoms [3]. A man with organic ED is considered at increased CVD risk until further workup suggests otherwise. ED can help to identify increased CVD risk in patients both with and without CVD symptoms or event history. The Panel recommends the risk assessments outlined in Table 22.2 [3], consistent with the 2010 ACCF/AHA guidelines [6], to identify men who may need further CVD workup. Therefore, a complete, noninvasive workup, managed by the primary care physician or cardiologist, is recommended, with invasive workup if necessary [33–36]. However, initial evaluation with more specialized tests may be warranted if symptoms suggest increased CVD risk [3].

Given the significant evidence that ED is predictive of future CVD, the Panel recommends that lifestyle modifications will not only improve cardiovascular health but also improve erectile function as shown in Table 22.3 [3, 38].

Several of the recommendations are aimed at preventing progression and even helping to reverse atherosclerotic and other CVD [3]. DM is associated with a twofold increase in CVD [45] and is a CAD equivalent. A recent study of 4,883 men and women 65 years and older followed for 10 years suggested that 90 % of new cases of DM were preventable if patients were in the low-risk group five lifestyle factors shown in Table 22.4 [46].

Waist circumference and waist to hip ratio are better predictors of cardiovascular outcomes than BMI [47, 48]. This is thought to be due to the secretion of excess free fatty acid, inflammatory cytokines, and reduced secretion of adiponectin from abdominal fat [49]. Chronic kidney disease also conveys significant cardiovascular morbidity and mortality. eGFR <60 ml/min and urinary albumin to creatinine ratios greater than 10 mg/g are associated with increased cardiovascular mortality independent of other traditional risk factors [50, 51].

Testosterone measurement has recently become controversial in men without symptoms of low testosterone. Testosterone plays important functions centrally and peripherally in erectile function in animal models [52–55]. This data has been consistent with clinical data. A single-center study of 1,050 men with new evaluation

Table 22.2 Recommendations for assessment of CVD in men with ED and no known CVD

Patient history	History, age, comorbid conditions (i.e., obesity, hypertension, dyslipidemia, prediabetes, OSA)
	Family history of premature atherothrombotic CVD (father aged <55 years or mother aged <65 years at cardiovascular event; ACCF/AHA class I, LOE B)
	Lifestyle factors (i.e., diet, alcohol use, sedentary lifestyle, and smoking)
Physical exam	BP, waist circumference (WC), body mass index (BMI)
	Cardiac auscultation, carotid bruits, and palpation of femoral and pedal pulses
	Fundal arterial changes
	ED severity (using the International Index of Erectile Function score or Sexual Health Inventory of Men) and duration
Laboratory testing	Fasting plasma glucose level
	Serum creatinine level (estimated glomerular filtration rate (eGFR))
	Albumin to creatinine ratio
	Total testosterone (TT) level before 11 AM
	Plasma lipid levels including total, low-density lipoprotein (LDL), and high-density lipoprotein cholesterol and triglyceride levels
	High-sensitivity C-reactive protein (hsCRP) (ACCF/AHA class IIb, LOE B in asymptomatic, intermediate-risk men ≤50 years) [6]
	Glycated hemoglobin (ACCF/AHA class IIb, LOE B in asymptomatic adults without diagnosis of DM) [6]
	Urinary albumin excretion (ACCF/AHA class IIa, LOE B in asymptomatic adults with hypertension or DM; ACCF/AHA class IIb, LOE B in asymptomatic, intermediate-risk adults without hypertension or DM) [6]
	Serum uric acid and lipoprotein-associated phospholipase A2 (ACCF/AHA class IIb, LOE B in asymptomatic, intermediate-risk adults) [6]
Invasive radiographic testing	Exercise stress testing (EST) (ACCF/AHA class IIb, LOE B in asymptomatic, intermediate-risk adults when nonelectrocardiogram markers are considered rather than ST-wave changes) [6, 37]
	Resting electrocardiogram (ACCF/AHA class IIa, LOE C in asymptomatic adults with hypertension or DM and ACCF/AHA class IIb, LOE C in asymptomatic adults without hypertension or DM)
	Carotid intima-media thickness (CIMT) (ACCF/AHA class IIa, LOE B in asymptomatic, intermediate-risk adults)
	Computed tomography for coronary artery calcium scoring (CACS) (ACCF/AHA class IIa, LOE B in asymptomatic, intermediate-risk men ≥40 years; ACCF/AHA class IIb, LOE B in low to intermediate risk [6–10 % 10-year risk] in men ≥40 years)
	Ankle-brachial index (ABI) (ACCF/AHA class IIa, LOE B in asymptomatic, intermediate-risk adults)
	CCTA (ACCF/AHA class III, LOE C in asymptomatic patients)
	Pulse wave velocity (PWV) (ACCF/AHA class III, LOE C in asymptomatic patients)
	Noninvasive assessment of endothelial function (i.e., brachial artery flow-mediated dilation) (ACCF/AHA class III, LOE B in asymptomatic adults)

Table 22.3 Lifestyle modifications shown to improve cardiovascular health

Modification	Clinical benefit
Smoking cessation	36 % decrease in mortality in CAD in a meta-analysis of prospective cohort studies [39]
Regular dynamic exercise	Reduced incidence of DM II and CAD by 30–50 % in physically active compared to sedentary patients [40–43]
Weight loss, dietary changes, and moderate alcohol consumption	Improved diet was shown to reduce CAD mortality by 36 % [44]

Table 22.4 Low-risk lifestyle factors linked to preventing DM [46]

Physical activity	Leisure-time activity
	Walking pace above the median
Diet	High-fiber intake
	High polyunsaturated to saturated fat ratio
	Low trans-fat intake and low mean glycemic index
Smoking	Never smoker
	Former smoker more than 20 years ago or for fewer than 5 pack-years,
Alcohol use	Predominately light or moderate
BMI and WC	BMI <25
	WC <88 cm and <92 cm for women and men, respectively

for sexual dysfunction found that 36 % had hypogonadism [56]. A meta-analysis of 7,000 men with ED in nine studies reported serum testosterone levels <300 ng/dL in 12 %. Hypogonadism is a potential cause of ED [57, 58], and testosterone replacement therapy (TRT) has been shown to improve response [58]. Recently, several large epidemiologic studies have associated low testosterone levels with increased all-cause and cardiovascular mortality shown in Table 22.5 [59–67]. However, caution should be advised, as there is no defined lower limit of normal TT.

Additionally, a 2010 meta-analysis of cohort studies in middle-aged men showed no association between endogenous TT levels and CVD risk in middle-aged men [68]. A more recent meta-analysis of 49 cross-sectional studies showed increased CVD in low TT levels and high estradiol levels [69]. However, a separate meta-analysis of 19 studies showed that low TT does not correlate with CVD in healthy men <70 years [68]. The same study, did however, show that low testosterone predicts increased risk for CVD and mortality in elderly men [68]. Nonetheless, the authors cautioned that low TT may be a marker of poor health, rather than testosterone being protective of CVD. This idea is consistent with studies that androgen deficiency is associated with insulin resistance, DM II, metabolic syndrome, and increased deposition of visceral fat [70–73]. The TIMES2 (Testosterone Replacement in Hypogonadal Men With Either Metabolic Syndrome or Type 2 DM) study, a randomized, placebo-controlled study of 6–12 months of transdermal TRT vs. placebo in hypogonadal men with DM II, resulted in improved insulin resistance and glycemic control (ACCF/AHA class Ib) [74]. Additionally, a meta-analysis of five other randomized controlled trials with

Table 22.5 Low testosterone levels and increased mortality rates in recent publications with populations greater than 500 men

Reference	HR (95 % CI)	Study design	Men (no.)	Avg follow-up (year)	Mortality
Shores et al. [59]	1.88 (1.34–2.63)	Retrospective	858	8.0	All-cause
Laughlin et al. [60]	1.40 (1.14–1.71)	Prospective	794	20.0	All-cause
	1.38 (1.02–1.85)				CVD
Khaw et al. [61]	2.29 (1.60–3.26)	Prospective	2,314 of 11,606	10.0	All-cause and CVD
Haring et al. [62]	2.32 (1.38–3.89)	Prospective	1,954	7.2	All-cause
	2.56 (1.15–6.52)				CVD
Malkin et al. [63]	2.27 (1.45–3.60)	Prospective	930	6.9	All-cause in men with CAD
Tivesten et al. [64]	1.65 (1.29–2.12)	Prospective	3,014	4.5	All-cause
Menke et al. [65]	1.43 (1.09–1.87)	Prospective	1,114	9.0	All-cause
Vikan et al. [66]	1.24 (1.01–1.54)	Prospective	1,568	11.2	All-cause
Corona et al. [67]	7.1 (1.8–28.6)	Prospective	1,687	4.3	CVD

mean follow-up of 58 weeks showed TRT to be associated with a significant reduction in glucose homeostasis model assessment of insulin resistance index, triglycerides, and WC and an increase in HDL levels [75]. Nonetheless, randomized controlled trials for TRT risks and benefits are needed to establish CVD risk and mortality.

The American College of Physicians recommends only testing for testosterone levels in men with ED when accompanied by the presence of other symptoms (decreased libido, decreased spontaneous erection) or other physical exam findings (testicular mass or muscle atrophy) [76]. Conversely, the Consensus recommends CVD risk and testosterone levels be measured in all men diagnosed with organic ED [3], especially for those who have failed PDE5 inhibitor therapy [6], consistent with British Society for Sexual Medicine [77], International Society for Sexual Medicine [78], Endocrine Society [79], and a combined proposal from the International Society of Andrology, International Society for the Study of the Aging Male, European Association of Urology European Academy of Andrology, and the American Society of Andrology [80] as outlined in Fig. 22.1 [81].

High sensitivity C reactive protein (hsCRP) is an independent predictor of coronary events after adjustment of traditional risk factors [6, 82–84] (i.e., age, total cholesterol, HDL, smoking, BMI, DM, hypertension, exercise level, and family history of CAD). Consequently, the Centers for Disease Control and Prevention and AHA recommended measurement of the hsCRP in addition to global risk prediction, especially those with intermediate risk [85]. The hsCRP level was also shown to improve the predictive value of the FRS in high-risk patients for CAD [86]. Similar evidence was also noted in a meta-analysis of 54 long-term prospective studies without history of vascular disease where high CRP was associated with increased risk of CAD, cerebrovascular disease, vascular mortality, and nonvascular mortality

```
┌─────────────────────────────────────────────┐
│   History & TT measurement in men with ED   │
└─────────────────────────────────────────────┘
   ┌──────────────────────────────────────────┐
   │ >350nd/dL                                │
 ──┤ • No supplementation                     │
   └──────────────────────────────────────────┘
   ┌──────────────────────────────────────────┐
   │ 230-350ng/dL                             │
 ──┤ • Four-six month trial of TRT with goal  │
   │   350-600ng/dL. Continue TRT if clinical │
   │   benefit after 6 months [81]            │
   └──────────────────────────────────────────┘
   ┌──────────────────────────────────────────┐
   │ <230ng/dL                                │
 ──┤ • Testosterone replacement therapy       │
   └──────────────────────────────────────────┘
```

Fig. 22.1 TRT algorithm in men with ED. Use caution in those with congestive heart failure due to fluid retention. Men >70 years and those with multiple comorbidities should be treated with easily titratable TRT such as gel, spray, or patch for rapid removal should adverse effects develop. Baseline prostate-specific antigen and hematocrit testing required every 6 months

[87]. Additionally, there is evidence that hsCRP correctly reclassifies patients from intermediate-risk CVD to low or high risk [88].

Serum uric acid levels in asymptomatic patients are not specifically addressed in the 2010 ACCF/AHA guidelines [6]; however, the Consensus recommends serum uric acid measurement due to recent evidence that increased levels are predictive of increased cardiovascular risk [89].

A recent analysis from the Atherosclerosis Risk in Communities Study found that the addition of glycated hemoglobin to prediction models with traditional risk factors improved CAD risk prediction in nondiabetic patients with no previous history of CVD [90]. A meta-analysis of 26 cohort studies showed that microalbuminuria was associated with a 50 % increased risk of CAD. Macroalbuminuria more than doubled CAD risk [91]. However, overall there is inconsistency regarding adding glycated hemoglobin and urinary albumin to traditional risk factors in reassessing CVD risk.

Lipoprotein-associated phospholipase A2 levels were shown to be independent predictors of CVD in healthy adults after adjustment for hsCRP and standard risk factors [92–95]. Measurement of lipoprotein-associated phospholipase A2 is consistent with the 2010 ACCF/AHA guidelines for intermediate-risk adults [6].

EST may prove particularly beneficial to evaluate silent CAD risk in patients with ED and DM. In patients with DM II, 33.8 % of men with silent CAD had ED, while only 4.7 % of men had ED without silent CAD [10]. Chemical stress testing (with dipyrimadole or adenosine with nuclear imaging) is appropriate for patients who cannot undergo EST due to disabling condition [3]. If the baseline EKG makes EST unequivocal, the Panel recommends referral to a cardiologist [3].

The 2010 ACCF/AHA guidelines state that it is reasonable to perform CIMT, CACS, and ABI during CVD assessment of intermediate-risk patients [6]. This was further supported by the Society for Heart Attack Prevention and Eradication task force that stated all asymptomatic men 45–75 years and women 55–75 years who do not have very-low-risk characteristics or a documented history of CVD be evaluated with CACS or CIMT for subclinical CAD [96]. Analysis from the Atherosclerosis Risk in Communities Study, CIMT, and plaque detection with ultrasound added to traditional risk factors improved CAD detection [97]. The Multi-Ethnic Study of Atherosclerosis showed that CACS has better predictive value of CVD than CIMT [98]. A meta-analysis of 16 population-based cohort studies showed that ABI ≤ 0.90 was associated with twice the 10-year overall mortality, cardiovascular mortality, and cardiovascular events than each FRS category [99]. Recent meta-analysis of 17 longitudinal studies with 7.7-year average follow-up found that patients with high aortic PWV were also at higher risk for overall mortality, cardiovascular mortality, and cardiovascular events [100].

Although endothelial dysfunction has yet to be thoroughly studied in men with ED, endothelial dysfunction was found to be an independent predictor of cardiac death, MI, revascularization, or cardiac hospitalization in symptomatic outpatients over 7-year follow-up [101]. Additionally, brachial artery endothelial function assessed by flow-mediated dilation [102, 103] or in the forearm microvasculature assessed by Doppler flow [104] predicted poor cardiovascular outcome independent of the FRS.

22.3 Management of ED in the Patient with Known CVD

Previous recommendations from the prior two Princeton Consensus Conferences stratified patients into low-, intermediate-, and high-risk categories, where risk is defined as the likelihood of morbidity and mortality while engaged in or shortly after sexual activity [1, 2]. A number of groups were stratified into different groups in the most recent Conference. Patients with New York Heart Association (NYHA) class II CHF are low risk rather than intermediate risk, NYHA class III CHF are intermediate risk rather than high risk, and patients with mild, stable angina, and those with past MI (>6–8 weeks) are intermediate risk rather than low risk.

As discussed previously, a sexual inquiry into all men with ED should be undertaken to identify potential cardiovascular risk factors and incorporate lifestyle and therapeutic interventions as needed [3]. Exercise tolerance should be evaluated in all patients with ED [105]. A recent meta-analysis of ten studies showed that episodic activity was associated with an increased risk of MI and sudden cardiac death (SCD). However, this effect was attenuated in those with high habitual levels of activity. For every hour per week exposed in physical activity, the relative risk for MI and SCD was decreased by 45 % and 30 %, respectively [106]. This may aid in physicians to estimate cardiovascular risk associated with sexual activity in patients. Patients are placed in appropriate groups for treatment based on symptoms and recent cardiovascular events with appropriate treatment regimens outlined in Fig. 22.2 [3].

Exercise ability: equivalent to walking 1 mile on a flat surface in 20 minutes or briskly climbing 2 flights of stairs in 10 seconds

Low-risk: moderate exercise without symptoms
- Asymptomatic & <3 CAD risk factors (excluding gender)
- Succesful revascularization via coronary artery bypass grafting (CABG), stenting or angioplasty
- Asymptomatic, controlled hypertension
- Mild valvular disease
- Left ventricular dysfunction/NYHA class I & II CHF who achieve 5 metabolic equivalents of the task (Mets) without ischemia
- **Low risk patients can resume or initiate sexual activity with ED treatment without further testing or evaluation.**

Intermediate-risk: require evaluation using EST to determine appropriate risk stratification (low- or high-risk) before resuming sexual activity. Chemical stress tests (i.e. dipyrimadole or adenosine with nuclear imaging) is sufficient in those who cannot complete exercise tests due to debilitating physical factors.
- Asymptomatic & ≥ 3 CAD risk factors (excluding gender)
- Mild to moderate stable angina
- Past MI (2-8 weeks) without intervention awaiting EST
- CHF NYHA class III
- Noncardiac manifestations of atherosclerotic disease (PAD, history of stroke or TIA)
- **The ability to complete 4 minutes of the standard Bruce treadmill protocol (5-6 Mets) without symptoms, arrhythmias or a fall in systolic BP is sufficient evidence to resume sexual activity [1,2,7]. Failure is equivalent to hish-risk patients.**

High-risk: cardiac conditions severe enough to pose significant risk for a cardiovascular event during sexual activity. Typically these patients are moderately to severely symptomatic.
- Unstable or refractory angina
- Uncontrolled hypertension
- CHF NYHA class IV
- Recent MI without intervention (<2 weeks)
- High-risk arrhythmia (exercise-induced ventricular tachycardia, implanted automatic internal cardioverter defibrillator (AICD) with frequent shocks and poorly controlled atrial fibrillation),
- Obstructive hypertrophic cardiomyopathy with severe symptoms
- Moderate to severe valve disease.
- **High-risk patients should defer all sexual activity until their cardiac condition is stabilized. Require referralto a cardiologist for evaluation and collaborative management. Follow up and further reassessment of CVD is recommended.**

Fig. 22.2 Management of men with ED and known CVD

Interventions for the management of ED should not compromise cardiovascular function. The second Princeton Recommendations highlighted the pharmacologic treatment of ED [2]. PDE5 inhibitors have been safely shown to improve ED as the first-line treatment without new significant cardiovascular events in recent analysis of placebo-controlled and postmarketing surveillance data [107, 108]. It is important to educate patients on the interaction between organic nitrates, used for angina treatment, and PDE5 inhibitors. Due to the possibility of marked systemic hypotension, organic nitrates and PDE5 inhibitors are absolutely contraindicated [109–111]. If angina should develop with a PDE5 inhibitor present, at least 24 h for a short-acting PDE5 inhibitor (sildenafil, vardenafil) must elapse [112] prior to nitrate therapy, and at least 48 h must elapse for a long-acting PDE5 inhibitor (tadalafil) [113].

Alpha-blockers have varying degrees of interaction with PDE5 inhibitors that warrants starting at low dose of alpha-blockers until patients can adjust [2, 114]. Vardenafil has increased QTc by 6–9 ms and is not recommended in men taking type 1A or type 3 antiarrhythmic agents or men with known congenital prolonged QT interval [109]. The beta-blocker nebivolol is less likely to cause ED than other beta-blockers due to direct vasodilating properties [115–117]. Angiotensin receptor blockers have also been shown to less likely cause ED than diuretics [118, 119]. Additionally, statins have been reported to improve erectile function in men both with and without PDE5 inhibitors [120–123]. However, recent data showed that men reported new onset ED in 22 % of 93 high-risk men after 6 months of statin use [124]. Overall, there is a lack of placebo-controlled studies on erectile function in men taking medications to treat CVD.

In addition to their well-known treatment of ED, studies have actually shown a possible role for PDE5 inhibitors in the management of hypertension [125–128] and endothelial dysfunction [129–131] in patients at risk for CVD. This is not entirely surprising given their initial design for the treatment of pulmonary hypertension. In addition to PDE5 inhibitors, TRT should be incorporated for men as discussed previously. This can be incorporated initially or after PDE5 failure [58, 132]. Other nonpharmacologic approaches [2] such as exercise, weight loss [133, 134], and acknowledging partner and relationship factors [135–138] should be incorporated at all points.

Due to the evidence that suggests there is a window where ED presents prior to symptomatic CAD, ED may serve as a valuable identifier for men who should undergo a more extensive cardiovascular risk assessment [3]. This workup should be performed prior to resuming sexual activity with appropriate interventions as needed. A patient's cardiovascular health must be properly evaluated and optimized prior to beginning therapy for ED as well. Lifestyle modifications are beneficial not only to improving cardiovascular health but also erectile function. The Princeton Consensus Panel recommends a collaborative, multidisciplinary approach to the management of all men with ED with primary care, cardiologic, endocrine, and urologic specialists [3].

References

1. DeBusk R, Drory Y, Goldstein I et al (2000) Management of sexual dysfunction in patients with cardiovascular disease: recommendations of The Princeton Consensus Panel. Am J Cardiol 86(2):175–181
2. Kostis JB, Jackson G, Rosen R et al (2005) Sexual dysfunction and cardiac risk (the Second Princeton Consensus Conference). Am J Cardiol 96(2):313–321
3. Nehra A, Jackson G, Miner M et al (2012) The Princeton III consensus recommendations for the management of erectile dysfunction and cardiovascular disease. Mayo Clin Proc 87(8):766–778
4. Montorsi F, Briganti A, Salonia A et al (2003) Erectile dysfunction prevalence, time of onset and association with risk factors in 300 consecutive patients with acute chest pain and angiographically documented coronary artery disease. Eur Urol 44(3):360–365
5. Hodges LD, Kirby M, Solanki J et al (2007) The temporal relationship between erectile dysfunction and cardiovascular disease. Int J Clin Pract 61(12):2019–2025
6. Greenland P, Alpert JS, Beller GA et al (2010) 2010 ACCF/AHA guideline for assessment of cardiovascular risk in asymptomatic adults: a report of the American College of Cardiology Foundation/American Heart Association Task Force on practice guidelines. Circulation 122(25):e584–e636
7. Jackson G, Boon N, Eardley I et al (2010) Erectile dysfunction and coronary artery disease prediction: evidence-based guidance and consensus. Int J Clin Pract 64(7):848–857
8. Thompson IM, Tangen CM, Goodman PJ et al (2005) Erectile dysfunction and subsequent cardiovascular disease. JAMA 294(23):2996–3002
9. Araujo AB, Travison TG, Ganz P et al (2009) Erectile dysfunction and mortality. J Sex Med 6(9):2445–2454
10. Gazzaruso C, Giordanetti S, De Amici E et al (2004) Relationship between erectile dysfunction and silent myocardial ischemia in apparently uncomplicated type 2 diabetic patients. Circulation 110(1):22–26
11. Solomon H, Man JW, Wierzbicki AS, Jackson G (2003) Relation of erectile dysfunction to angiographic coronary artery disease. Am J Cardiol 91(2):230–231
12. Vlachopoulos C, Rokkas K, Ioakeimidis N et al (2005) Prevalence of asymptomatic coronary artery disease in men with vasculogenic erectile dysfunction: a prospective angiographic study. Eur Urol 48(6):996–1003
13. Montorsi P, Ravagnani PM, Galli S et al (2006) Association between erectile dysfunction and coronary artery disease: role of coronary clinical presentation and extent of coronary vessels involvement: the COBRA trial. Eur Heart J 27(22):2632–2639
14. Johannes CB, Araujo AB, Feldman HA et al (2000) Incidence of erectile dysfunction in men 40 to 69 years old: longitudinal results from the Massachusetts male aging study. J Urol 163(2):460–463
15. Moinpour CM, Lovato LC, Thompson IM Jr et al (2000) Profile of men randomized to the prostate cancer prevention trial: baseline health-related quality of life, urinary and sexual functioning, and health behaviors. J Clin Oncol 18(9):1942–1953
16. Araujo AB, Hall SA, Ganz P et al (2010) Does erectile dysfunction contribute to cardiovascular disease risk prediction beyond the Framingham Risk Score? J Am Coll Cardiol 55(4):350–356
17. Batty GD, Li Q, Czernichow S et al (2010) Erectile dysfunction and later cardiovascular disease in men with type 2 diabetes: prospective cohort study based on the ADVANCE (Action in Diabetes and Vascular Disease: Preterax and Diamicron Modified-Release Controlled Evaluation) trial. J Am Coll Cardiol 56(23):1908–1913
18. Blumentals WA, Gomez-Caminero A, Joo S, Vannappagari V (2004) Should erectile dysfunction be considered as a marker for acute myocardial infarction? Results from a retrospective cohort study. Int J Impot Res 16(4):350–353

19. Bohm M, Baumhakel M, Teo K et al (2010) ONTARGET/TRANSCEND Erectile Dysfunction Substudy Investigators. Erectile dysfunction predicts cardiovascular events in high-risk patients receiving telmisartan, ramipril, or both: the Ongoing Telmisartan Alone and in combination with Ramipril Global Endpoint Trial/Telmisartan Randomized Assessment Study in ACE intolerant subjects with cardiovascular disease (ON- TARGET/TRANSCEND) Trials. Circulation 121(12):1439–1446
20. Gazzaruso C, Solerte SB, Pujia A et al (2008) Erectile dysfunction as a predictor of cardiovascular events and death in diabetic patients with angiographically proven asymptomatic coronary artery disease: a potential protective role for statins and 5-phosphodiesterase inhibitors. J Am Coll Cardiol 51(21):2040–2044
21. Schouten BW, Bohnen AM, Bosch JL et al (2008) Erectile dysfunction prospectively associated with cardiovascular disease in the Dutch general population: results from the Krimpen Study. Int J Impot Res 20(1):92–99
22. Dong JY, Zhang YH, Qin LQ (2011) Erectile dysfunction and risk of cardiovascular disease meta-analysis of prospective cohort studies. J Am Coll Cardiol 58(13):1378–1385
23. Polonsky TS, Taillon LA, Sheth H et al (2009) The association between erectile dysfunction and peripheral arterial disease as determined by screening ankle-brachial index testing. Atherosclerosis 207(2):440–444
24. Ponholzer A, Temml C, Obermayr R et al (2005) Is erectile dysfunction an indicator for increased risk of coronary heart disease and stroke? Eur Urol 48(3):512–518
25. Inman BA, Sauver JL, Jacobson DJ et al (2009) A population-based, longitudinal study of erectile dysfunction and future coronary artery disease. Mayo Clin Proc 84(2):108–113
26. Chew KK, Finn J, Stuckey B et al (2010) Erectile dysfunction as a predictor for subsequent atherosclerotic cardiovascular events: findings from a linked-data study. J Sex Med 7(1):192–202
27. Marma AK, Berry JD, Ning H, Lloyd-Jones DM et al (2010) Distribution of 10-year and lifetime predicted risks for cardiovascular disease in US adults: findings from the National Health and Nutrition Examination Survey 2003 to 2006. Circ Cardiovasc Qual Outcomes 3(1):8–14
28. Billups KL, Bank AJ, Padma-Nathan H et al (2005) Erectile dysfunction is a marker for cardiovascular disease: results of the Minority Health Institute Expert Advisory Panel. J Sex Med 2(1):40–52
29. Hall SA, Shackelton R, Rosen RC, Araujo AB (2010) Sexual activity, erectile dysfunction, and incident cardiovascular events. Am J Cardiol 105(2):192–197
30. Salem S, Abdi S, Mehrsai A et al (2009) Erectile dysfunction severity as a risk predictor for coronary artery disease. J Sex Med 6(12):3425–3432
31. Greenstein A, Chen J, Miller H et al (1997) Does severity of ischemic coronary disease correlate with erectile function? Int J Impot Res 9(3):123–126
32. Wilson PW, D'Agostino RB, Levy D et al (1998) Prediction of coronary heart disease using risk factor categories. Circulation 97(18):1837–1847
33. Perrone-Filardi P, Achenbach S, Mohlenkamp S et al (2011) Cardiac computed tomography and myocardial perfusion scintigraphy for risk stratification in asymptomatic individuals without known cardiovascular disease: a position statement of the Working Group on Nuclear Cardiology and Cardiac CT of the European Society of Cardiology. Eur Heart J 32(16):1986–1993
34. Dewey M, Dubel HP, Schink T et al (2007) Head-to-head comparison of multislice computed tomography and exercise electrocardiography for diagnosis of coronary artery disease. Eur Heart J 28(20):2485–2490
35. Henneman MM, Schuijf JD, van Werkhoven JM et al (2008) Multi-slice computed tomography coronary angiography for ruling out suspected coronary artery disease: what is the prevalence of a normal study in a general clinical population? Eur Heart J 29(16):2006–2013
36. Jackson G, Padley S (2008) Erectile dysfunction and silent coronary artery disease: abnormal computed tomography coronary angiogram in the presence of normal exercise ECGs. Int J Clin Pract 62(6):973–976
37. Gibbons RJ, Balady GJ, Bricker JT et al (2002) ACC/AHA 2002 guideline update for exercise testing: summary article: a re- port of the American College of Cardiology/American

Heart Association Task Force on practice guidelines (Committee to Update the 1997 Exercise Testing Guidelines). Circulation 106(14):1883–1892
38. Gupta BP, Murad MH, Clifton MM et al (2011) The effect of lifestyle modification and cardiovascular risk factor reduction on erectile dysfunction: a systematic review and meta-analysis. Arch Intern Med 171(20):1797–1803
39. Critchley JA, Capewell S (2003) Mortality risk reduction associated with smoking cessation in patients with coronary heart disease: a systematic review. JAMA 290(1):86–97
40. Thompson PD, Buchner D, Pina IL et al (2003) Exercise and physical activity in the prevention and treatment of atherosclerotic cardiovascular disease: a statement from the Council on Clinical Cardiology (Subcommittee on Exercise, Rehabilitation, and Prevention) and the Council on Nutrition, Physical Activity, and Metabolism (Subcommittee on Physical Activity). Circulation 107(24):3109–3116
41. Netz Y, Wu MJ, Becker BJ, Tenenbaum G (2005) Physical activity and psychological well-being in advanced age: a meta-analysis of intervention studies. Psychol Aging 20(2):272–284
42. Bassuk SS, Manson JE (2005) Epidemiological evidence for the role of physical activity in reducing risk of type 2 diabetes and cardiovascular disease. J Appl Physiol 99(3):1193–1204
43. Mozaffarian D, Wilson PW, Kannel WB (2008) Beyond established and novel risk factors: lifestyle risk factors for cardiovascular disease. Circulation 117(23):3031–3038
44. Cloutier M, Adamson E (2004) The Mediterranean diet – newly revised and updated. HarperCollins Publishers
45. Sarwar N, Gao P, Seshasai SR et al (2010) Diabetes mellitus, fasting blood glucose concentration, and risk of vascular disease: a collaborative meta-analysis of 102 prospective studies. Lancet 375(9733):2215–2222 [published correction appears in Lancet 376(9745):958]
46. Mozaffarian D, Kamineni A, Carnethon M et al (2009) Lifestyle risk factors and new-onset diabetes mellitus in older adults: the cardiovascular health study. Arch Intern Med 169(8):798–807
47. Walls HL, Stevenson CE, Mannan HR et al (2011) Comparing trends in BMI and waist circumference. Obesity (Silver Spring) 19(1):216–219
48. Lee CM, Huxley RR, Wildman RP, Woodward M (2008) Indices of abdominal obesity are better discriminators of cardiovascular risk factors than BMI: a meta-analysis. J Clin Epidemiol 61(7):646–653
49. Bray GA, Clearfield MB, Fintel DJ, Nelinson DS (2009) Overweight and obesity: the pathogenesis of cardiometabolic risk. Clin Cornerstone 9(4):30–42
50. van der Velde M, Matsushita K, Coresh J et al (2011) Lower estimated glomerular filtration rate and higher albuminuria are associated with all-cause and cardiovascular mortality: a collaborative meta-analysis of high-risk population cohorts. Kidney Int 79(12):1341–1352
51. Matsushita K, van der Velde M, Astor BC et al (2010) Association of estimated glomerular filtration rate and albuminuria with all-cause and cardiovascular mortality in general population cohorts: a collaborative meta-analysis. Lancet 375(9731):2073–2081
52. Goglia L, Tosi V, Sanchez AM et al (2010) Endothelial regulation of eNOS, PAI-1 and t-PA by testosterone and dihydrotestosterone in vitro and in vivo. Mol Hum Reprod 16(10):761–769
53. Traish AM, Park K, Dhir V et al (1999) Effects of castration and androgen replacement on erectile function in a rabbit model. Endocrinology 140(4):1861–1868
54. Morelli A, Filippi S, Mancina R et al (2004) Androgens regulate phosphodiesterase type 5 expression and functional activity in corpora cavernous. Endocrinology 145(5):2253–2263
55. Zhang XH, Morelli A, Luconi M et al (2005) Testosterone regulates PDE5 expression and in vivo responsiveness to tadalafil in rat corpus cavernous. Eur Urol 47(3):409–416
56. Guay AT, Velasquez E, Perez JB (1999) Characterization of patients in a medical endocrine-based center for male sexual dysfunction. Endocr Pract 5(6):314–321
57. Blute M, Hakimian P, Kashanian J et al (2009) Erectile dysfunction and testosterone deficiency. Front Horm Res 37:108–122
58. Buvat J, Montorsi F, Maggi M et al (2011) Hypogonadal men non-responders to the PDE5 inhibitor tadalafil benefit from normalization of testosterone levels with a 1 % hydroalco-

holic testosterone gel in the treatment of erectile dysfunction (TADTEST study). J Sex Med 8(1):284–293
59. Shores MM, Matsumoto AM, Sloan KL, Kivlahan DR (2006) Low serum testosterone and mortality in male veterans. Arch Intern Med 166(15):1660–1665
60. Laughlin GA, Barrett-Connor E, Bergstrom J (2008) Low serum testosterone and mortality in older men. J Clin Endocrinol Metab 93(1):68–75
61. Khaw KT, Dowsett M, Folkerd E et al (2007) Endogenous testosterone and mortality due to all causes, cardiovascular disease, and cancer in men: European prospective investigation into cancer in Norfolk (EPIC-Norfolk) Prospective Population Study. Circulation 116(23):2694–2701
62. Haring R, Volzke H, Steveling A et al (2010) Low serum testosterone levels are associated with increased risk of mortality in a population-based cohort of men aged 20–79. Eur Heart J 31(12):1494–1501
63. Malkin CJ, Pugh PJ, Morris PD et al (2010) Low serum testosterone and increased mortality in men with coronary heart disease. Heart 96(22):1821–1825
64. Tivesten A, Vandenput L, Labrie F et al (2009) Low serum testosterone and estradiol predict mortality in elderly men. J Clin Endocrinol Metab 94(7):2482–2488
65. Menke A, Guallar E, Rohrmann S et al (2010) Sex steroid hormone concentrations and risk of death in US men. Am J Epidemiol 171(5):583–592
66. Vikan T, Schirmer H, Njolstad I, Svartberg J (2009) Endogenous sex hormones and the prospective association with cardiovascular disease and mortality in men: the Tromso Study. Eur J Endocrinol 161(3):435–442
67. Corona G, Monami M, Boddi V et al (2010) Low testosterone is associated with an increased risk of MACE lethality in subjects with erectile dysfunction. J Sex Med 7(4):1557–1564
68. Ruige JB, Mahmoud AM, De Bacquer D, Kaufman JM (2011) Endogenous testosterone and cardiovascular disease in healthy men: a meta-analysis. Heart 97(11):870–875
69. Corona G, Rastrelli G, Monami M et al (2011) Hypogonadism as a risk factor for cardiovascular mortality in men: a meta-analytic study. Eur J Endocrinol 165(5):687–701
70. Grossmann M, Thomas MC, Panagiotopoulos S et al (2008) Low testosterone levels are common and associated with insulin resistance in men with diabetes. J Clin Endocrinol Metab 93(5):1834–1840
71. Laaksonen DE, Niskanen L, Punnonen K et al (2003) Sex hormones, inflammation and the metabolic syndrome: a population- based study. Eur J Endocrinol 149(6):601–608
72. Osuna JA, Gomez-Perez R, Arata-Bellabarba G, Villaroel V (2006) Relationship between BMI, total testosterone, sex hormone- binding-globulin, leptin, insulin and insulin resistance in obese men. Arch Androl 52(5):355–361
73. Kapoor D, Aldred H, Clark S et al (2007) Clinical and biochemical assessment of hypogonadism in men with type 2 diabetes: correlations with bioavailable testosterone and visceral adiposity. Diabetes Care 30(4):911–917
74. Jones TH, Arver S, Behre HM et al (2011) Testosterone replacement in hypogonadal men with type 2 diabetes and/or metabolic syndrome (the TIMES2 study). Diabetes Care 34(4):828–837
75. Corona G, Monami M, Rastrelli G et al (2011) Testosterone and metabolic syndrome: a meta-analysis study. J Sex Med 8(1):272–283
76. Qaseem A, Snow V, Denberg TD et al (2009) Hormonal testing and pharmacologic treatment of erectile dysfunction: a clinical practice guideline from the American College of Physicians. Ann Intern Med 151(9):639–649
77. Hackett G, Kell P, Ralph D et al (2008) British Society for Sexual Medicine guidelines on the management of erectile dysfunction. J Sex Med 5(8):1841–1865
78. Montorsi F, Pierce C, Khoury S (2010) Advancing science in the interest of patient care. In: Proceedings from the third international consultation on Sexual Medicine, Paris, July 2013. J Sex Med 7(1):311–631
79. Bhasin S, Cunningham GR, Hayes FJ et al (2010) Testosterone therapy in men with androgen deficiency syndromes: an Endocrine Society clinical practice guideline. J Clin Endocrinol Metab 95(6):2536–2559

80. Wang C, Nieschlag E, Swerdloff R et al (2009) Investigation, treatment, and monitoring of late-onset hypogonadism in males: ISA, ISSAM, EAU, EAA, and ASA recommendations. Eur Urol 55(1):121–130
81. Buvat J, Maggi M, Gooren L et al (2010) Endocrine aspects of male sexual dysfunctions. J Sex Med 7(4):1627–1656
82. Ridker PM, Rifai N, Rose L et al (2002) Comparison of C-reactive protein and low-density lipoprotein cholesterol levels in the prediction of first cardiovascular events. N Engl J Med 347(20):1557–1565
83. Ridker PM, Glynn RJ, Hennekens CH (1998) C-reactive protein adds to the predictive value of total and HDL cholesterol in determining risk of first myocardial infarction. Circulation 97(20):2007–2011
84. Ridker PM (2001) High-sensitivity C-reactive protein: potential adjunct for global risk assessment in the primary prevention of cardiovascular disease. Circulation 103(13):1813–1818
85. Pearson TA, Mensah GA, Alexander RW et al (2003) Markers of inflammation and cardiovascular disease: application to clinical and public health practice: a statement for healthcare professionals from the Centers for Disease Control and Prevention and the American Heart Association. Circulation 107(3):499–511
86. Nozaki T, Sugiyama S, Koga H et al (2009) Significance of a multiple biomarkers strategy including endothelial dysfunction to improve risk stratification for cardiovascular events in patients at high risk for coronary heart disease. J Am Coll Cardiol 54(7):601–608
87. Kaptoge S, Di Angelantonio E, Lowe G et al (2010) C-reactive protein concentration and risk of coronary heart disease, stroke, and mortality: an individual participant meta-analysis. Lancet 375(9709):132–140
88. Ridker PM (2007) C-reactive protein and the prediction of cardio- vascular events among those at intermediate risk: moving an inflammatory hypothesis toward consensus. J Am Coll Cardiol 49(21):2129–2138
89. Krishnan E, Sokolove J (2011) Uric acid in heart disease: a new C-reactive protein? Curr Opin Rheumatol 23(2):174–177
90. Selvin E, Steffes MW, Zhu H et al (2010) Glycated hemoglobin, diabetes, and cardiovascular risk in nondiabetic adults. N Engl J Med 362(9):800–811
91. Perkovic V, Verdon C, Ninomiya T et al (2008) The relationship between proteinuria and coronary risk: a systematic review and meta-analysis. PLoS Med 5(10):e207
92. Madjid M, Ali M, Willerson JT (2010) Lipoprotein-associated phospholipase A2 as a novel risk marker for cardiovascular disease: a systematic review of the literature. Tex Heart Inst J 37(1):25–39
93. Jenny NS, Solomon C, Cushman M et al (2010) Lipoprotein-associated phospholipase A(2) (Lp-PLA(2)) and risk of cardio- vascular disease in older adults: results from the Cardiovascular Health Study. Atherosclerosis 209(2):528–532
94. Daniels LB, Laughlin GA, Sarno MJ et al (2008) Lipoprotein-associated phospholipase A2 is an independent predictor of incident coronary heart disease in an apparently healthy older population: the Rancho Bernardo Study. J Am Coll Cardiol 51(9):913–919
95. Koenig W, Khuseyinova N, Lowel H et al (2004) Lipoprotein-associated phospholipase A2 adds to risk prediction of incident coronary events by C-reactive protein in apparently healthy middle-aged men from the general population: results from the 14-year follow-up of a large cohort from southern Germany. Circulation 110(14):1903–1908
96. Naghavi M, Falk E, Hecht HS et al (2006) SHAPE Task Force. From vulnerable plaque to vulnerable patient, part III: executive summary of the Screening for Heart Attack Prevention and Education (SHAPE) Task Force report. Am J Cardiol 98(2A):2H–15H
97. Nambi V, Chambless L, Folsom AR et al (2010) Carotid intima-media thickness and presence or absence of plaque improves prediction of coronary heart disease risk: the ARIC (Atherosclerosis Risk In Communities) study. J Am Coll Cardiol 55(15):1600–1607
98. Folsom AR, Kronmal RA, Detrano RC et al (2008) Coronary artery calcification compared with carotid intima-media thickness in the prediction of cardiovascular disease incidence: the Multi- Ethnic Study of Atherosclerosis (MESA). Arch Intern Med 168(12):1333–1339

99. Fowkes FG, Murray GD, Butcher I et al (2008) Ankle brachial index combined with Framingham Risk Score to predict cardiovascular events and mortality: a meta-analysis. JAMA 300(2):197–208
100. Vlachopoulos C, Aznaouridis K, Stefanadis C (2010) Prediction of cardiovascular events and all-cause mortality with arterial stiffness: a systematic review and meta-analysis. J Am Coll Cardiol 55(13):1318–1327
101. Rubinshtein R, Kuvin JT, Soffler M et al (2010) Assessment of endothelial function by non-invasive peripheral arterial tonometry predicts late cardiovascular adverse events. Eur Heart J 31(9):1142–1148
102. Yeboah J, Crouse JR, Hsu FC et al (2007) Brachial flow-mediated dilation predicts incident cardiovascular events in older adults: the Cardiovascular Health Study. Circulation 115(18):2390–2397
103. Yeboah J, Folsom AR, Burke GL et al (2009) Predictive value of brachial flow-mediated dilation for incident cardiovascular events in a population-based study: the multi-ethnic study of atherosclerosis. Circulation 120(6):502–509
104. Anderson TJ, Charbonneau F, Title LM et al (2011) Microvascular function predicts cardiovascular events in primary prevention: long-term results from the Firefighters and Their Endothelium (FATE) study. Circulation 123(2):163–169
105. Levine GN, Steinke EE, Bakaeen FG et al (2012) Sexual activity and cardiovascular disease: a scientific statement from the American Heart Association. Circulation 125(8):1058–1072
106. Dahabreh IJ, Paulus JK (2011) Association of episodic physical and sexual activity with triggering of acute cardiac events: systematic review and meta-analysis. JAMA 305(12):1225–1233
107. Giuliano F, Jackson G, Montorsi F et al (2010) Safety of sildenafil citrate: review of 67 double-blind placebo-controlled trials and the postmarketing safety database. Int J Clin Pract 64(2):240–255
108. Kloner RA, Jackson G, Hutter AM et al (2006) Cardiovascular safety update of tadalafil: retrospective analysis of data from placebo-controlled and open-label clinical trials of tadalafil with as needed, three times-per-week or once-a-day dosing. Am J Cardiol 97(12):1778–1784
109. Bayer Health Care, GlaxoSmithKline (2013) Levitra® (vardenafil HCL) prescribing information. https://www.gsksource.com/gskprm/en/US/images/gsk_content/LEVITRA/Levitra_PI.PDF. Accessed 14 Feb 2014
110. Pfizer (2014) Viagra prescribing information. http://labeling.pfizer.com/ShowLabeling.aspx?id=652. Accessed 14 Feb 2014
111. Lilly ICOS LLC (2013) Cialis (tadalafil) prescribing information. http://pi.lilly.com/us/cialis-pi.pdf. Accessed 14 Feb 2014
112. Cheitlin MD, Hutter AM Jr, Brindis RG et al (1999) ACC/AHA expert consensus document. Use of sildenafil (Viagra) in patients with cardiovascular disease. American College of Cardiology/American Heart Association. J Am Coll Cardiol 33:273–282
113. Kloner RA, Hutter AM, Emmick JT et al (2003) Time course of the interaction between tadalafil and nitrates. J Am Coll Cardiol 42:1855–1860
114. Kloner RA, Jackson G, Emmick JT et al (2004) Interaction between the phosphodiesterase 5 inhibitor, tadalafil, and the two alpha blockers: doxazosin, tamsulosin in healthy normotensive men. J Urol 172:1935–1940
115. Boydak B, Nalbantgil S, Fici F et al (2005) A randomised comparison of the effects of nebivolol and atenolol with and without chlorthalidone on the sexual function of hypertensive men. Clin Drug Investig 25(6):409–416 [published correction appears in Clin Drug Investig. 2007; 27(12):864]
116. Brixius K, Middeke M, Lichtenthal A et al (2007) Nitric oxide, erectile dysfunction and beta-blocker treatment (MR NOED study): benefit of nebivolol versus metoprolol in hypertensive men. Clin Exp Pharmacol Physiol 34(4):327–331
117. Doumas M, Tsakiris A, Douma S et al (2006) Beneficial effects of switching from beta-blockers to nebivolol on the erectile function of hypertensive patients. Asian J Androl 8(2):177–182

118. Baumhakel M, Schlimmer N, Bohm M, DO-IT Investigators (2008) Effect of irbesartan on erectile function in patients with hypertension and metabolic syndrome. Int J Impot Res 20(5):493–500
119. Llisterri JL, Lozano Vidal JV, Aznar Vicente J et al (2001) Sexual dysfunction in hypertensive patients treated with losartan. Am J Med Sci 321(5):336–341
120. Bank AJ, Kelly AS, Kaiser DR et al (2006) The effects of quinapril and atorvastatin on the responsiveness to sildenafil in men with erectile dysfunction. Vasc Med 11(4):251–257
121. Saltzman EA, Guay AT, Jacobson J (2004) Improvement in erectile function in men with organic erectile dysfunction by correction of elevated cholesterol levels: a clinical observation. J Urol 172(1):255–258
122. Dadkhah F, Safarinejad MR, Asgari MA et al (2010) Atorvastatin improves the response to sildenafil in hypercholesterolemic men with erectile dysfunction not initially responsive to sildenafil. Int J Impot Res 22(1):51–60
123. Gokkaya SC, Ozden C, Levent Ozdal O et al (2008) Effect of correcting serum cholesterol levels on erectile function in patients with vasculogenic erectile dysfunction. Scand J Urol Nephrol 42(5):437–440
124. Solomon H, Samarasinghe YP, Feher MD (2006) Erectile dysfunction and statin treatment in high cardiovascular risk patients. Int J Clin Pract 60(2):141–145
125. Kloner R (2007) Erectile dysfunction and hypertension. Int J Impot Res 19(3):296–302
126. Scranton RE, Lawler E, Botteman M et al (2007) Effect of treating erectile dysfunction on management of systolic hypertension. Am J Cardiol 100(3):459–463
127. Oliver JJ, Melville VP, Webb DJ (2006) Effect of regular phosphodiesterase type 5 inhibition in hypertension. Hypertension 48(4):622–627
128. Patterson D, McInnes GT, Webster J et al (2006) Influence of a single dose of 20 mg tadalafil, a phosphodiesterase 5 inhibitor, on ambulatory blood pressure in subjects with hypertension. Br J Clin Pharmacol 62(3):280–287
129. Kimura M, Higashi Y, Hara K et al (2003) PDE5 inhibitor sildenafil citrate augments endothelium-dependent vasodilation in smokers. Hypertension 41(5):1106–1110
130. Gillies HC, Roblin D, Jackson G (2002) Coronary and systemic hemodynamic effects of sildenafil citrate: from basic science to clinical studies in patients with cardiovascular disease. Int J Cardiol 86(2–3):131–141
131. Katz SD, Balidemaj K, Homma S et al (2000) Acute type 5-phosphodiesterase inhibition with sildenafil enhances flow-mediated vasodilation in patients with chronic heart failure. J Am Coll Cardiol 36(3):845–851
132. Buvat J, Gilbert BJ (2008) Combination therapy with phosphodiesterase type V inhibitors and testosterone. Curr Sex Health Rep 5:135–140
133. Esposito K, Giugliano F, Di Palo C et al (2004) Effect of lifestyle changes on erectile dysfunction in obese men: a randomized controlled trial. JAMA 291(24):2978–2984
134. Wing RR, Rosen RC, Fava JL et al (2010) Effects of weight loss intervention on erectile function in older men with type 2 diabetes in the Look AHEAD trial. J Sex Med 7(1):156–165
135. Fisher WA, Eardley I, McCabe M, Sand M (2009) Erectile dysfunction (ED) is a shared sexual concern of couples II: association of female partner characteristics with male partner ED treatment seeking and phosphodiesterase type 5 inhibitor utilization. J Sex Med 6(11):3111–3124
136. Riley A (2002) The role of the partner in erectile dysfunction and its treatment. Int J Impot Res 14(suppl 1):S105–S109
137. Riley A (2008) When treating erectile dysfunction, do not forget the partner. Int J Clin Pract 62(1):6–8
138. Westheimer RK (2000) Partner and relationship issues in the treatment of erectile dysfunction. Am J Manag Care 6(12):S639–S640

Sexual Counseling for Patients with Cardiovascular Disease

Athanasios Manolis, Andreas Pittaras, Antonios Lazaridis, and Michael Doumas

23.1 Introduction

Sexuality is a very important characteristic of human beings, both at the reproductive and the recreational level. Therefore, sexual activity is not only essential for the human reproduction but is also an essential component of life quality. For years, it was believed that sexuality is not important among older or the diseased individuals. However, it is currently recognized that sexuality is maintained even in the very elderly and keeps playing an important role in patients with overt cardiovascular disease [1].

"Sexual championship" is the most significant physiological and sociological problem of sexuality nowadays. Males engage in sports such as soccer, basketball, football, baseball, or tennis in order to enjoy themselves without finding it essential to be champions [2]. However, when it comes to sex, everyone feels the need to be a champion in this, to be the Michael Jordan, Joe DiMaggio, Bjorn Borg, or Usain Bolt. Moreover, men feel the need to compare their sexual ability with the former men of their sexual partners and beat them in every aspect.

Another significant problem is the difficulty in communication, both from the patients and the physician's side. Sexuality was for centuries a "taboo" issue with

---

A. Manolis (✉) • A. Pittaras
Cardiology Department, Asklepeion General Hospital, Athens, Greece
e-mail: ajmanol@otenet.gr; andreaspittaras@gmail.com

A. Lazaridis
2nd Propedeutic Department of Internal Medicine, Aristotle University, Thessaloniki, Greece
e-mail: spanbiol@hotmail.com

M. Doumas
Internal Medicine, Aristotle University, Thessalonik, Greece

George Washington University, Washington, DC, USA
e-mail: michalisdoumas@yahoo.co.uk

several cultural, religious, and societal factors dictating a secrecy and intimacy in discussing these issues. From the other part of the hill, physicians are frequently reluctant to open a discussion about sexuality due to several factors including intimacy, lack of familiarity, and lack of training on and knowledge about sexual function [3].

Erectile dysfunction is highly prevalent among males with overt cardiovascular disease or cardiovascular risk factors [4–6]. Erectile dysfunction exerts a significant negative impact on the quality of life of patients and their sexual partners. Two factors are of major clinical importance and need to be highlighted: (a) reduced sexual activity is frequently encountered in patients following a cardiovascular event and (b) erectile dysfunction is frequently underreported, under-recognized, and undertreated [7, 8]. Therefore, sexual counseling in patients with cardiovascular disease is of utmost importance both for patients and their sexual partners.

This review aims to summarize the topics that need to be addressed during sexual counseling in patients with cardiovascular disease and critically discuss the problems observed in everyday clinical practice.

23.2 Sexual Counseling

Patients suffering a major cardiovascular event (myocardial infarction, stroke), undergoing a cardiac procedure (percutaneous coronary intervention, coronary artery bypass graft, and defibrillator), or having cardiovascular disease (heart failure, angina) many times experience fear in engaging to sexual activities [9]. Therefore, sexual counseling need not only to appropriately identify and manage patients with erectile dysfunction but also to adequately address factors limiting sexual activity in patients with cardiovascular disease [10, 11].

Sexual counseling is a complex process during which a health-care professional advises patients regarding the initiation of sexual activity following an acute cardiovascular event; discusses with the patient any concerns, fear, or distress regarding sexual activity; and involves the sexual partner of the patient in order to diminish any potential problems regarding a safe and enjoyable sexual life in patients with cardiovascular disease [12–14]. Sexual counseling might be a short-term or long-term process, either provided once immediately after an acute event or as a part of prolonged counseling when concerns are still present and not adequately addressed [12, 13]. The importance of sexual counseling in patients with cardiovascular disease was recently highlighted by the publication of a joint scientific statement from the American Heart Association and the European Society of Cardiology [14].

Sexual counseling covers a wide range of topics, which should be addressed in patients with cardiovascular disease, trying to provide answers in the most clinically meaningful and usual questions patients usually ask, such as the following: (a) Is it safe to engage in sexual intercourse? (b) When (following an acute event)? (c) How intense? (d) Which sexual position is better? (e) Is sexual activity affected by concomitant drugs or disease? (f) Is it safe to use phosphodiesterase-5 (PDE-5) inhibitors?

23.3 Safety of Sexual Activity

Several lines of evidence strongly indicate that exercise capacity is associated with reduced risk for cardiovascular morbidity, cardiovascular mortality, and all-cause mortality in health and in disease [15–22]. The benefits of regular exercise have been also shown in several studies. However, some evidence suggests that acute vigorous exercise might in fact trigger an acute cardiac event [23–26]. Acute cardiac events may occur during or immediately after sexual intercourse and are defined as sexually induced or coital acute cardiac events. Coital angina or "angina d'amour" is not very common since it consists less than 5 % of angina events [27].

A recent systematic review and meta-analysis evaluated the association of episodic physical and sexual activity with triggering of acute cardiac events (myocardial infarction, acute coronary syndrome, sudden cardiac death) [28]. It was found that episodic sexual activity was associated with a significantly increased risk of myocardial infarction (relative risk, 2.70; 95 % CI, 1.48–4.91). Two points need, however, to be highlighted. First, the absolute rate of events is substantially low due to the infrequent and transient nature of sexual activity. It has been estimated that the absolute rate of myocardial infarction is 2–3 per 10,000 person-years (1 per 10,000 person-years for sudden cardiac death) for every 1 h of additional sexual activity per week. Second, the association between sexual activity and acute cardiac events greatly depends on habitual physical activity. It has been estimated that the relative risk for myocardial infarction and sudden cardiac death is reduced by 45 and 30 %, respectively, for every additional time per week an individual is engaged in physical activity.

An individual who achieves more than 3–5 METs during treadmill exercise test without development of symptoms (angina, excessive dyspnea), ischemia at electrocardiogram, hypotension, or arrhythmia is likely to engage in sexual intercourse without significant risk [29]. Therefore, it seems prudent to recommend an exercise stress test in patients who are at intermediate and especially at high cardiovascular risk [30–35].

23.4 Re-initiation of Sexual Activity

No hard data exist determining the right time to engage in sexual activity following an acute event. In the absence of robust evidence-based recommendations, it is essential to provide clinical-based recommendations according to a rational interpretation of available data using clinical judgment and common sense [36]. In addition, advice should be disease specific as different time intervals seem to apply in different forms of cardiovascular disease.

Following an acute myocardial infarction, it seems reasonable to recommend re-initiation of sexual activity after 1 week, in the case that the patient had no significant complications during hospital stay (heart failure, arrhythmias, recurrent angina, etc.), and mild-to-moderate physical activity is not accompanied by angina or dyspnea. The recommendation reflects our current approach regarding physical activity following an acute myocardial infarction, although specific data regarding the safe re-initiation of sexual activities is missing.

Following a cardiovascular operation, either coronary artery bypass grafting or noncoronary open-heart operation, it seems reasonable to re-initiate sexual activity after 6–8 weeks. This requires that no severe complications occurred following the operation and the surgical trauma is adequately healed.

23.5 Intensity of Sexual Activity

The intensity of sexual activity depends on the type of sexual activities and the duration of sex.

The energy expenditure is low during sexual foreplay (hugging, kissing, caressing), increases with sexual activities other than intercourse (oral sex, masturbation), and peaks with sexual intercourse. The effects of different sexual activities were assessed in one study by measuring the rate-pressure product and oxygen uptake. It was found that noncoital sexual activities (noncoital stimulation of male by female and male self-stimulation) were associated with lower energy expenditures than coital activities [37].

Sexual activity is more or less a form of exercise. Blood pressure reaches a peak during the beginning of plateau phase of sexual cycle and returns to baseline at 10 min after orgasm, while heart rate peaks at the beginning of orgasm and drops to baseline after 10–20 min [38]. It has been shown that sexual activity provides modest physical stress, which is comparable to the energy expenditure observed with Stage II of the Bruce treadmill exercise protocol for men and Stage I for women. In addition, the duration of treadmill exercise predicts the duration of sexual activity. In a study of 32 middle-aged individuals, per minute of treadmill exercise duration, an increase of 2.3 min in sexual activity duration has been observed [39].

The duration of sexual intercourse obviously matters. Patients with premature ejaculation (<1 min following vaginal penetration) require less energy than patients with normal and especially delayed ejaculation (>20–30 min). It seems rationale to tailor the intensity of sexual activities according to individual's exercise capacity and symptomatology. Coital angina or dyspnea during sexual intercourse should guide the engagement to sexual activities.

Heart failure is a very good example of individualized sexual counseling. Sexual problems are very common in patients with heart failure, especially in decompensated forms [40]. Individuals suffering from heart failure often experience shortness of breath and fatigue [41], limiting their sexual ability. It is therefore not surprising that patients with heart failure ask for clear and specific information; they are not content with general and vague advice; they are absolutely unsatisfied by the failure of treating physicians to appropriately discuss this issue and provide relevant information [40, 42].

Patients with advanced or even decompensated heart failure (classes III and IV according to New York Heart Association) should defer from sexual intercourse until their condition is improved or at least stabilized with medical therapy. Patients with milder forms of heart failure (classes I and II) may participate in sexual activities depending on their symptoms and exercise capacity. In case dyspnea or angina occurs with intense sexual activities, alternative forms of sexual activity, convenient positioning, and prolonged relaxation before activities might be extremely helpful and provide sexual satisfaction.

23.6 Sexual Positioning

Sexual positions seem to affect the energy expenditure of sexual intercourse. Some sexual positions require less energy (man on bottom, side by side) than others (man on top, man on the back, anal sex), and the energy expenditure is usually less with long-time sexual partners than with new partners, young partners (especially with large age-difference), and extramarital affairs.

A small study evaluated the effects of sexual positioning by measuring the rate-pressure product and oxygen uptake. It was found that the man on top positioning required higher expenditure than the man on bottom positioning [37]. Although available data do not allow for definite conclusions, it seems rationale to recommend convenient and less stressful positions in patients with cardiovascular disease and impaired exercise capacity. Sexual positioning is also important in some occasions, such as in patients with coronary artery bypass graft, pacemakers, implantable defibrillators, or left ventricular assist devices.

Extramarital sex needs to be highlighted. A Japanese study reported that 47 out of 67 deaths directly related to sexual activity occurred in the context of extramarital relations, mostly in brothels or hotel rooms [43]. A retrospective, postmortem study from Germany confirms the risks of extramarital sex. Almost 27,000 forensic autopsies were performed during a 27-year period, and 48 deaths occurred during sexual activity (0.18 %). Deaths occurred almost exclusively in men (45/48 cases), and the vast majority occurred during an extramarital intercourse (36/48 cases), usually with prostitutes at unfamiliar environments (brothels, hotels) [44]. Similarly, death was preceded by extramarital intercourse in 23 out of 30 fatal events in a forensic autopsy study from Berlin [45]. In another small study from Korea, only one out of 14 cases of sexual activity-related sudden death occurred with a marital partner, while the others occurred at an extramarital context [46].

23.7 Comorbidities: Concomitant Medication

Erectile dysfunction is a vascular disease and frequently encountered in patients with traditional cardiovascular risk factors, especially hypertension and diabetes mellitus [3–6]. However, other factors are also implicated in erectile dysfunction, beyond cardiovascular risk factors, including chronic pain, arthritis, depression, and anxiety [47, 48]. The impact of concomitant disease is significant in patients with cardiovascular disease, and especially in stroke patients [49].

Stroke survivors may experience functional disability (hemiparesis) or speaking problems (aphasia, dysphasia) that may significantly impair the ability for sexual activities, verbal intimacy, and overall sexual satisfaction. Stroke patients are usually old with several concomitant disease conditions that may contribute to sexual dysfunction. Moreover, patients with stroke may have low self-esteem and emotional problems that are frequently associated with depression and anxiety [50]. The latter psychological factors are associated with sexual problems as shown by several lines of evidence [review depression, anxiety]. Specific tools to overcome physical disability and verbal communication problems may be extremely helpful in stroke patients [51, 52].

The impact of concomitant medication is also very significant. Patients with cardiovascular disease frequently use drugs that may affect erectile function [53, 54]. Diuretics and beta-blockers are the most implicated drug categories, while some agents might exert even beneficial effects [55, 56]. It has to be noted, however, that the treating physician has to balance the necessity of administering the implicated drug for the primary condition, the probability of the drug to cause sexual problems, and the potential benefit of switching therapy, taking into account patient's wish. Regarding beta-blockers, the "true" detrimental effects on erectile function have been recently questioned [57]; however, the vast majority of available evidence point towards a negative effect of this drug category on erectile function, excluding nebivolol [58].

23.8 PDE-5 Inhibitors

PDE-5 inhibitors revolutionized the management of patients with erectile dysfunction. PDE-5 inhibitors have vasorelaxant properties, which must be taken into account when these agents are administered in patients with cardiovascular disease. Accumulating data indicate that PDE-5 inhibitors can be safely administered in patients on multiple, perplexed therapeutic regimes, even in patients with cardiovascular risk factors or overt cardiovascular disease [59, 60]. However, one exception and one precaution apply. Coadministration with nitrates is contraindicated, while precaution is needed with alpha-blockers [3–6].

Indeed, potentially life-threatening episodes of symptomatic hypotension have been observed with coadministration of PDE-5 inhibitors with organic nitrates [61]. Coadministration with alpha-blockers is no longer contraindicated. However, the risk of excessive hypotension (especially orthostatic) calls for special care. It seems rationale to recommend administration of low-dose PDE-5 inhibitors in patients receiving alpha-blockers and vice versa initiation of low-dose alpha-blockers in patients receiving PDE-5 inhibitors [54], with close patient monitoring.

> **Conclusions**
> To conclude, sexual dysfunction, although frequently underreported, underrecognized, or underdiagnosed, is still an issue of great importance that overshadows the quality of everyday life of the patients regardless their gender or

age. As such, individualized sexual counseling aiming to establish a healthy sexual life for both patients and their sexual partners should be properly provided. Patients with overt cardiovascular disease or existing cardiovascular risk factors constitute a frail group calling for such particular sexual counseling. In this context, safety concerns regarding the initiation of sexual activity according to baseline cardiovascular profile, the reestablishment of sexual intercourse after an acute cardiovascular event, and the appropriate intensity of sexual activity depending on the type and the duration of sexual intercourse, proper sexual positioning, comorbidities, and concomitant medications including the therapeutic utility of PDE-5 inhibitors are some essential aspects that must be always addressed when approaching sexual dysfunction in a patient with cardiovascular disease or risk factors.

References

1. Manolis A, Doumas M (2009) Hypertension and sexual dysfunction. Arch Med Sci 5:S337–S350
2. Hoch Z (1976) Sexual counselling and therapy. Sexual counselling and therapy. J Fam Counseling 4:7–13
3. Viigimaa M, Doumas M, Vlachopoulos C et al (2011) European Society of hypertension working group on sexual dysfunction. Hypertension and sexual dysfunction: time to act. J Hypertens 29:403–407
4. Doumas M, Douma S (2006) Sexual dysfunction in essential hypertension: myth or reality? J Clin Hypertens 8:269–274
5. Manolis A, Doumas M (2008) Sexual dysfunction: the 'prima ballerina' of hypertension-related quality-of-life complications. J Hypertens 26:2074–2084
6. Doumas M, Tsakiris A, Douma S et al (2006) Factors affecting the increased prevalence of erectile dysfunction in Greek hypertensive compared with normotensive subjects. J Androl 27:469–477
7. Manolis AJ, Doumas M, Viigimaa M, Narkiewitz K (2011) Hypertension and sexual dysfunction. European Society of Hypertension Scientific Newsletter: Update on Hypertension Management. Eur Soc Hyp 32:1–2
8. Douma S, Doumas M, Tsakiris A, Zamboulis C (2007) Male and female sexual dysfunction: is hypertension an innocent bystander or a major contributor? Rev Bras Hypertens 14:139–147
9. Mosack V, Steinke E (2009) Trends in sexual concerns after myocardial infarction. J Cardiovasc Nursing 24:162–170
10. Nikolai MPJ, Both S, Liem SS et al (2013) Discussing sexual function in the cardiology practice. Clin Res Cardiol 102:329–336
11. O'Donovan K (2007) Addressing the taboos: resuming sexual activity after myocardial infarction. Br J Card Nurs 2:165–175
12. Steinke EE, Mosack V, Barnason S, Wright DW (2011) Progress in sexual counseling by cardiac nurses, 1994 to 2009. Heart Lung 40:e15–e24
13. Steinke EE (2013) How can heart failure patients and their partners be counseled on sexual activity? Curr Heart Fail Rep 10:262–269
14. Steinke EE, Jaarsma T, Barnason SA et al (2013) Sexual counseling for individuals with cardiovascular disease and their partners. A consensus document from the American Heart Association and the ESC council on Cardiovascular Nursing and Allied Professions (CCNAP). Circulation 128:2075–2096
15. Kokkinos P, Myers J, Kokkinos JP et al (2008) Exercise capacity and mortality in black and white men. Circulation 117:614–622

16. Kokkinos P, Manolis A, Pittaras A et al (2009) Exercise capacity and mortality in hypertensive men with and without additional risk factors. Hypertension 53:494–499
17. Blair SN, Kampert JB, Kohl HW III et al (1996) Influences of cardiorespiratory fitness and other precursors on cardiovascular disease and all-cause mortality in men and women. JAMA 276:205–210
18. Kokkinos P, Myers J, Doumas M et al (2009) Exercise capacity and all-cause mortality in prehypertensive men. Am J Hypertens 22:735–741
19. Kokkinos P, Doumas M, Myers J et al (2009) A graded association of exercise capacity and all-cause mortality in males with high-normal blood pressure. Blood Press 18:261–267
20. Kokkinos P, Myers J, Faselis C et al (2010) Exercise capacity and mortality in older men: a 20-year follow-up study. Circulation 122:790–797
21. Faselis C, Doumas M, Kokkinos JP et al (2012) Exercise capacity and progression from prehypertension to hypertension. Hypertension 60:333–338
22. Myers J, Prakash M, Froelicher V et al (2002) Exercise capacity and mortality among men referred for exercise testing. N Engl J Med 346:793–801
23. Gunby P (1979) Snow falls; ischemic heart deaths rise. JAMA 241:1987
24. Glass RI, Zack MM Jr (1979) Increase in deaths from ischemic heart disease after blizzards. Lancet 8114:485–487
25. Trichopoulos D, Katsouyanni K, Zavitsanos X et al (1983) Psychological stress and fatal heart attack: the Athens (1981) earthquake natural experiment. Lancet 8322:441–444
26. Moller J, Theorell T, de Faire U et al (2005) Work related stressful life events and the risk of myocardial infarction: case-control and case-crossover analyses within the Stockholm Heart Epidemiology Programme (SHEEP). J Epidemiol Community Health 59:23–30
27. DeBusk RF (2003) Sexual activity in patients with angina. JAMA 290:3129–3132
28. Dahabreh IJ, Paulus JK (2011) Association of episodic physical and sexual activity with triggering of acute cardiac events. Systematic review and meta-analysis. JAMA 305:1225–1233
29. Drory Y (2002) Sexual activity and cardiovascular risk. Eur Heart J Suppl 4:H13–H18
30. Levine GN, Steinke EE, Bakaeen FG et al (2012) Sexual activity and cardiovascular disease. A scientific statement of the American Heart Association. Circulation 125:1058–1072
31. Jackson G, Nehra A, Miner M et al (2013) The assessment of vascular risk in men with erectile dysfunction: the role of the cardiologist and general physician. Int J Clin Pract 67:1163–1172
32. Vlachopoulos C, Jackson G, Stefanadis C, Montorsi P (2013) Erectile dysfunction in the cardiovascular patient. Eur Heart J 34:2034–2046
33. Jackson G, Montorsi P, Adams MA et al (2010) Cardiovascular aspects of sexual medicine. J Sex Med 7:1608–1626
34. Miner M, Nehra A, Jackson G et al (2014) All men with vasculogenic erectile dysfunction require a cardiovascular workup. Am J Med 127:174–182
35. Nehra A, Jackson G, Miner M et al (2012) The Princeton III consensus recommendations for the management of erectile dysfunction and cardiovascular disease. Mayo Clin Proc 87:766–778
36. Sniderman AD, LaChapelle KJ, Rachon NA, Furberg CD (2013) The necessity for clinical reasoning in the era of evidence-based medicine. Mayo Clin Proc 88:1108–1114
37. Bohlen JG, Held JP, Sanderson MO, Patterson RP (1984) Heart rate, rate-pressure product, and oxygen uptake during four sexual activities. Arch Intern Med 144:1745–1748
38. Xue-Rui T, Ying L, Da-Zhong Y, Xiao-Jun C (2008) Changes of blood pressure and heart rate during sexual activity in healthy adults. Blood Press Monit 13:211–217
39. Palmeri ST, Kostis JB, Casazza L, Sleeper LA, Lu M, Nezgoda J, Rosen RS (2007) Heart rate and blood pressure response in adult men and women during exercise and sexual activity. Am J Cardiol 100(12):1795–1801
40. Hoekstra T, Jaarsma T, Sanderman R, van Veldhuisen DJ, Lesman-Leegte I (2012) Perceived sexual difficulties and associated factors in patients with heart failure. Am Heart J 163:246–251
41. Hoekstra T, Lesman-Leegte I, Luttik ML, Sanderman R, van Veldhuisen DJ, Jaarsma T (2012) Sexual problems in elderly male and female patients with heart failure. Heart 98:1647–1652

42. Medina M, Walker C, Steinke EE, Wright DW, Mosack V, Farhoud MH (2009) Sexual concerns and sexual counseling in heart failure. Prog Cardiovasc Nurs 24:141–148
43. Ueno M (1963) The so-called coital death. Jpn J Legal Med 17:330–340
44. Parzeller M, Bux R, Raschka C, Bratzke H (2006) Sudden cardiovascular death associated with sexual activity: a forensic autopsy study (1972–2004). Forensic Sci Med Pathol 2:109–114
45. Krauland W (1976) Unerwarterer tod – Herzinfarct und sexualitat aus der sicht des rechtsmediziners. Sexual-medizin 10:20–23
46. Lee S, Chae J, Cho Y (2006) Causes of sudden death related to sexual activity: results of a medicolegal postmortem study from 2001 to 2005. J Korean Med Sci 21:995–999
47. Anyfanti P, Pyrpasopoulou A, Triantafyllou A et al (2013) The impact of frequently encountered cardiovascular risk factors on sexual dysfunction in rheumatic disorders. Andrology 1(4):556–562
48. Gkaliagkousi E, Gavriilaki E, Doumas M et al (2012) Cardiovascular risk in rheumatoid arthritis: pathogenesis, diagnosis, and management. J Clin Rheumatol 18:422–430
49. Kautz DD, Van Horn ER, Moore C (2009) Sex after stroke: an integrative review and recommendations for clinical practice. Crit Rev Phys Rehabil Med 21:99–115
50. Thompson SB, Walker L (2011) Sexual dysfunction after stroke: underestimating the importance of psychological and physical issues. Webmed Cent Phys Med 2:WMC002281
51. Kautz DD (2007) Hope for love: practical advice for intimacy and sex after stroke. Rehabil Nurs 32:95–103
52. Lemieux L, Cohen-Schneider R, Holzapfel S (2001) Aphasia and sexuality. Sex Disabil 19:253–266
53. Doumas M, Douma S (2006) The effect of antihypertensive drugs on erectile function: a proposed management algorithm. J Clin Hypertens 8:359–364
54. Manolis A, Doumas M (2012) Antihypertensive treatment and sexual dysfunction. Curr Hypertens Rep 14:285–292
55. Dusing R (2003) Effect of the angiotensin II antagonist valsartan on sexual function in hypertensive men. Blood Press 12:S29–S34
56. Doumas M, Tsakiris A, Douma S et al (2006) Beneficial effects of switching from beta-blockers to nebivolol on the erectile function of hypertensive patients. Asian J Androl 8:177–182
57. Silvestri A, Galetta P, Cerquetani E et al (2003) Report of erectile dysfunction after therapy with beta-blockers is related to patient knowledge of side effects and is reversed by placebo. Eur Heart J 24:1928–1932
58. Douma S, Doumas M, Petidis K, Triantafyllou A, Zamboulis C (2008) Beta blockers and sexual dysfunction: bad guys – good guys. In: Endo M, Matsumoto N (eds) Beta blockers: new research. Nova Science Publishers Inc., Hauppauge, NY, pp 1–13
59. Pickering TG, Shepherd AM, Puddey I et al (2004) Sildenafil citrate for erectile dysfunction in men receiving multiple antihypertensive agents: a randomized controlled trial. Am J Hypertens 17:1135–1142
60. Kloner RA, Sadovsky R, Johnson EG et al (2005) Efficacy of tadalafil in the treatment of erectile dysfunction in hypertensive men on concomitant thiazide diuretic therapy. Int J Impot Res 17:450–454
61. Webb DJ, Muirhead GJ, Wulff M et al (2000) Sildenafil citrate potentiates the hypotensive effects of nitric oxide donor drugs in male patients with stable angina. J Am Coll Cardiol 36:25–31

Management of Erectile Dysfunction: Therapeutic Algorithm

Charalambos Vlachopoulos and Nikolaos Ioakeimidis

24.1 Erectile Dysfunction in Hypertension: Disease- or Drug-Related?

The relationship between arterial hypertension and erectile dysfunction (ED) has raised an important clinical issue: is hypertension per se, antihypertensive drug therapy, or a combination of these associated with impaired erectile function in hypertensive patients? Recently, the European Society of Hypertension in a seminal position paper highlighted that current evidence regarding the influence of antihypertensive drugs on erectile function is limited, usually addresses monotherapy, and mainly comes from observational studies [1]. Worsening of erectile function after identifying a hypertensive patient at risk for future cardiovascular events is more likely to be due to atherosclerosis progression and hypertension per se rather than due to antihypertensive drugs [2, 3]. Furthermore, in a recent study it was shown that the presence of "nondipper" pattern on ambulatory blood pressure (BP) monitoring among treated hypertensive patients was strongly related to worst erectile function independently of the number or the class of antihypertensive drugs in use [4].

Compared with older antihypertensive drugs (beta-blockers, diuretics), newer agents (vasodilating beta-blockers, calcium channel antagonists) have neutral or even beneficial effects on erectile function [5]. Patients frequently blame the medication for their ED, particularly if there seems to be a temporal relationship and if ED is mentioned as a side effect in the product insert. This is an important point since patient concerns about the adverse effects of drugs on erectile function might limit the use of essential medications (e.g., beta-blockers) in cardiovascular high-risk hypertensive patients, such as men with coronary artery disease [6]. It is recommended to explain

C. Vlachopoulos (✉) • N. Ioakeimidis
1st Cardiology Department, Athens Medical School, Hippokration Hospital, Athens, Greece
e-mail: cvlachop@otenet.gr; nioakim@gmail.com

to patients in detail the effect of drug treatment on erectile function and the association between vasculogenic ED and cardiovascular disease in order to improve adherence to evidence-based treatment of hypertension [7].

24.2 Selecting Initial Antihypertensive Drug Therapy

Beta-blockers are frequently associated with impairment of sexual desire, libido, and especially ED [2, 5, 6]. In contrast and considering the strong correlation and pathophysiological links between endothelial and erectile function, beta-blockers with beneficial effects on nitric oxide synthase and oxidative stress such as nebivolol have been suggested to improve erectile function [2, 5, 8]. There is no clinical trial evaluating the effect of calcium channel antagonists on erectile function with an adequate assessment of ED, but they are generally reported to have no relevant effect on erectile function [5]. For drugs that act over renin-angiotensin system, most evidence suggests that there was no influence on erectile function, and some authors indicate a beneficial effect [5]. However, in 1549 cardiovascular high-risk patients included in ONTARGET/TRANSCEND trial, there was neither a beneficial nor an unfavorable effect of the angiotensin-converting enzyme inhibitor ramipril, the angiotensin receptor blocker telmisartan, and the combination of both on erectile function [9].

Overall, although no class of antihypertensive agents presents a clearly superior effect over the others in terms of quality of life, the current impression is that nebivolol, angiotensin-converting enzyme inhibitors, and angiotensin II receptor antagonists may offer some advantage, at least in regard to effects on sexual activity [10].

The presence of comorbidities (coronary artery disease, diabetes) and the concomitant administration of other drugs (statins), a common situation in older hypertensive subjects, as well as the lack of diagnostic standardization concerning tools to access erectile function, impair a reliable analysis of trials about the relationship between ED and hypertension and derivation of robust conclusion about deleterious action of antihypertensive drugs on erectile function [3]. Therefore, search for new evidence on basic mechanisms underlying ED development in hypertensive individuals is an actual need. On an individual basis, sexual activity and erectile function quality should be part of anamnesis before initiation of antihypertensive therapy and seems to play a central role in the follow-up, as it would allow a scalable monitoring of erectile function, help the selection of better classes of antihypertensive drugs, facilitate the identification of adverse sexual events, and even improve therapeutic compliance [11].

24.3 Phosphodiesterase-5 Inhibitors

Phosphodiesterase-5 (PDE-5) inhibitors are very effective in treating ED; however, their safety was questioned in hypertensive patients, due to the vasodilatory effect of PDE-5 [12, 13]. However, concerns seem to be outdated, since BP reductions observed both in hypertensive patients and normotensive individuals are usually small and clinically insignificant [14]. Several lines of evidence indicate that PDE-5 inhibitors are not associated with significantly higher incidence of adverse events in hypertensive patients, even on a concomitant multidrug regimen [15, 16]. Therefore, PDE-5 inhibitors may be effectively and safely co-administered with antihypertensive drugs, with alpha-blockers and nitrates being the only exception [12].

Poor adherence to antihypertensive drug therapy is a critical contributor to unsatisfactory BP control rates. The contribution of ED in poor adherence to antihypertensive drug therapy has been highlighted in a study of hypertensive ED patients [17]. The interesting finding is that sildenafil use for ED resulted in significant improvements in adherence rates (from 48 to 66 %). Indeed, PDE-5 inhibitor use in men with hypertension is associated with initiation rather than withdrawal, and addition rather than rejection, of antihypertensive treatment. It should be noted, however, that initiation of PDE-5 inhibitors in hypertensive patients should follow adequate BP stabilization and is therefore contraindicated in patients with untreated, poorly controlled, accelerated, or malignant hypertension; these patients are considered "high-risk" for cardiovascular events and should be evaluated carefully before prescribing PDE-5 inhibitors [18, 19].

By virtue of their vascular effects [20], PDE-5 inhibitors are an appealing class of agents for the treatment of hypertension. Thus, despite the small acute BP-lowering effect reported in treated hypertensive patients [14], their potential as antihypertensive agents has not been thoroughly explored. Active mid-term treatment with sildenafil reduced ambulatory and clinic BP to a similar extent as that observed with other classes of antihypertensive drugs [12]. An incremental antihypertensive effect of a single dose of tadalafil has been demonstrated in uncontrolled hypertensive subjects on multiple agents [21]. However, at this stage, the use of current PDE-5 inhibitors as antihypertensive agents cannot be advocated. Other long-lasting PDE-5 inhibitors currently under development may prove to be more efficacious in this setting.

24.4 Testosterone Therapy

Testosterone deficiency defined as total testosterone below 3.0 ng/ml is highly prevalent among hypertensive men, and it is also a common pathogenetic mechanism linking arterial hypertension and vasculogenic ED [19, 22]. Several studies suggest that testosterone deficiency is a risk factor for reduced response to PDE-5 inhibitors in men with ED [18]. A relatively high prevalence (30–40 %) of low testosterone levels (mean total testosterone; 1.7–2.3 ng/ml) has been reported in non-responders to sildenafil or tadalafil ED patients [22]. Therefore, additional considerations for treatment of ED in men with arterial hypertension should include testosterone therapy for patients who have biochemical evidence of testosterone deficiency and they are symptomatic (ED or reduced libido) of testosterone deficiency. Addition of testosterone to PDE-5 inhibitor therapy after PDE-5 inhibitor failure is an appealing option. In fact, the use of testosterone as an adjunctive therapy to PDE-5 inhibitors for the treatment of ED and hypogonadism has resulted in successful outcomes in patients in whom PDE-5 inhibitor therapy alone has failed [18, 22].

Realization that low serum testosterone levels may contribute significantly to the pathogenesis of arterial hypertension reinforces search of testosterone deficiency as part of the investigation. Currently available evidence derived from a meta-analysis of 30 trials [23] supported a neutral effect of testosterone supplementation on BP that was consistent across trials. However, in a recent prospective, observational study, the use of injectable long-acting testosterone undecanoate showed an antihypertensive effect of testosterone replacement therapy [24]. Additional work on the impact of testosterone therapy on BP levels in treated and untreated hypertensive patients with testosterone deficiency remains to be done.

24.5 Proposed Therapeutic Algorithm

24.5.1 Step 1: Cardiac Risk Assessment

Sexual activity doubles the risk of a cardiac event [18, 19]. However, as the absolute risk for a cardiac event is extremely low in individuals without cardiovascular risk factors (one in a million), it seems rational to assume that sexual activity is rather safe in low-risk individuals. The Princeton III Guidelines offer a comprehensive and at the same time clinically friendly guidance of stratifying risk, and the proposed algorithm is complemented by recent review articles [18, 19, 25] (Fig. 24.1). Particular emphasis is given to linking the recommendations to clinical practice for the effective management of hypertensive patients. According to these recommendations, patients with controlled hypertension are considered low-risk patients and may safely proceed to sexual intercourse. On the contrary, high-risk patients have a tenfold increased risk for a cardiac event during sexual intercourse and the following 2 h. Patients with untreated, poorly controlled, accelerated, or malignant hypertension are considered high-risk patients, and sexual activity should be deferred until the patient's condition has been stabilized by treatment and a decision has been made by a cardiologist and/or internist that sexual activity may be safely resumed.

24.5.2 Step 2: The Use of Biomarkers in the Therapy of ED

The key question that must be answered is whether the use of a new biomarker (vascular or circulating) can determine a therapeutic approach (e.g., choice of drug, dose of drug) or the likelihood of response to an agent [18, 19, 25, 26]. In a man with arterial hypertension who is starting therapy with PDE-5 inhibitors for the first time, baseline testosterone levels in conjunction with penile Doppler evaluation can potentially aid in the prediction of response to treatment. As mentioned above, regarding baseline testosterone, it has been shown that a low testosterone level may inhibit the effectiveness of PDE-5 inhibitors [22]. Aging and cardiovascular risk factors (i.e., hypertension, diabetes) are associated with several changes in arterial structure and function, part of them related to

A. Patients without established CVD or diabetes		
Low SCORE/FRS	Moderate SCORE/FRS	High or Very high SCORE/FRS
exercise ability lifestyle advice or intervention treatment of RFs PDE5i	exercise ability or stress test (in higher scores) lifestyle intervention consider drug intervention if RF uncontrolled PDE5i	cardiologist referral stress test lifestyle intervention RF drug intervention PDE5i Tth‡
Biomarker abnormal / hypogonadism exercise ability or stress test lifestyle intervention RF drug intervention PDE5i Tth‡	**Biomarker abnormal / hypogonadism** stress test lifestyle intervention RF drug intervention PDE5i Tth‡	

B. Patients with established CVD or diabetes			
Low risk*	Indeterminate risk**		High risk***
	Low risk (negative stress test)	High risk (positive stress test)	
exercise ability or stress test lifestyle intervention RF drug intervention PDE5i Tth‡	lifestyle intervention RF drug intervention PDE5i Tth‡	deferral of sexual activity cardiologist referral	deferral of sexual activity cardiologist referral

Fig. 24.1 Management of hypertensive patients with CVD (**a**) or without known CVD (**b**). *Low-risk patients include those with complete revascularization (e.g., via coronary artery bypass grafting, stenting, or angioplasty), patients with asymptomatic controlled hypertension, those with mild valvular disease, and patients with left ventricular dysfunction/heart failure (NYHA classes I and II) who achieved five metabolic equivalents of the task (*METS*) without ischemia on recent exercise testing. **Indeterminate risk patients include diabetics, those with mild or moderate stable angina pectoris, past myocardial infarction (2–8 weeks) without intervention awaiting exercise electrocardiography, congestive heart failure (NYHA class III), and noncardiac sequelae of atherosclerotic disease (e.g., peripheral artery disease and a history of stroke or transient ischemic attack); this patient with ED may require assessment for additional vascular disease using carotid intima-media thickness or ankle-brachial index and subsequent reclassification to low or high risk. ***High-risk patients include those with unstable or refractory angina pectoris, uncontrolled hypertension, congestive heart failure (NYHA class IV), recent myocardial infarction without intervention (2 weeks), high-risk arrhythmia (exercise-induced ventricular tachycardia, implanted internal cardioverter defibrillator with frequent shocks, and poorly controlled atrial fibrillation), obstructive hypertrophic cardiomyopathy with severe symptoms, and moderate to severe valve disease, particularly aortic stenosis. ‡Where appropriate *CVD* cardiovascular disease, *FRS* Framingham risk score, *PDE5i* phosphodiesterase type 5 inhibitors, *RF* risk factor, *Tth* testosterone therapy; *NYHA* New York Heart Association. From Vlachopoulos et al. [19]

decline of circulating levels of testosterone [19, 22, 25, 26]. These changes may be responsible, to an extent, for the lack of efficacy of ED treatments in men with low androgen level as an important component of vasculogenic ED. Furthermore, the dynamic penile color duplex Doppler ultrasonography (using 20 μg intracavernous prostaglandin E1 and audiovisual stimulation) is required for secure diagnosis of vasculogenic ED. Importantly, sporadic studies have shown that non-responders to PDE-5 inhibitors have ultrasonographically documented severe penile vascular disease [27].

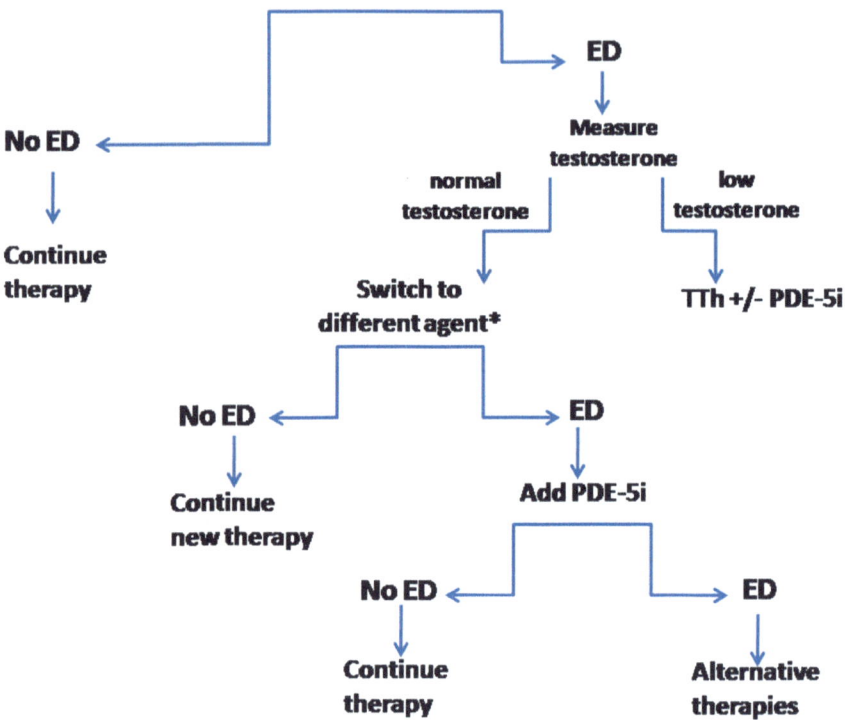

Fig. 24.2 Proposed algorithm for the management of erectile dysfunction in hypertensive patients who take antihypertensive drugs. *ED* erectile dysfunction, *PDE-5i* phosphodiesterase-5 inhibitors, *unless contraindicated or current antihypertensive drug therapy is absolutely indicated

24.5.3 Step 3: Treatment Strategies

Figure 24.2 shows the flow chart for the proposed treatment algorithm. Treatment of ED in hypertensive patients requires certain steps. First, in hypertensive men with ED resulting from antihypertensive drugs, the physician may substitute current treatment with drugs with a better profile regarding sexual side effects (nebivolol or renin-angiotensin system blocker) [28]. If ED persists, the combination of PDE-5 inhibitors and antihypertensive drugs with favorable effect on sexual function [16, 20] is the next choice [29]. Testosterone replacement therapy should be reserved for ED patients who have biochemical evidence of testosterone deficiency [18, 22]. Often such a hormonal disorder is revealed in patients who are non-responders to PDE-5 inhibitors. Intracavernous self-injection, penile prostheses, low-intensity extracorporeal shock wave therapy, and stent implantation in focal atherosclerotic lesions of the internal pudendal arteries with endovascular stents constitute also common path for men with ED refractory to PDE-5 inhibitors [30–32].

It should be emphasized that (a) data regarding combination antihypertensive drug therapy are remarkably lacking. As the majority of hypertensive patients take two or more drugs, it seems to be of great importance to know the effect of different combination regimens [29, 33]. (b) Although most data obtained during a formal evaluation, comprising of medical history, questionnaires, physical examination, and first-line tests (testosterone levels, penile Doppler), are very important in assessing the patient's characteristics and ED etiology, they do not help in selecting the best PDE-5 inhibitor for a given patient. (c) Finally, ED patients should be informed about the correct way of sexual medication usage. Although it sounds obvious, it is important to emphasize that improper drug usage is a common reason for lack of efficacy.

Conclusion

A comprehensive approach is needed both for identifying sexual dysfunction earlier and individualizing treatment. It is important to recognize that ED contributes to a reduction of therapeutic compliance and aggravates further the quality of life among men who already suffer from essential hypertension and other comorbidities. Available data point towards significant benefits in erectile function when prior antihypertensive drug therapy is switched to either nebivolol or renin-angiotensin system blockers. PDE-5 inhibitors, a class of agents that has offered new perspectives in the management of ED, are effective and safe in hypertensive patients, but their use should follow appropriate consultation. Testosterone deficiency should be searched for and therapy should be offered in hypertensive males with clinical evidence of this disorder. Further evidence is warranted to elucidate the effects of antihypertensive drug therapy on erectile function, especially regarding the combination of antihypertensive drugs and the combination of antihypertensive drugs with PDE-5 inhibitors.

References

1. Viigimaa M, Doumas M, Vlachopoulos C et al (2011) European Society of Hypertension working group on sexual dysfunction. Hypertension and sexual dysfunction: time to act. J Hypertens 29(2):403–407
2. Manolis A, Doumas M (2012) Antihypertensive treatment and sexual dysfunction. Curr Hypertens Rep 14:285–292
3. Düsing R (2005) Sexual dysfunction in male patients with hypertension: influence of antihypertensive drugs. Drugs 65:773–786
4. Erden I, Ozhan H, Ordu S et al (2010) The effect of non-dipper pattern of hypertension on erectile dysfunction. Blood Press 19:249–253
5. Baumhäkel M, Schlimmer N, Kratz M et al (2011) Cardiovascular risk, drugs and erectile function—a systematic analysis. Int J Clin Pract 65:289–298
6. Silvestri A, Galetta P, Cerquetani E et al (2003) Report of erectile dysfunction after therapy with beta-blockers is related to patient knowledge of side effects and is reversed by placebo. Eur Heart J 24:1928–1932
7. Scranton RE, Goldstein I, Stecher VJ (2013) Erectile dysfunction diagnosis and treatment as a means to improve medication adherence and optimize comorbidity management. J Sex Med 10:551–561

8. Toblli J, Cao G, Casas G et al (2006) In vivo and in vitro effects of nebivolol on penile structures in hypertensive rats. Am J Hypertens 19:1226–1232
9. Böhm M, Baumhäkel M, Teo K et al (2010) Erectile dysfunction predicts cardiovascular events in high-risk patients receiving telmisartan, ramipril, or both: the ongoing telmisartan alone and in combination with ramipril global endpoint trial/telmisartan randomized assessment study in ace intolerant subjects with cardiovascular disease (ontarget/transcend) trials. Circulation 121:1439–1446
10. Mancia G, Fagard R, Narkiewicz K et al (2013) 2013 ESH/ESC guidelines for the management of arterial hypertension: the task force for the management of arterial hypertension of the European Society of Hypertension (ESH) and of the European Society of Cardiology (ESC). Eur Heart J 34(28):2159–2219
11. Fogari R, Zoppi A (2004) Effect of antihypertensive agents on quality of life in the elderly. Drugs Aging 21:377–393
12. Vlachopoulos C, Terentes-Printzios D, Ioakeimidis N et al (2009) PDE5 inhibitors in non-urological conditions. Curr Pharm Des 15:3521–3539
13. Ioakeimidis N, Kostis JB (2014) Pharmacologic therapy for erectile dysfunction and its interaction with the cardiovascular system. J Cardiovasc Pharmacol Ther 19:53–64
14. Oliver JJ, Melville VP, Webb DJ (2006) Effect of regular phosphodiesterase type 5 inhibition in hypertension. Hypertension 48:622–627
15. Pickering TG, Shepherd AM, Puddey I et al (2004) Sildenafil citrate for erectile dysfunction in men receiving multiple antihypertensive agents: a randomized controlled trial. Am J Hypertens 17:1135–1142
16. Lee JH, Chae MR, Park JK et al (2012) The effects of the combined use of a PDE5 inhibitor and medications for hypertension, lower urinary tract symptoms and dyslipidemia on corporal tissue tone. Int J Impot Res 24:221–227
17. McLaughlin T, Harnett J, Burhani S et al (2005) Evaluation of erectile dysfunction therapy in patients previously nonadherent to long-term medications: a retrospective analysis of prescription claims. Am J Ther 12:605–611
18. Nehra A, Jackson G, Miner M et al (2012) The Princeton III consensus recommendations for the management of erectile dysfunction and cardiovascular disease. Mayo Clin Proc 87:766–778
19. Vlachopoulos C, Jackson G, Stefanadis C et al (2013) Erectile dysfunction in the cardiovascular patient. Eur Heart J 34:2034–2046
20. Toblli JE, Cao G, Lombraña A et al (2007) Functional and morphological improvement in erectile tissue of hypertensive rats by long-term combined therapy with phosphodiesterase type 5 inhibitor and losartan. J Sex Med 4:1291–1303
21. Patterson D, McInnes GT, Webster J et al (2006) Influence of a single dose of 20 mg tadalafil, a phosphodiesterase 5 inhibitor, on ambulatory blood pressure in subjects with hypertension. Br J Clin Pharmacol 62:280–287
22. Buvat J, Maggi M, Guay A et al (2013) Testosterone deficiency in men: systematic review and standard operating procedures for diagnosis and treatment. J Sex Med 10:245–284
23. Haddad RM, Kennedy CC, Caples SM et al (2007) Testosterone and cardiovascular risk in men: a systematic review and meta-analysis of randomized placebo-controlled trials. Mayo Clin Proc 82:29–39
24. Zitzmann M, Mattern A, Hanisch J et al (2013) IPASS: a study on the tolerability and effectiveness of injectable testosterone undecanoate for the treatment of male hypogonadism in a worldwide sample of 1,438 men. J Sex Med 10:579–588
25. Jackson G, Nehra A, Miner M et al (2013) The assessment of vascular risk in men with erectile dysfunction: the role of the cardiologist and general physician. Int J Clin Pract 67:1163–1172
26. Miner M, Seftel AD, Nehra A et al (2012) Prognostic utility of erectile dysfunction for cardiovascular disease in younger men and those with diabetes. Am Heart J 164:21–28
27. Wespes E, Rammal A, Garbar C (2005) Sildenafil non-responders: haemodynamic and morphometric studies. Eur Urol 48:136–139

28. Doumas M, Douma S (2006) The effect of antihypertensive drugs on erectile function: a proposed management algorithm. J Clin Hypertens (Greenwich) 8:359–364
29. Doumas M, Viigimaa M, Papademetriou V (2013) Combined antihypertensive therapy and sexual dysfunction: terra incognita. Cardiology 125:232–234
30. Shamloul R, Ghanem H (2013) Erectile dysfunction. Lancet 381:153–165
31. Vardi Y, Appel B, Kilchevsky A et al (2012) Does low intensity extracorporeal shock wave therapy have a physiological effect on erectile function? Short-term results of a randomized, double-blind, sham controlled study. J Urol 187:1769–1775
32. Rogers JH, Goldstein I, Kandzari DE et al (2012) Zotarolimus-eluting peripheral stents for the treatment of erectile dysfunction in subjects with suboptimal response to phosphodiesterase-5 inhibitors. J Am Coll Cardiol 60:2618–2627
33. Yang L, Yu J, Ma R et al (2013) The effect of combined antihypertensive treatment (felodipine with either irbesartan or metoprolol) on erectile function: a randomized controlled trial. Cardiology 125:235–241

The manufacturer's authorised representative in the EU is Springer Nature Customer Service Centre GmbH, Europaplatz 3, 69115 Heidelberg, Germany. If you have any concerns regarding our products, please contact ProductSafety@springernature.com

Printed and bound by CPI Group (UK) Ltd, Croydon, CR0 4YY

23/03/2026
02076666-0015